Advances in Alzheimer's Research
(Volume 2)

Editor

Debomoy K. Lahiri

Departments of Psychiatry and of Medical & Molecular Genetics
Indiana University School of Medicine, Institute of Psychiatric Research
Neuroscience Research Center, 320 W. 15th Street
Indianapolis, IN-46202
USA

Bentham Science Publishers
Executive Suite Y - 2
PO Box 7917, Saif Zone
Sharjah, U.A.E.
subscriptions@benthamscience.org

Bentham Science Publishers
P.O. Box 446
Oak Park, IL 60301-0446
USA
subscriptions@benthamscience.org

Bentham Science Publishers
P.O. Box 294
1400 AG Bussum
THE NETHERLANDS
subscriptions@benthamscience.org

CONTENTS

PREFACE

Alzheimer's disease (AD) is an incurable, progressive, degenerative and fatal disease that afflicts over 36 million people worldwide, and this figure is expected to quadruple by 2050. Epidemiologic data indicate we are on the precipice of a global epidemic of AD; yet, unfortunately, current treatment options are only provide short term symptomatic relief.

The major aim of the series *Advances in Alzheimer's Research*, from Volume 1 and continuing to Volume 2, is to present a combined approach to AD from mechanistic, clinical and translational research and discuss the important information on the cause, progression and prevention of AD. This volume is not meant to report exhaustively on the many other research efforts in the broader AD research arena. Its primary objective is to discuss and highlight improvements toward the diagnosis and potential treatment of AD using both recognized and novel strategies. This book series, including the present volume, offers a unique platform to a range of scientific interests and expertise, specifically focused on AD and related disorders. A major attempt is undertaken to disseminate the most current knowledge on recent advances in AD research.

The volume 2 compiles selected articles previously published in *Current Alzheimer Research* (CAR) and are updated for this volume. The selection of subject matter comprises a collection of diverse research articles that are representative publications in CAR. They cover forward-thinking and provocative ideas, enthralling to read for those both in the AD field and outside of it. It is pleasing to obtain 15 exceptional contributions that create the present issue to skillfully achieve this.

The etiology of AD is being slowly understood. The contribution of gene and environment, including education, physical activity and lifestyle, are important for the most common cases of sporadic AD. Another heavily investigated aspect is mechanism(s) of amyloid plaque deposition. One of the most noteworthy recent approaches to amyloid plaque involved removal of brain amyloid-β peptide (Aβ) using anti-Aβ antibodies. Aβ immunotherapy emerged as a promising treatment strategy based on human neuropathology and preclinical studies. The characteristic deposition of parenchymal and vascular amyloid-β peptide (Aβ) pathology detected in the brains of AD subjects suggested a logical target. However, there were several recent setbacks at the clinical trial stage, and some these issues and other developments have been discussed recently in *Current Alzheimer Research* (Vol. 11, 2014).

This volume comprises 15 chapters written by a group of eminent experts in various aspects of AD research. In short these chapters capture recent advances that can be broadly grouped into eight major important areas. 1) memory and consciousness, 2) proliferation (cancer) *vs*. degeneration (AD), 3) risk factors for AD (such as dietary, *e.g.*, cholesterol, and environmental, *e.g.*, metals), 3) pharmacological intervention (*e.g.,* cholinesterase inhibitors), 4) non-pharmacological approaches (*e.g.*, music), 5) neuroprotective strategies (*e.g.*, heme oxygenase-1 suppression), 6) biomarkers (*e.g.*, Cytochrome C) and detection, 7) Morphological studies(such as spine pathology and laterality of the affected AD brain , and 8) Caregivers' perspectives.

The first chapter deals with memory, awareness and consciousness relevant to AD. Specifically, the authors (Souchay and Moulin) provide an overview of the brain regions supporting conscious experience of memory and suggest that the memory and awareness deficits observed in AD may be viewed as a deficit in autonoetic consciousness. At the cellular level, Behrens *et al*. describe common biological mechanisms in AD and cancer. For example, epidemiological data suggest an inverse association between AD and cancer, such that the risk of developing cancer is significantly lower in AD patients, while cancer patients have a lower risk of developing AD. At the molecular level, Behrens and colleagues discuss the roles of some specific signaling pathway, and the process of adult neurogenesis as potential candidates, which may explain an inverse association between AD and cancer.

Several risk factors are known for AD, and some are controversial. A provocative chapter (Stefani and Liguri) discusses the role of cholesterol as a susceptibility factor or a protective agent in neurodegeneration and, especially in the context of amyloid-induced cytotoxicity. Epidemiological studies on the hypercholesterolemia-AD risk relation and beneficial outcomes of statin therapy studies suggest cholesterol as a susceptibility factor in AD. However, reduction of cellular cholesterol favors co-localization of BACE1 and APP in non-raft membrane domains and inhibits production of the Aβ-degrading enzyme plasmin. There is also a reduction of the cholesterol/phospholipid ratio in aged and AD brains. Stefani and colleagues ably tackle both sides in this field by supporting both roles of cholesterol either as a susceptibility factor or as a protective agent in AD. Apart from cholesterol, environmental factors, such as metals, can play a role in the etiology of AD. AD fits to a major class of diseases, called amyloidoses, in which endogenous proteins or peptides undertake a misfolding process changing from soluble physiological configurations to a pathological fibrillar insoluble state. A significant role is played in these processes by transition metals (such as copper and zinc) that were detected in fairly great amounts in senile plaques of AD subjects. Using a combination of modern spectroscopic techniques and numerical simulations, the authors Morante and Rossi shows that different metals can rival in peptide binding, which suggest that metal dyshomeostasis may be important in the development of AD.

Deciphering the role of specific molecular pathways may help elucidate disease progression. Further, such studies are useful to propose and develop specific biomarker(s) and targets for the disease. Collapsin response mediator protein-2 (CRMP-2) plays an important role in neuronal development and polarity and in axon growth and guidance. CRMP-2 is a physiological substrate for GSK3 and Cdk5, two protein kinases that exhibit significant activity in AD. Herein, authors Soutar *et al.* examine the function of CRMP-2; and how it is controlled by phosphorylation, what changes in molecular mechanisms could lead to the abnormally high CRMP-2 phosphorylation in AD. This is important if CRMP-2 plays a specific role in AD and not in other forms of neurodegeneration. In the context of biomarker, the role of CSF cytochrome C levels and auditory event-related potentials (AERPs) in the progress of mild cognitive impairment (MCI) to AD is an important development. Authors Papaliagkas *et al.* suggest that MCI to AD conversion is associated with markedly elevated N200 latency at baseline and a high elevation of cytochrome C levels in the course of a relatively short period of time. The authors argue that both parameters could be possibly considered as candidate markers to differentiate between AD converters and MCI stable patients.

Regarding the pharmacological strategies, cholinesterase inhibitors (ChEIs) and related drugs form the subject matter of another chapter. As the authors Pepeu and Giovannini have rightly pointed out, whereas an increase in brain acetylcholine and an improvement of cognitive deficits have been reliably proven in animal models of AD, from aging rats to transgenic mice, the clinical effectiveness of ChEIs is still controversial. The possibility still exists of ChEIs exerting their effects through mechanisms other than cholinesterase inhibition. Diverging opinions on clinical efficacy do not discourage researchers from developing new ChEIs, particularly multifunctional ChEIs. They still exemplify the future of cholinergic therapy, not only for AD but also for vascular dementia and MCI.

Another hallmark of AD is oxidative stress resulting from the body's inability to neutralize excessive reactive oxidizing species (ROS). The mechanisms responsible for oxidative damage include iron deposition and mitochondrial insufficiency in brains of AD subjects. Heme oxygenase-1 (HO-1) is a 32 kDa stress protein, which is significantly over-expressed in AD-affected temporal cortex and hippocampus relative to control preparations. Targeted destruction of glial HO-1 hyperactivity may prove to be a logical and effective neurotherapeutic intervention in AD and related neurodegenerative disorders. Authors Schipper *et al.* describe efforts to determine whether systemic administration of a novel, selective and brain-permeable inhibitor of HO-1 activity improves cognitive dysfunction and neuropathology in a transgenic mouse model of AD, and such research has a great translational impact.

Regarding non-pharmacological strategies, authors Raglio and Gianelli focuses on the potential use of music therapy in a specific application distinct from generic use of music in a variety of pathologies. The authors highlight the therapeutic nature proper to music therapy with specific reference to the domain of the dementias. Apart from its controversy music therapy accelerates expression, communication and interpersonal relationship in a non-verbal context.

Regarding mechanistic and drug target developmental studies, it is important to use and develop an appropriate model that closely mimics the features of (human) AD. The most common animal models currently used for AD research are transgenic mice that express a mutant form of human Aβ precursor protein (APP) and/or some of the enzymes and molecules implicated in their metabolic processing, such as BAC1 and presenilins. However, these transgenic mice carry their own endogenous APP and APP-processing enzymes, which may interfere in the production of different Aβ peptides encoded by the human transgenes. In this context, authors Sarasa and Pesini suggest that important information on the physiopathology of AD could be obtained from other natural non-transgenic models. They have analyzed the chick embryo and the dog, which may be better experimental models, as their enzymatic and cellular machinery for processing APP is almost identical to that of humans.

Regarding improvement in diagnostics, *post mortem* identification of amyloid plaques, consisting of the Aβ peptide, and of neurofibrillary tangles in the brains of AD patients is still the gold standard for diagnosis for AD. Significant attempts have been made to detect reliable biomarkers for AD that can be used for early diagnosis. For example, body fluids, such as CSF and plasma, of AD patients are used to detect levels of total or soluble Aβ peptides. Here, authors Funke *et al.* present an updated overview of the current status of development of assays for Aβ aggregate specific detection and quantification. Apart from detection of soluble Aβ peptides, it is increasingly recognized that several neurodegenerative diseases, including Alzheimer's, Parkinson's, and prion diseases, are characterized by intra- and/or extracellular deposition of fibrillar proteinaceous aggregates and by extensive neuron loss. However, the dynamic and metastable nature of Aβ oligomers makes their study difficult. Herein authors Rahimi and Bitan review structural, functional, and biological experiments that are employed to study non-fibrillar Aβ assemblies. They point out challenges and highlight future research prospects in this important field relevant to not only to AD but other neurodegenerative disorders also.

Two chapters cover morphological aspect of the disease. First, dendritic spines are important sites of neuronal contacts, and alterations in the activity of neurons directly affect spine morphology. Indeed, spines are greatly dynamic structures and spine shape correlates with the power of synaptic transmission. Investigators Brandt *et al.* provide an overview on spine morphology and function, and describe different experimental models to analyze spine changes and dynamics. The review discusses potential mechanisms of how disease-relevant factors influence dendritic spines and how spine alterations could be therapeutically blocked or overturned.

The second morphological chapter deals Zach *et al.* with the examinations of alterations in brain asymmetry, which often focus on the planum temporale of patients with schizophrenia. Notably, recent data also suggest changes in laterality of demented patients associated with a more marked impairment of the left hemisphere. The plana temporalia were assessed using a new volumetric method with dental resin matter. Interestingly, shifts to left/right laterality of areas and volumes were detected in all demented groups. In the more prevalent AD group, the change in laterality of an area was associated with a mild decrease on the right and a mild increase on the left side.

Finally, authors Lu and Haase present experience and perspectives of caregivers of spouses with MCI. They describe commonalities of the lived experience of being a spouse caregiver of a person with MCI.

In short, the volume 2 captures a window, in the form of 15 exciting chapters, of stimulating ideas dedicated to the latest advances in AD research, diagnosis and treatment. This effort would enable the researchers in identifying the most critical gaps in our knowledge that require filling. We plan to prepare the future volumes of the series *Advances in Alzheimer's Research* that will discuss, debate and report several other pivotal hypothesis-driven strategies and thought-provoking ideas, which would help us in understanding the neurobiology of AD, and in potentially halting the progression of AD, perhaps a combination of approaches that may ultimately prove to be most effective, as found in other diseases.

Finally, I express my sincere gratitude to the authors for the value of their excellent contributions, their perseverance for the peer review process, and their patience for publication. Both the publisher and I appreciate the researchers who assisted in the peer review process, checking and correcting various chapters and the editorial. I sincerely appreciate the authors, publisher and staff of *Current Alzheimer Research* for their advice, efforts and support in the creating of this eBook series, specifically this volume.

Debomoy K. Lahiri

Departments of Psychiatry and of Medical & Molecular Genetics
Indiana University School of Medicine, Institute of Psychiatric Research
Neuroscience Research Center, 320 W. 15th Street,
Indianapolis, IN-46202
USA

List of Contributors

Adam R. Cole
Medical Research Institute, University of Dundee, Ninewells Hospital, Dundee DD1 9SY, Scotland, United Kingdom

Adnan Ghori
Department of Neurobiology, University of Osnabrück, Barbarastrasse 11, 49076 Osnabrück, Germany

Ajay Gupta
Osta Biotechnologies Inc., Montreal, Quebec, Canada

Alfredo Raglio
Sospiro Foundation, Piazza Libertà, 2 – 26048 Sospiro, Cremona, Italy

Calum Sutherland
Medical Research Institute, University of Dundee, Ninewells Hospital, Dundee DD1 9SY, Scotland, United Kingdom

Catherine M. Roe
Department of Neurology and the Charles F. and Joanne Knight Alzheimer Disease Center Washington, University School of Medicine in St Louis

Céline Souchay
LEAD CNRS UMR 5022, Université de Bourgogne, Dijon, France

Chris J.A. Moulin
LEAD CNRS UMR 5022, Université de Bourgogne, Dijon, France

Christian Tackenberg
Department of Neurobiology, University of Osnabrück, Barbarastrasse 11, 49076 Osnabrück Germany and Division of Psychiatry Research, University of Zurich, Wagistrasse 12, 8952 Schlieren, Switzerland

Daniela P. Ponce
Instituto de Ciencias Biomédicas, Facultad de Medicina, Universidad de Chile, Chile

Daniela Řípová
Prague Psychiatric Center, Czech Republic

Dieter Willbold
Forschungszentrum Jülich, ICS-6, D-52425 Jülich, Germany

Emerich Majer
Psychiatric Hospital Bohnice, Czech Republic

Eva Birkmann
Forschungszentrum Jülich, ICS-6, 52425 Jülich, Germany and Institut für Physikalische Biologie, Heinrich-Heine-Universität, 40225 Düsseldorf, Germany

Farid Rahimi
Research School of Biology, Division of Biomedical Science and Biochemistry, College of Medicine, Biology, and Environment, The Australian National University, Canberra, ACT Australia

Felipe Salech
Instituto de Ciencias Biomédicas, Facultad de Medicina, Universidad de Chile

Filip Španiel
Prague Psychiatric Center, Czech Republic, Chile

Gal Bitan
Department of Neurology, David Geffen School of Medicine, Brain Research Institute, and Molecular Biology Institute, University of California at Los Angeles, USA

Georgios A. Anogianakis
Department of Experimental Physiology, Faculty of Medicine, Aristotle University of Thessaloniki, Greece

Giancarlo Pepeu
Department of Preclinical and Clinical Pharmacology, University of Florence, Viale Pieraccini 6, 50139 Florence, Italy

Giancarlo Rossi
Dipartimento di Fisica, Università di Roma "Tor Vergata" and INFN, Sezione di Roma "Tor Vergata", Via della Ricerca Scientifica, 00133 Roma, Italy

Gianfranco Liguri
Department of Biochemical Sciences and Research Centre on Neurodegeneration (CIMN), University of Florence, Florence, Italy

Hyman M. Schipper
Bloomfield Centre for Research in Aging, Lady Davis Institute for Medical Research, Jewish General Hospital, McGill University, Montreal, Quebec, Canada

Jana Kenney
Czech Academy of Science, Czech Republic

Jana Mrzílková
Institute of Anatomy, Third Faculty of Medicine, Charles University, Czech Republic

Joan E. Haase
Emily Holmquist Professorship in Pediatric Oncology Nursing, Indiana University School of Nursing, Indianapolis, IN. 1111 Middle Drive, NUE421, Indiana University School of Nursing Indianapolis, IN 46202, USA

Magda N. Tsolaki
Third Department of Neurology, "G. Papanikolaou" Hospital, Aristotle University of Thessaloniki, Exohi Thessaloniki, Greece

Manuel Sarasa
Araclon Biotech S.L., 50009 Zaragoza, Spain

Marc P.M. Soutar
Medical Research Institute, University of Dundee, Ninewells Hospital, Dundee DD1 9SY, Scotland, United Kingdom

Maria G. Giovannini
Department of Preclinical and Clinical Pharmacology, University of Florence, Viale Pieraccini 6, 50139 Florence, Italy

Maria I. Behrens
Departamento de Neurología y Neurocirugía, Hospital Clínico Universidad de Chile, Santos Dumont 999, Clínica Alemana de Santiago, Chile

Maria V. Gianelli
University of Genova, Italy and INTERDEM Group, (Psycho-Social Interventions in Dementia) EU, Italy

Martina Kutová
Institute of Anatomy, Third Faculty of Medicine, Charles University, Czech Republic

Massimo Stefan
Department of Biochemical Sciences and Research Centre on Neurodegeneration (CIMN), University of Florence, Florence, Italy

Paul Thornhill
Medical Research Institute, University of Dundee, Ninewells Hospital, Dundee DD1 9SY, Scotland, United Kingdom

Pavel Selinger
Faculty Hospital Bulovka, Czech Republic

Pedro Pesini
Araclon Biotech S.L., 50009 Zaragoza, Spain

Petr Zach
Institute of Anatomy, Third Faculty of Medicine, Charles University at Prague, Ruská 87, Prague 10, 100 00, Czech Republic

Roland Brandt
Department of Neurobiology, University of Osnabrück, Barbarastrasse 11, 49076 Osnabrück, Germany

Silvia Morante
Dipartimento di Fisica, Università di Roma "Tor Vergata" and INFN, Sezione di Roma "Tor Vergata", Via della Ricerca Scientifica, 00133 Roma, Italy

Susanne A. Funke
Forschungszentrum Jülich, ICS-6, 52425 Jülich, Germany and Hochschule für Angewandte Wissenschaften, Bioanalytik, 96450 Coburg

Vasileios K. Kimiskidis
Clinical Neurophysiology Department, AHEPA University Hospital, Thessaloniki, Greece

Vasileios T. Papaliagkas
Third Department of Neurology, "G. Papanikolaou" Hospital, Aristotle University of Thessaloniki, Exohi Thessaloniki, Greece

Walter A. Szarek
Department of Chemistry, Queen's University, Kingston, Ontario, Canada

Yueh-Feng Y. Lu
Adult Health Nursing, Indiana University School of Nursing, 1111 Middle Drive, NUW407 Indiana University School of Nursing, Indianapolis, IN 46202, USA

Zdena Krištofiková
Prague Psychiatric Center, Czech Republic

CHAPTER 1

Memory, Awareness and Consciousness in Alzheimer's Disease

Céline Souchay* **and Chris J.A. Moulin**

LEAD CNRS UMR 5022, Université de Bourgogne, Dijon, France

Abstract: Human memory can be split into familiarity and recollection processes which contribute to different aspects of memory function. These separate processes result in different experiential states. In this review, we examine how this dominant theoretical framework can explain the subjective experience of people with Alzheimer's disease, the profile of their memory impairments and their inability to reflect on their performance metacognitively. We conclude with a brief overview of the brain regions supporting conscious experience of memory, and propose that the memory and awareness deficits seen in Alzheimer's disease could be primarily conceived of as a deficit in autonoetic consciousness. We briefly introduce how these these robust constructs are being incorporated into research programmes examining rehabilitation and pharmacological intervention.

Keywords: Awareness, familiarity, metacognition, recollection.

1. OVERVIEW

People with Alzheimer's disease seem to have information which is inaccessible to recall, such as an inability to name the president of France, but which is available for recognition, such as correctly picking out *Francois Hollande* from a set of alternatives. Such a discrepancy between recall and recognition has been cited as evidence of a specific form of memory deficit in AD since patients have memory for a word (*recognising* it as the correct answer), and yet they cannot retrieve it spontaneously, or *recall* it. Clinically, tests of recall are more sensitive to Alzheimer brain changes than are tests of recognition [1].

Considering this difference in recall and recognition, the relationship between consciousness and memory is in question. How is it that the patient cannot on the one hand report something, but know it when prompted? In this review we aim to

***Corresponding author Céline Souchay:** LEAD CNRS UMR 5022, Pole AAFE, Université de Bourgogne, DIJON 21065, France; Tel: +33 (0)3 80 39 90 25; Fax: +33 (0)3 80 39 57 67; E-mail: celine.souchay@u-bourgogne.fr

D.K. Lahiri (Ed)

illustrate that there exists a complex relationship between consciousness and memory, and that in Alzheimer's disease, this relationship breaks down, according to known patterns of neuropathology. We propose that Alzheimer's disease results in a disconnection between medial temporal and frontal areas and that this leads to a specific deficit in *recollection*, which is characterised by certain subjective feelings, and evocative, associated and personal information coming to mind during memory retrieval (See Table **1**).

The concept of recollection is a relatively recent theoretical development [2] and helps us understand other issues in memory and awareness more generally in Alzheimer's. In short, the emergent view is that memory function is supported by conscious states, and that a full understanding of memory function is only possible through understanding the experience of what comes to mind in memory [3]. We examine to what extent consciousness and awareness influence memory function and real world behaviours.

Table 1: A contemporary overview of memory: Recollection and familiarity processes

	Brain Region	**Conscious State**	**Mental Resources**	**Contextual Information**	**Status in AD**
Recollection	Hippocampus; Frontal lobes	'remembering'	Effortful, Slow	Some	Impaired
Familiarity	Peri-Hippocampal Regions	'knowing' or finding familiar	Relatively automatic, Quick	None	Equivocal

2. MEMORY IN ALZHEIMER'S DISEASE

In Alzheimer's disease, memory impairment is the earliest and most severe cognitive deficit. The commonest means of demonstrating this deficit is to evaluate the number of previously encountered items that can be recovered after a retention interval [1, 4, 5]. Such tests have been shown to be particularly sensitive at detecting pre-clinical changes in memory in people who develop Alzheimer's disease [6-8]. Additionally, neuroimaging studies have converged on temporo-parietal and hippocampal areas as being particularly involved in Alzheimer's disease. These regions are known to be crucial in learning of new information [9]. Convit *et al.* [10] demonstrated with volumetric MRI that atrophy in the medial occipito-temporal and the middle and inferior temporal gyri are associated with progression to Alzheimer's disease. Similarly, pre-morbid volumetric measurements of the hippocampus predict progression [11].

Thus, a large literature points to the fact that people with Alzheimer's have particular difficulties in retrieving material learnt in previous episodes, and this relates to underlying neuropathology. Cognitive Neuropsychologists see this memory deficit as episodic, relating to a specific study episode. That is, people with Alzheimer's disease have particular difficulties in learning and recalling recently encountered information, as opposed to material encountered and acquired premorbidly. However, rather than considering the types of materials and tasks which delineate different forms of memory impairment, a contemporary focus is the experiential state during memory retrieval – the state of awareness associated with the act of remembering. Because this conceptualisation opens up new fields of research and has utility in understanding disorders such as Alzheimer's disease, it is this emergent field that we review here.

This subjective approach was developed by Tulving [12]. He classified memory on the basis of experience, arguing that without considering experience you could not investigate cognition [13]. 'Self knowing' or 'autonoetic' memory described a memory where the first person experience was of 'remembering'. Memory without self-knowledge 'noetic' is often described as 'knowing' (See Table **1**). Episodic memories are self-knowing – that is, some aspect of the memory includes its source, an awareness of its origin, a feeling of pastness, a conscious evaluation of itself, what Koriat and Goldsmith [13] call 'contextual detail'. As an example, the memory of what one had for breakfast and the circumstances surrounding it, is episodic. Semantic memories concern conceptual knowledge, or facts, such as *Kelloggs is a brand of breakfast cereal.* Using these concepts of remembering and knowing yields many insights into memory dysfunction [14], education [15] and the aging process [16] (For reviews see [17, 18]). Henson *et al.* [19] have demonstrated that these two subjective states derive from separate brain regions. In particular, hippocampal structures are preferentially engaged for memory decisions based on this form of recollection [20] and hippocampal structures are more active for items which are more strongly 'remembered' [21].

One implication of this view is that memory proficiency is dependent upon conscious processes; healthy memory is influenced by reflective monitoring processes and guided by experiential states. For instance, the feeling of remembering arguably guides memory processes acting at retrieval, and influences how confident one feels about that memory, and whether the experient searches for extra detail. If information is retrieved with only a vague feeling of familiarity, one will be less certain of its veracity and less able to draw on information in support of that memory [22]. As developed below, vague feelings may lead the experient to produce false memories.

3. MEMORY AND CONSCIOUSNESS IN ALZHEIMER'S DISEASE

3.1. Memory Awareness

Pinker [23] suggests that consciousness comprises three distinct parts: Sentience, Access to Information and Self-Knowledge. Sentience describes subjective experience, phenomenal awareness, feelings of what something seems like. Access to information considers the ability to report ongoing mental experience or operations. Self-knowledge considers whether an organism can know itself and its impact on the world. These concepts are somewhat difficult to measure because of their subjective nature, but the memory literature has focussed on one easily operationalised measure – the accuracy of people's predictions of their memory, and memory awareness. Each type of prediction is reviewed in turn and the main findings summarized in Table **2**.

In everyday life, the ability to know, or to be aware, that one will be able or not to retrieve information is very well described by the tip-of-the-tongue phenomenon (TOT). The TOT is a striking state of awareness – a common and dramatic word-finding failure where a person is temporarily unable to produce a well-known word, despite feeling certain that one knows the word [24]. This phenomenon has not been widely explored in Alzheimer's disease and the studies have found contradictory results; one study shows that Alzheimer's disease patients have more TOT states [25] and the other shows that Alzheimer's patients do not produce more [26]. This issue is one which should be a priority for future research: people who have TOT experiences can be worried that they are a sign of dementia.

Other measures have received more attention in the Alzheimer's disease literature [22], and are more concrete. If consciousness is impaired in Alzheimer's disease one would expect that the access to information or self awareness would be impaired. This is easily measured by examining how estimates of performance relate to actual performance. The most common measure consists of asking a participant to predict their future memory performance [27] for currently inaccessible information, the Feeling-of-Knowing (FOK) paradigm. In this task, participants are asked to estimate the likelihood with which they will recognize an item which they have failed to recall [27-30]. A FOK state thus occurs when one believes that one knows a piece of information, and given that the information is not forthcoming, believes that they would be able to identify it if it were shown at a later point in time. Prediction accuracy is obtained by comparing predictions to subsequent recognition of targets [31]; healthy participants make reliably non-chance judgements of future performance; they show self-awareness in their judgements.

The FOK can be measured on newly learned information (Episodic FOK, [29, 30, 32, 33]) or for general knowledge (Semantic FOK [34, 35]). Researchers have found that Alzheimer's disease patients do not present a uniform profile of performance across tasks and materials. Souchay *et al.* [33] found striking deficits in episodic FOK. Alzheimer's disease patients were unable to accurately gauge whether they would be able to recognise recently learned but currently non-retrievable items. In contrast, Bäckman and Lipinska [34, 35] gave patients a test using general knowledge questions. Pronounced deficits in fact retrieval among the Alzheimer's disease patients were observed but no reliable group differences in semantic FOK accuracy were found: patients were able to accurately predict which non recallable general knowledge items they would be able to recognise. Overall, these findings show that AD patients have accurate FOKs for semantic material but not for episodic tests. Given that the FOK measures a form of conscious awareness of memory processing, it might be suggested that awareness of *episodic* processes is impaired in Alzheimer's Disease, whereas the ability to make inferences about general knowledge is unimpaired (at least early in the disease, [36]).

Finally, another measure called either the judgment-of-knowing or judgment-of-learning refers to predictions made during or immediately after the learning phase

[37]. A few studies have examined Alzheimer's Disease patients' ability to predict their memory performance on an episodic memory task using these judgements [38], finding that patients have some difficulty predicting their likelihood of future memory performance. For example, Moulin *et al.* [38] demonstrated that whereas memory performance increased over several repetitions of a learning event, the people with Alzheimer's Disease, unlike controls, did not demonstrate a corresponding shift in their predictions. Whereas memory performance was improved by repetition, the patients lacked the reflective abilities to consciously report this in their predictions.

Table 2: Memory awareness: A summary of the literature

Study	Method/Material	Findings
Tip-of-the-tongue states (TOT)		
Astell *et al.* (1996) [25]	General knowledge	More TOT states in AD
Delazer *et al.* (2003) [26]	Famous people	No differences between AD patients and older adult control
Feeling-of-knowing judgments (FOK)		
Backman *et al.* (1993) [34]	Semantic FOK (general knowledge)	Accurate FOK in AD
Lipinska *et al.* (1996) [35]	Semantic FOK (dated *Vs.* contemporary knowledge)	Accurate FOK in AD AD Gammas*:.31 (dated information);.55 (contemporary information) / Control Gammas:.40 (dated information);.45 (contemporary information)
Pappas *et al.* (1993) [36]	Semantic FOK (general knowledge)	Non accurate FOK in AD
Souchay *et al.* (2002) [33]	Episodic FOK (word pairs)	Non accurate FOK in AD AD Gammas: -.12 Control Gammas:.33
Judgment-of-Learning (JOL)		
Moulin *et al.* (2000) [38]	JOL on list of words	AD Gammas:.14 Gamma accuracy scores for patients not different from zero suggesting a difficulty to predict memory performance Control Gammas:.54

*Gamma scores are presented when available. Gamma scores are used to calculate prediction accuracy and are a measure of association that allows the comparison of performance for high and low predictions. This index ranges from –1 to +1, with large positive values corresponding to a strong association between memory performance and predictions, while negative values show an inverse relationship.

Thus far, it seems that people with Alzheimer's disease are unable to reflect upon their performance during an episodic task [*e.g.*, 38]. Furthermore, people with Alzheimer's disease have a particular deficit in predicting the recognition of a non-recallable item in an episodic memory task [33]. These empirical findings suggest that one feature of the episodic deficit is a lack of awareness of the processing of this form of memory. No studies on the neural correlates of episodic metacognitive judgements have been carried out in Alzheimer's disease; this remains a priority for future research.

3.2 Recollection

Another concept related to consciousness is sentience, in this case, what memory functioning feels like. This concept links to the notion of recollection, and the examination of mental contents during an act of remembering. Different theories have been proposed describing the nature of the information processed within the episodic system, and what constitutes 'remembering' [2]. For example, according to the *fuzzy-trace theory* [39], it involves both *detail information* such as characteristics of the material presented, contextual or source information, and *gist information* defined as the general meaning conveyed by the information. Similarly, one can distinguish between *item memory* and *source memory*, source memory pertaining to the contextual information associated to the item (such as a spatial location or timing of a prior event). As in Table **1**, episodic memory has also been associated with the process of *recollection* in opposition to *familiarity* [40, 41]. Familiarity is the sense that an item has been encountered earlier but without the recall of any contextual detail about this item, while recollection involves the recall of specific details about the event. Thus it is possible to complete some memory tasks when recollection is impaired or unavailable, merely on a sense of whether material is a familiar or not. The terms recollection and familiarity are used differently by different researchers and in different paradigms. However, there is consensus that recollection and familiarity differ in terms of the type of information they provide. Familiarity is described as an index of memory strength whereas recollection reflects the retrieval of specific traces, contextual details or source information linked to the study event [42, 43].

The final view is that remembering does not only involve recalling information with its context but also involves feelings. Recently, Conway [44] suggested that remembering was 'a process and a state'. The process refers to the construction of a mental representation while the state is 'a state of conscious awareness distinguished by a specific type of mental content an a particular *cognitive feeling.*' According to Conway [44] these feelings can be conceptualised as *autonoetic consciousness* or *recollective experience*. Recollective experience, or 'remembering' occurs when a rememberer has a sense or feeling of the self in the past. Images (often visual), feelings, thoughts and verbal statements directly related to the recalled episode also often come to mind during recollective remembering.

These frameworks are all somewhat different, with some emphasising subjective feelings, and others, the nature of a retrieved memory by the nature of the material. For instance, the process of recollection is inferred if someone is able to state not only that the word 'garage' was presented to them in a memory test, but also that it was presented in blue ink, or with a female voice, *etc.* For others, the process of recollection is a direct statement about the quality of the experience of remembering. Authors often cite the different frameworks interchangeably, and whilst the field would clearly benefit from some precision [2], for the purposes of this review, we might think of recollection as any form of rich, evocative retrieval based on a subjective state and containing contextual information. One reason that we adopt this view is that, as will be shown, people with Alzheimer's disease have deficits in this form of rich, evocative retrieval but not such the weaker, less self-knowing form of retrieval. The studies reviewed below clearly point to a recollection deficit, but they do not discriminate between theoretical positions.

3.3. Measuring Recollection in Alzheimer's Disease

Specific paradigms have been developed to explore recollection and familiarity directly and some of these methods have been used in Alzheimer's disease. These measures can be classified into three categories. The first category refers to the procedures used to estimate recollection and measures one of the main functions of recollection – the ability to minimize memory errors and avoid 'illusions of familiarity' [45]. For instance, if you had experienced a crime, and had seen two faces, one of a bystander and one the perpetrator, you would want to be able to recall the information about who was who in order to not be 'seduced' by the overwhelming sensation of familiarity of the bystander. This ability has been termed *recollection rejection* [46] and consists in correctly rejecting errors on the basis of recollection, *e.g. remembering that the man with glasses was the man who was sat opposite you on the bus, and not the one who ran off with the handbag*. Recollection is also involved in reducing susceptibility to memory distortions such as misattribution (*i.e.* the act of attributing a recollection or idea to an incorrect source). The second category refers to the subjective states associated with memory retrieval by directly asking the participants to say whether or not the information is familiar or if they can remember it. Finally, the last category refers to paradigms assessing participants' abilities to retrieve specific information linked to the target event and measure another function of recollection: *source monitoring (i.e. attributing the correct source to a particular item)* [47]. Results from each type of category are reviewed in turn and the main findings summarized in Table **3**.

3.3.1 Estimation Methods

Several paradigms have been proposed in which recollection is essential to minimize memory errors. With these paradigms the correct use of recollection is necessary to select or retrieve the correct answer. In the paradigm proposed by Deese, Roediger and McDermott [48], recollection is used to reduce familiarity-based false recognition. Several studies have used this paradigm to estimate *memory for gist* and *memory for details*. In this paradigm, participants are presented with lists of words related to a non-presented critical lure [49]. For example, participants study different categorised lists, *e.g. thread, haystack, pin, cotton*. Then in the recognition phase, participants are presented with studied items (targets; *thread, pin*) and non-studied items (critical lures; such as *needle*) and non-related lures, such as other categorised items, like *red, blue*). At test, critical lures are likely to be falsely recognized because they match the gist information formed at study about related concepts [50]. Detail information is measured as the ability to distinguish between studied items and non-presented critical lures, requiring conscious awareness of the specifics of encoding [51].

Memory for both gist and detail information decreases in Alzheimer's disease [51-54]. Budson *et al.* [51] suggest that Alzheimer's disease patients demonstrate low levels of false recognition because they cannot create gist information. However, after repeated trials, gist memory is improved and patients' sensitivity to false alarms increases as they fail to accumulate contextual recollection over repeated presentation of the list. These results thus suggest that Alzheimer's patients have difficulties in suppressing false recognition of semantic associates using recollection. Pierce *et al.* [55] used a different paradigm, originally proposed by Smith *et al.* [56] in which recollection of source information is needed to avoid intruding presented exemplars from categorized lists. Alzheimer's patients were unable to use recollection to avoid intrusions. Thus, people with Alzheimer's disease have cognitions which are more likely to be on the basis of gist. In social situations, as one example, this might lead to inappropriate interpretations of events. The extension of this recollection deficit into real world behaviours remains an interesting priority for future research.

Another procedure used to estimate recollection is the process dissociation procedure [57]. In this paradigm participants complete two different memory tasks, one where they merely have to identify whether or not they studied the item before, and one where, additionally, they have to specifically declare where or when the item was studied. By comparing performance on the test assessing specifics (which requires recollection) and the test asking for a simple old/new distinction (which merely requires familiarity) it is possible to estimate the separate contributions of familiarity and recollection. Several studies using different variations of this procedure have showed that Alzheimer's patients' memory difficulties are attributable to a deficiency in effortful memory processes (*i.e.* recollection requiring specifics) but also had some reduced automatic processing (*i.e.* familiarity) [58-61]. Recently, this paradigm has been applied to Mild Cognitive Impairment, demonstrating that whereas familiarity is not impaired relative to controls, recollection is [62]. This procedure, therefore, might be suitable for early diagnosis of memory impairment in dementia.

3.3.2 Subjective States

The second category regards reports of subjective experience. With the remember/know procedure, participants are asked to report directly whether or not they recognize items on the basis of remembering or knowing, having been given definitions of the concepts, and/or examples. This method therefore asks for conscious self-evaluations of memory 'feelings'. So far, only three studies have used the remember/know paradigm in Alzheimer's disease. Della Barba [63] showed that patients produced fewer remember and the same amount of know responses compared to control participants. More recently, Rauchs, Piolino, Mezenge *et al.* [64] showed that Alzheimer's disease patients give fewer remember but more know responses than controls. Rauchs *et al.* also asked participants to justify their responses. For each remember response, the participants were invited to give contextual details related to the target; Alzheimer's disease patients were less able to justify their remember responses and they reported fewer details about the learning context. Finally, the fact that Alzheimer's disease patients report fewer remember responses has also been observed using an autobiographical memory task, where participants retrieve memories from their own past life [65].

These results clearly suggest that the subjective feelings associated with recollection are impaired in Alzheimer's disease. Alzheimer's patients report being in a state of remembering less often than controls and this is the case for newly learned information (episodic memory) or more remote personal information (autobiographical memory). In short, it appears that people with Alzheimer's disease are less likely to experience the sensation of remembering: they are impaired in terms of consciousness in that they do not re-experience pervious events with the same quality as healthy older adults.

3.3.3 Source Memory: Contextual Details

The final category considers the specific information that can be produced during a memory test. Item *vs.* associative recognition methods have been used to explore the retrieval of contextual information associated with recollection. In this approach, pairs are given at study, such as *apple-table, monkey-tennis, radio-head.* Participants are later asked to discriminate intact pairs (words studied in the same pair, *apple-table*) from rearranged pairs (words studied but in different pairs, *monkey-head*). The ability to correctly reject the rearranged pairs depends on recollection [41, 66, 67], because both of the items will feel familiar – they have both been encountered recently, but only recollection can produce information specific enough to correctly judge which item was presented with which other item. Gallo *et al.* [68] used such a task and showed that Alzheimer's disease patients recognized fewer intact pairs and made more false alarms to rearranged pairs compared to control participants.

In other versions of recognition tasks, with a similar rationale, participants are asked to decide whether the word was spoken by a male or female voice or where the item was presented. With this type of task participants are thus asked to retrieve the context, or the source in which they learnt the information. Several studies with slightly different procedures have demonstrated that source memory is impaired in Alzheimer's disease [69-73]. Mitchell *et al.* [69] asked Alzheimer's patients to identify words from a sentence they had read or from a sentence for which they had generated the ending; Dick *et al.* [70] asked whether participants had performed an act or whether the experimenter did it; Dalla Barba *et al.* [71] asked participants to discriminate seen from imagined objects; Multhaup and Balota [72] asked participants to discriminate words they had read from words they had generated and words they had generated from words generated by the experimenter. Finally, Tendolkar *et al.* [73]. asked participants to recall the colour in which words where printed when presented at study.

This research points to deficits in the specificity of recall: people with Alzheimer's disease may be able to retrieve one piece of information, but arguably due to a failure of other aspects of the study phase to reach consciousness, they are unable to make sophisticated judgements about its source, or the specifics of encoding. Thus, in our view, the pattern of deficits in memory in Alzheimer's disease are explained by the relative difficulty with recollection compared to familiarity. It is important to note that familiarity is probably impaired in Alzheimer's disease but to a lesser extent than recollection [58-61]. Clearly there will be cases where both fail: and complete forgetting occurs.

Both *familiarity* and *recollection* are involved in successful retrieval, and some authors suggest that they may act sequentially [74] (See Fig. **1**). The idea is that a fast familiarity response guides retrieval processes until recollection provides a subjective feeling of remembering, and additional contextual information [75].

Table 3: Recollection: A summary of the literature

Study	Paradigm	Findings
Estimation Methods		
Budson *et al.* 2000, 2001, 2001 [51-53]	DRM* paradigm	Decreased memory for gist and detail in AD
Hudon *et al.* 2006 [54]	DRM paradigm and text memory task	Decreased memory for gist and detail in AD
Adam *et al.*, 2005; Hudson and Robertson, 2007; Knight, 1998; Koivisto *et al.*, 1998. [58-61]	PDP* paradigm	Impaired controlled processes (recollection) in AD Reduced automatic processes (familiarity) in AD
Subjective States		
Della Barba (1997) [63]	R/K* paradigm	Fewer R (recollection) responses in AD
Rauchs *et al.* (2007) [64]	R/K paradigm with justification for R responses	Fewer R responses in AD and fewer justification (contextual details)
Piolino *et al.* (2003) [65]	R/K paradigm on an autobiographical memory task	Fewer R responses
Source Memory		
Gallo *et al.* (2004) [68]	Discrimination between intact word pairs and rearranged word pairs	More false alarms to rearranged pairs in AD
Mitchell *et al.* (1986) [71]	Discrimination between words read *vs.* generated	Impaired source discrimination in AD
Dick *et al.* (1989) [70]	Discrimination between words acted and words non-acted	Impaired discrimination in AD
Dalla Barba *et al.* (1999) [69]	Discrimination between seen from imagined objects	Impaired discrimination in AD
Multhaup *et al.* (1997) [72]	Discrimination between read *vs.* self of experimenter generated words	Impaired discrimination in AD
Tendolkar *et al.* (1999) [73]	Words presented in different colours	AD patients unable to recall the correct colours

*DRM = Deese-Roediger and McDermott procedure [48].
*PDP = Process dissociation procedure [57].
*R/K = Remember/Know procedure [12].

4. On the relationship between recollection, familiarity and metacognition.

The experient acts metacognitively upon these sensations of familiarity and recollection in order to reflect upon their mental operations. Thus, familiarity is used at a 'pre-retrieval stage' (cue-familiarity [73]) to trigger a rapid preliminary feeling which helps in the selection of the retrieval strategy. At a subsequent stage, the process underlying memory predictions may become more analytic, influenced by explicit consideration of the content of the cues (partial information, or contextual detail) that come to mind during the search of the target. This post-retrieval stage is based on both familiarity and recollection; familiarity and recollection are reflective states which enable one to process information in memory appropriately. We now turn to how such subjective sensations of memory drive more concrete concepts such as the feeling of knowing. We hypothesise that without recollection, someone with Alzheimer's disease will not be able to reflect upon their memory function.

In a recent study on young adults, Hicks and Marsh [76] showed that high FOK predictions (*i.e.* when participants are confident that they will recognize the target) were associated with making more remember judgments in a recognition task. This suggests that the feeling of 'knowing' experienced during a failed recall attempt leads to items being later recognised on the basis of remembering (and not familiarity). Souchay *et al.* [22] showed that FOK accuracy was significantly to correlated remember responses but not to know responses, confirming this link between FOK and recollection (demonstrated in Fig. **1**).

Research examining the basis of the FOK states also draws on concepts described above. According to Koriat [76], when healthy participants fail to retrieve a target they use some *partial information* related to this target to guide their predictions. This partial information induces the subjective feeling that the target will be recognized or recalled in the future. Our novel suggestion is that the partial information used to make metacognitive judgments depends on the type of states of consciousness associated to memory retrieval: noetic or autonoetic [12]. The use of noetic partial information would lead to a judgment based on familiarity whilst the use of autonoetic partial information would lead to a judgment based on recollection.

So far, two types of partial information have been proposed in the literature: structural-phonological and semantic. This has been supported by the studies showing that the tip of the tongue [77] and FOK states were associated with the retrieval of various types of information such as the initial letter of the missing word [32, 78] or the connotative meaning of this missing word [78-80]. We suggest that these cues are noetic cues. Our novel hypothesis is to suggest that, in particular for an episodic memory task, a third type of partial information needs to be added. This partial information is akin to the contextual information, feelings and self-awareness captured in Tulving's concept of autonoetic consciousness and the state of 'remembering' [16]. Thus, partial information can be of three types: structural-phonological (noetic), semantic (noetic) or episodic (autonoetic). This is similar to the different types of source information proposed by Johnson *et al.* [47]. Source memory information can be of different types: sensory/perceptual information (noetic), spatial and temporal information (autonoetic), semantic detail (noetic) and affect (autonoetic) [47]. We argue that people with Alzheimer's cannot reflect on their memory abilities when needing autonoetic consciousness to do so; the inability to correctly gauge performance in an FOK task is a consequence of a failure of recollection.

The disruption of recollection in Alzheimer's disease explains why there is impaired awareness of memory in some circumstances but not others. According to Koriat's model [74], recollection is involved at a post-retrieval stage, when patients are actively searching the target. Souchay *et al.* [16] suggest that the type of partial information used to estimate future retrieval differs according to the type of task and what autonoetic partial information (or contextual details) are specific to the memory task. In an episodic task, the sensation of recollection, which indicates the presence of contextual information in memory, is a powerful cue by which one can gauge how well something is learnt, and how likely it is that one will retrieve it again later; such cues are absent in Alzheimer's disease. In contrast, familiarity is relatively intact and this may actually lead to inappropriate evaluations of memory performance. Metcalfe *et al.* [75] suggest that *familiarity* leads people to 'approximate the uncertain quantity indirectly, rather than measuring the quantity itself', resulting in biases and errors. The fact that Alzheimer's patients have to rely more on familiarity than on recollection explains their difficulties in predicting future retrieval, but also the variability and lack of precision in their recall. In a general knowledge task, autonoetic partial information is not necessary to evaluate the state of memory and future performance – on such semantic tasks people with Alzheimer's disease are unimpaired.

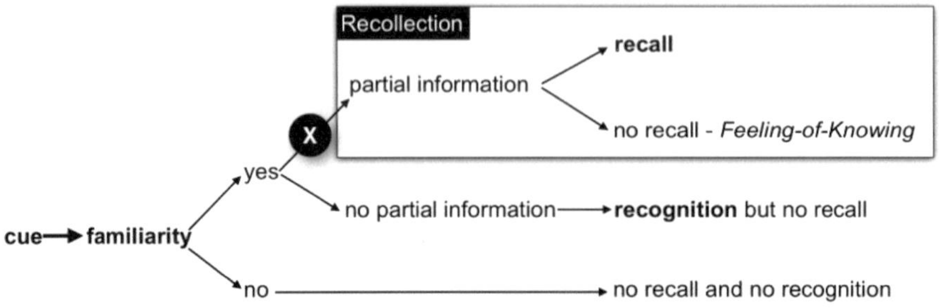

Figure 1: Figure to illustrate relationship between familiarity, recollection and feeling of knowing. Cross illustrates where disconnection occurs in Alzheimer's disease.
Note: Memory processes are cued by stimulus in the environment. A fast assessment of familiarity with cue is carried out, leading to a feeling of familiarity. If item is familiar a search for a target is started which activates associated partial information. If partial information is recovered item is either recalled or non-recalled. If item is not recalled, a 'feeling of knowing' is generated. If no partial information is generated, memory processes and awareness are based on familiarity alone. Dashed box illustrates processes and judgements reliant upon recollection.

4. MEMORY, CONSCIOUSNESS AND THE BRAIN IN ALZHEIMER'S DISEASE

We now turn our attention to the neural substrates of this recollection deficit. A few studies have explored the neural correlates of recollective experience in Alzheimer's disease. The cortical and neurochemical changes that characterize Alzheimer's disease could support impaired recollection in two ways [68]. As outlined above, damage to the medial-temporal lobe explain the deficits in recollection observed in Alzheimer's patients [81]. Consistent with this hypothesis Tendolkar *et al.* [73] showed that Alzheimer's patients who had smaller hippocampi showed more difficulties in recalling the study context (source memory). In a more recent study, Sperling *et al.* [82] found a decreased encoding activation in the hippocampal formation in a face name association task, suggesting a role of these regions in binding together contextual details.

Damage to the frontal lobes also explains Alzheimer's patients' difficulties in recollection. Neuropsychological studies suggest that damage to the frontal lobes disrupts recollection but leaves familiarity relatively intact. Frontal lobe patients have deficits in source memory [83], give fewer Remember responses [84, 85] and often present a very high rate of false alarms in recognition [86]. Recent neuroimaging studies on normal populations have confirmed the involvement of the frontal lobes in recollection [41]. Direct support for the role played by the frontal lobes in explaining the recollection deficits in Alzheimer's disease comes from a recent study published by Rauchs *et al.* [64]. Using correlations between memory performance and resting-state cerebral metabolism measured by positron emission tomography, these authors showed that the lack of remember responses in AD patients was supported by a dysfunction of frontal areas.

Despite the fact that no study has yet explored the neural correlates of the feeling of knowing in Alzheimer's disease, we suggest here that as with recollection, the cortical changes observed in the frontal lobes and in the medial-temporal lobe regions produce the feeling of knowing deficit. Patient and neuroimaging investigations suggest the existence of a network of brain regions implicated in awareness of memory including the mediotemporal lobe and the prefrontal regions [87]; a memory network that Conway [88] termed the fronto-temporal route (see [14] for a case showing impairment to this network, and disruption of memory awareness). Patients with frontal lobe damage are less accurate than control participants at predicting their memory performance when using FOK predictions, but as with Alzheimer's patients this was only on episodic and not semantic material [83, 87, 89, 90]. Neuroimaging studies on healthy groups have clearly confirmed the role of the frontal lobes in FOK judgments, by showing frontal lobe activation for FOK accuracy in both episodic and semantic memory tasks [91-94]. Functional magnetic resonance imaging studies studies also showed activation of the temporal lobes in FOK accuracy [91, 94] suggesting that FOK was related to a left hemisphere network of frontal and temporal cortical regions. The neural substrates of tip of the tongue states in healthy adults have also been investigated using functional magnetic resonance imaging revealing that this state was associated to the activation of the prefrontal cortex [93]. Some studies also suggest that the frontal lobes would be involved in judgements of learning made during study [95, 96, but also see 90, 97].

Our novel suggestion is that, in Alzheimer's disease, the deficit in conscious awareness of memory elucidated here could be due to a disconnection syndrome

[22]. Several neuroimaging studies show a structural disconnection between the prefrontal areas and the hippocampus [98, 99] in Alzheimer's disease. This would lead to two types of impairment underlying recollection and awareness. First, the network of regions involving the medial temporal lobe and the frontal lobes would be involved in the retrieval of partial, contextual or source information. Indeed, in healthy populations, retrieval of partial information related to the target is linked to the activity of the medial temporal lobe [100] and the ventral medial prefrontal cortex [97]. Thus, a disconnection of these brain regions would result in a decrease of partial information retrieved, lead to recollection deficits and difficulties in predicting future performance. Second, a disconnection of the mediotemporal regions and frontal regions could contribute to Alzheimer's patients' inaccuracy through the involvement of these brain regions in monitoring retrieval. This resonates with the studies showing that the ventral medial prefrontal cortex is involved in the assessment of 'felt-rightness' of a memory [101] and that the frontal lobes are involved in strategic control of memory outputs [14].

5. RECOLLECTION AND METAMEMORY: AN UPDATE

Using a search on the Web of Knowledge for articles published since this article was originally written (2009), with the search terms "Alzheimer" combined with "metamemory" or "recollection" returns 14 and 49 articles respectively[1]; this is a field which is still developing. The article here is not a systematic review, but clearly as the field develops, a more thorough synthesis of the literature will be critical.

Recent studies challenge our hypothesis that recollection is differentially impaired in Alzheimer's disease, and the emphasis in the field has shifted to consider whether there is an impairment of familiarity, given a consensus in the impairment of recollection. A growing number of studies suggest that familiarity is not spared in Alzheimer's disease (see Table **4**). Indeed one theoretical article, driven from a neuroanatomical viewpoint, even proposes that it is familiarity processes which are first impaired in Alzheimer's disease [109]. It is also

[1] Search conducted on 22 March 2013

suggested that tests of familiarity, not recollection, might be the best diagnostic tests for early detection of pre-Alzheimer cognitive change [110].

Table 4: An update. Examples of recent studies examining recollection and familiarity in Alzheimer's disease (AD) and Mild Cognitive Impairment (MCI)

	Recollection Impairment	**Familiarity Impairment**	**Group**	**Neuroimaging**
Algarabel *et al.* [102]	Not tested	Yes	AD, MCI	-
Ally *et al.* [103]	Yes	Yes	AD, MCI	-
Bastin *et al.*, [104]	Not tested	No	AD	-
Genon *et al.* [105]	Yes	No	AD	fMRI
Hudon *et al.* [106]	Yes	Yes	AD, MCI	-
van der Meulen, *et al.* [107]	Greater	Lesser	MCI	fMRI
Wolk *et al.* [108]	Yes	Yes	AD, MCI	MRI

Other studies still place an emphasis on strategic difficulties in using recollection to overcome feelings of familiarity [111], and the inability to use item-specific recollection in order to avoid false recognition [112, 113], or the impairment of recollection relative to other more automatic processes such as habit-based memory [114]. A nuanced view of the field is that there may well be deficits in familiarity as well as recollection, but the value of considering separable processes in memory has the benefit of describing how people with Alzheimer's strategically regulate (or not) their memory system.

Given this emphasis on the interplay between memory systems, memory awareness and its role in regulation continues to be a topic of major interest in the Alzheimer's literature. Researchers continue to examine awareness using questionnaires. Recent studies have confirmed that even at the early states, AD patients have a tendency to overestimate their cognitive ability (see [115] for a review and a model).

Experimental studies using predictions of performance have taken different directions. One new theme is that of recollection-based metamemory; a test of our original idea that recollection deficits in AD could, at least partly, explain awareness deficits as measured by predictions such as the Feeling-of-knowing. Dodson *et al.* [116] examined AD patients' ability to predict the likely accuracy of source judgments. Participants listened to statements spoken by a male or a female voice and gave recognition and source judgments. For both recognition and source judgments, AD patients were found to assign identical confidence ratings to correct and incorrect judgments, thus showing deficits. Thus showing a deficit, Dodson *et al.* [116] suggested a 'Remembrance-Evaluation model of monitoring'.

According to this model, high confidence misrecollection (falsely remembered information given high confidence) drives the impairment observed for source judgments. To explore further the idea that memory awareness and metacognitive judgments would be more impaired in AD on tasks requiring participants to recollect specific details, Gallo *et al.* [117] presented patients with studied objects as coloured photos or as line drawings. At recognition participants were presented two picture labels and participants had to choose the word that was studied with a coloured picture. They showed that AD patients had accurate judgments of confidence and could thus estimate the accuracy of their response on a recollection test (see [36] for similar findings). Thus, the Gallo *et al.* [116] and Dodson *et al.* [117] studies provide conflicting results. Clearly, the impact of recollection deficits on awareness of memory in AD is still a matter of debate.

Another direction taken by the researchers in the field concentrates not on item judgements but on general memory awareness and whether AD patients update their evaluation of their memory ability. Several recent studies have used global predictions of performance to measure memory awareness in AD. Of particular interest, a recent study [118] showed that despite being able to revise their global predictions during a test, AD patients were not able to maintain this information; after a 1h delay, their estimate had returned to a previous (inaccurate) level. Such findings lead Morris and Mograbi [115] to suggest that a lack of memory awareness in AD is caused by 'a decline in specific mnenomic processes leading to a loss of personal knowledge' (see also the 'Petrified Self' hypothesis [119]), in line with the thesis of the current article.

Finally, a novel a evolution in this field consists of moving away from explicit predictions and self-ratings to examine behavioural responses. Mograbi *et al.* [120] report a study in which AD patients were presented with memory tasks in a success or a failure condition. Explicit awareness was measured by asking patients to predict their performance and 'implicit awareness' was measured by ratings of filmed facial expression. AD patients had preserved emotional reactivity to failure despite their impaired awareness as measured by predictions. These findings reinforce the idea of a fractionation of memory awareness deficits in Alzheimer's disease, with graded levels of awareness depending of the task and the measure used. In fact we would like to suggest that AD patients can often monitor online their performance, but maybe not when the task relies heavily on recollection.

6. CONCLUDING REMARKS

This review has described a pattern of deficits in Alzheimer's patients involving the relationship between awareness of memory and a state of consciousness, recollection. There is the possibility that further investigations into this disease can illuminate current hot topics in psychology; the complex interaction between self and memory [88] and more subjective disorders of memory awareness, such as déjà vu [14, 121]. Our view is that Alzheimer's disease results in a disconnection between experience and process in the operation of memory. In giving an overview of recollection and familiarity processes in human memory there is a clear explanation of the differences in recall and recognition, and one based on emergent research in the neuroscience of memory; recall requires recollection processes, whereas recognition can be completed on the basis of familiarity alone.

From a clinical point of view, further studies should determine how to improve memory rehabilitation and differential diagnosis in this population. The role of awareness has been explored in relation to rehabilitation in Alzheimer's [122]; however, studies have not yet explored how to use the relatively spared familiarity in Alzheimer's patients to potentially improve awareness of memory abilities. Awareness of memory abilities is a crucial issue as it is linked to the correct use of memory strategies and recent work showed that Alzheimer's patients failed to use appropriate memory strategies [123]. Research [124] has considered whether it is possible to train recollection (which is possible in healthy older adults with memory difficulties; [125]): there is a transfer from recollection training to other domains of memory. It would be interesting to see whether this improvement in recollection would also improve awareness of memory.

One critical issue in Alzheimer's disease is early diagnosis. Interestingly, Mild Cognitive Impairment (MCI), which represents a preclinical phase of this disease [126] has attracted little or no attention from researchers investigation awareness of memory abilities or recollection (but see Table **4**). One study suggests that measuring MCI patient's abilities to predict their memory abilities might be a useful tool for differential diagnosis [127] where another has shown that assessing recollection can help to differentiate Alzheimer's patients from MCI patients [54]. As a consequence, knowing more about MCI in this regard is a research priority.

Finally, the more that is understand about the specifics of memory impairment in Alzheimer's disease, and its underlying brain basis, the better our understanding of pharmacological interventions will be. In this regard, Winstein *et al.* [128] have researched the impact of donepezil on declarative and non-declarative memory in Alzheimer's and showed that this medication had beneficial effects on both. Declarative memory can be further sub-divided into the separate recollection and familiarity processes discussed here. Following, Winstein *et al.*'s lead, the further fractionation of memory in Alzheimer's disease and its treatment remains a priority for current Alzheimer research.

ACKNOWLEDGEMENTS

This paper was produced directly from discussions held at the 2nd Recollection, Remembering and the Complex Nature of the Self ERSC/CNRS workshop RES-170-25-0008 in Tours, France, in May 2008.

CONFLICT OF INTEREST

The authors confirm that this chapter content has no conflict of interest.

DISCLOSURE

This chapter is an update of our previous publication in CAR "Memory and Consciousness in Alzheimer's Disease" published in "CAR, Volume 6, Number 3, June, pp. 186 to 195".

REFERENCES

[1] Welsh K, Butters N, Hughes J, Mosh R, Heyman A. Detection of abnormal memory decline in mild cases of Alzheimer's disease using CERAD neuropsychological measures. Archives of Neurology 48: 278-281 (1991).

[2] Mandler G. Familiarity Breeds Attempts. Perspectives on Psychological Sciences 3: 390-399 (2008).

[3] Gennaro RJ, Herrmann DJ, Sarapata M. Aspects of the unity of consciousness and everyday memory failures. Consciousness and Cogn, 15: 372-385 (2006).

[4] Greene JD, Baddeley AD, Hodges JR. Analysis of the episodic memory deficit in early Alzheimer's disease: evidence from the doors and people test. Neuropsychologia 34 (6): 537-51 (1996).

[5] Moulin CJA, James N, Freeman JE, Jones RW Deficient acquisition and consolidiation: Intertrial Free Recall Performance in Alzheimer's diseas and Mild Cognitive Impairment. Journal of Clinical and Experimental Neuropsychology 26: 1-10 (2004).

[6] Grober E, Kawas C. Learning and retention in preclinical and early Alzheimer's disease. Psychology and Aging, 12: 183-188 (1997).

[7] Hodges JR. Memory in the dementias. In E Tulving & F.I.M Craik (Eds). The Oxford Handbook of Memory (pp. 441-459). Oxford, United Kingdom: Oxford University Press (2000).

[8] Chen P, Ratcliff G, Belle SH, Cauley JA, DeKosky ST, Ganguli M Cognitive tests tat best discriminate between presymptomatic AD and those who remain nondemented. Neurology 55(12): 1847-53 (2000).

[9] Kopelman MD, Steven, TG, Foli S, Grasby P. PET activation of the medial temporal lobe in learning. Brain 121: 875-887 (1998).

[10] Convit A, de Asis J., de Leon M.J, Tarshish C.Y., De Santi S, Rusinek H. Atrophy of the medial occipitotemporal, inferior, and middle temporal gyri in non-demented elderly predict decline to Alzheimer's disease. Neurobiology of Aging, 21: 19-26 (2000).

[11] Jack C.R., Petersen R.C., Xu Y.C., O'Brien P.C., Smith G.E., Ivnik R.J., Boeve B.F., Waring S.C., Tangalos *E.G.* and Kokmen E. Prediction of AD with MRI-based hippocampal volume in mild cognitive impairment. Neurology, 52: 1397-1403 (1999).

[12] Tulving E. How many memory systems are there ? American Psychologist 40: 385-398 (1985).

[13] Koriat A, Goldsmith M. Monitoring and control processes in the strategic regulation of memory accuracy. Psychological review 103: 490-517 (1996).

[14] Moulin CJA, Conway MA, Thompson RG, James N, Jones RW. Disordered Memory Awareness: Recollective Confabulation in Two Cases of Persistent Deja Vecu. Neuropsychologia 43: 1362-1378 (2005).

[15] Conway MA, Gardiner JM, Perfect TJ, Anderson, SJ Cohen G. Changes in memory awareness during learning: The acquisition of Knowledge by psychology undergraduates. Journal of Experimental Psychology: Learning, Memory and Cognition 126(4): 1-21 (1997).
[16] Souchay C, Moulin CJA, Clarys D, Taconnat L, Isingrini M. Diminished episodic memory awareness in older aadults: Evidence from Feeling of knowing and Recollection. Consciousness and Cognition 16(4): 769-84 (2007).
[17] O'Connor AR, Moulin CJA, Cohen G. Memory and Consciousness. In Cohen G. & Conway M.A (eds) Memory and the Real World (3rd Edition) Hove UK: Psychology Press (2008).
[18] Gardiner JM, Richardson-Klavehn A. Remembering and knowing. In E. Tulving & F.I.M. Craik (Eds.), Handbook of Memory. New York, Oxford University Press, p. 229-244 (2000).
[19] Henson RN, Rugg MD, Shallice T, Josephs O, Dolan RJ. Recollection and familiarity in recognition memory: an event-related functional magnetic resonance imaging study. Journal of Neuroscience, 19: 3962-3972 (1999).
[20] Eldridge LL, Knowlton BT, Furmanski CS, Bookheimer SYand Engel SA. Remembering episodes: a selective role for the hippocampus during retrieval. Nature Neuroscience 3: 1149-1152 (2000).
[21] Shrager Y, Kirwan CB and Squire LR. Activity in both hippocampus and perirhinal cortex predicts the memory strength of subsequently remembered information. Neuron 59: 547-553 (2008).
[22] Souchay C. (2007) Metamemory in Alzheimer's disease. Cortex 43: 987-1003 (2007).
[23] Pinker S. How the mind works. New York, USA: W.W. Norton. (1997)
[24] Brown R, McNeill D. The 'Tip of the Tongue' Phenomenon. Journal of verbal learning and verbal Behavior 5: 325-337 (1966).
[25] Astell A, Harley T. Tip-of-the-tongue States and Lexical Access in Dementia. Brain and Language 54: 196-215 (1996).
[26] Delazer M, Semanza C, Reiner M, Hofe R, Benke T. Anomia for people names in DAT-evidence for semantic and post-semantic impairments. Neuropsychologia 41: 1593-1598 (2003).
[27] Hart JT. Memory and the Feeling-Of-Knowing Experience. Journal of Educational Psychology 56: 208-216 (1965).
[28] Nelson T and Narens L. Metamemory: A Theoretical Framework and New findings. The Psychology of Learning and motivation 26: 125-322 (1990).
[29] Schacter DL. Feeling of Knowing in Episodic Memory. Journal of Experimental Psychology: Learning, Memory, and Cognition 9: 39-54 (1983).
[30] Souchay C, Isingrini M and Espagnet L. Relations between Feeling-of-knowing and Frontal lobe functioning in older adults, Neuropsychology 14: 299-309 (2000).
[31] Nelson TO. A comparison of current measures of the accuracy of feeling-of-knowing predictions. Psychological Bulletin 95,: 109-133 (1984).
[32] Blake M. Prediction of Recognition when Recall Fails: Exploring the Feeling of Knowing Phenomenon, Journal of Verbal Learning and Verbal Behavior 12: 311-319 (1973).
[33] Souchay C, Isingrini M, Gil R. Alzheimer's disease and Feeling-of-knowing in Episodic Memory, Neuropsychologia 40: 2386-2396 (2002).

[34] Bäckman L, Lipinska B. Monitoring of General Knowledge: Evidence For Preservation in Early Alzheimer's disease, Neuropsychologia 31: 335-345 (1993).

[35] Lipinska B, Bäckman L. Feeling-of-knowing in fact retrieval: further evidence for preservation in early Alzheimer's disease. Journal of the International Neuropsychological Society 2: 350-358 (1996).

[36] Pappas B, Sunderland T, Weingartner H, Vitiello B, Martinson H, Putman, K. Alzheimer's Disease and Feeling-of-Knowing for Knowledge and Episodic Memory. Journal of Gerontology: Psychological Science 47: 159-164 (1992).

[37] Arbuckle T and Cuddy L. Discrimination of item strength at time of presentation. Journal of Experimental Psychology 81: 126-131 (1969).

[38] Moulin CJA, Perfect T, Jones RW. The effect of repetition on allocation of study time and judgments of learning in Alzheimer's disease, Neuropsychologia 38: 748-756 (2000).

[39] Reyna VF, Brainerd CJ. Fuzzy-trace theory: An interim synthesis. Learning and Individual Differences 7: 1-75 (1995).

[40] Mandler G. Recognizing: the judgment of previous occurrence. Psychological Review 87: 252-271 (1980).

[41] Yonelinas A.P. The nature of recollection and familiarity: A review of 30 years of research. Journal of Memory and Language 46: 441-517 (2002).

[42] Jacoby L Perceptual enhancement. Persistent effects of an experience. Journal of Experimental Psychology: Learning, Memory, and Cognition 9: 21-38 (1983)

[43] Yonelinas AP Receiver-operating characteristics in recognition memory: evidence for a dual-process model. Journal of Experimental Psychology: Learning, Memory and Cognition 20(6): 1341-54 (1994).

[44] Conway M.A Remembering. In H. Roediger jnr III, D. Yadi & E. Tulving (eds). The Science of Memory: Concepts (2006).

[45] Jacoby L, Kelley C, Dywan J. Memory Attributions. In H.L. Roediger, F.Craik, Varieties of Memory and Consciousness, p 391-422 (1989).

[46] Brainerd CJ, Reyna VF, Wright R, Mojarding AH Recolllection rejection: false-memory editing in children and adults. Psychol Rev, 110(4): 762-84 (2003)

[47] Johnson M, Hastroudi S and Lindsay S. Source Monitoring. Psychological Bulletin 113(1): 3-28 (1993)

[48] Roediger HL, McDermott KB. Creating false memories: Remembering words not presented in lists. Journal of Experimental Psychology: Learning, Memory, and Cognition 21: 803-814 (1995).

[49] Stadler M. A, Roediger H. L. 3rd and McDermott K. B. Norms for word lists that create false memories. Memory & Cognition 27(3): 494-500 (1999).

[50] Brainerd C. J and Reyna V. F. Fuzzy-trace theory and children's false memories. Journal of Experimental Child Psychology 71: 81-129 (1998).

[51] Budson A. E, Daffner K. R, Desikan R, Schacter DL. When false recognition is unopposed by true recognition: gist-based memory distortion in Alzheimer's disease. Neuropsychology 14(2): 277-287 (2000).

[52] Budson AE, Desikan R, Daffner KR, Schacter DL. Perceptual false recognition in Alzheimer's disease. Neuropsychology 15(2): 230-243 (2001).

[53] Budson A. E, Sitarski J, Daffner K. R and Schacter D. L. False recognition of pictures *vs.* words in Alzheimer's disease: the distinctiveness heuristic. Neuropsychology 16(2): 163-173 (2002).

[54] Hudon C, Belleville S, Souchay C, Lepage E and Gely-Nargeot M-C. Memory for gist information in Alzheimer's disease and Mild cognitive Impairment. Neuropsychology 20(5): 266-77 (2006).

[55] Pierce B, Sullivan A, Schacter D and Budson A Comparing Source-based and Gist-based False Recognition in Aging and Alzheimer's disease. Neuropsychology 19(4): 411-419 (2005).

[56] Smith S, Tindell D, Pierce B, Gilliland T and Gerkens D The use of source memory to identify one's own episodic confusion errors. Journal of Experimental Psychology: Learning, Memory and Cognition 27: 386-395 (2001).

[57] Jacoby L. (1991). A process dissociation framework: Separating automatic from intentional influences of memory, Journal of memory and language 30: 513-54 (1991)

[58] Adam S, Van der Linden M, Collette F, Lemauvais L and Salmon E Further Exploration of Controlled and Automatic Memory Processes in Early Alzheimer's disease. Neuropsychology 19(4): 420-427 (2005).

[59] Hudson J and Robertson C Automatic and Controlled use of Memory in Alzheimer's disease. Cortex 43: 524-530 (2007).

[60] Knight R.G Controlled and automatic memory processes in Alzheimer's disease. Cortex 34: 427-435 (1998).

[61] Koivisto M, Portin R and Rinne J Automatic influences of memory in Alzheimer's disease. Cortex 34: 209-219 (1998).

[62] Anderson N, Ebert P, Jennings J, Grady C, Cabeza R and Simon J. Recollection- and familiarity-based memory in healthy aging and amnestic mild cognitive impairment. Neuropsychology 22(2): 177-187 (2008).

[63] Della Barba G Recognition memory and recollective experience ini Alzheimer's disease. Memory 5: 657-692 (1997).

[64] Rauchs G, Piolino P, Mezenge F, Landeau B, Lalevee C *et al.* Autonoetic Consciousness in Alzheimer's disease: Neuropsychological and PET findings using an episodic learning and recognition task. Neurobiology of Aging 28: 1410-1420 (2007).

[65] Piolino P, Desgranges B, Belliard S, Matuszewski V *et al.* Autobiographical memory and autonoetic consciousness: triple dissociation in neurodegenerative disease. Brain 126: 2203-19 (2003)

[66] Hockley W.E and Consoli A Familiarity and Recollection in item and associative recognition. Memory and Cognition 27: 657-664 (1999).

[67] Kelley R and Wixted J.T On the nature of associative information in recognition memory. Journal of Experimental Psychology: Learning, Memory and Cognition 27: 701-722 (2000).

[68] Gallo D, Sullivan A, Daffner K, Schacer D and Budson A. Associative Recognition iin Alzheimer's disease: Evidence for Impaired Recall-to-Reject. Neuropsychology 18 (3): 556-563 (2004).

[69] Mitchell DB, Hunt RR, Schmitt FA. The generation effect and reality monitoring: evidence from dementia and normal aging. Journal of Gerontology 41(1): 79-84 (1986).

[70] Dick MB, KEan ML, and Sand D. Memory for internally generated words in Alzheimer's disease: Breakdown in encoding and semantic memory. Brain and Cognition 9(1): 88-108 (1989).

[71] Dalla Barba G, Nedjam Z, Dubois B. Confabulation, executive functions, and source memory in Alzheimer's disease. Cognitive Neuropsychology 27: 1-16 (1999).

[72] Multhaup K, Balota D. Generation effects and Source Memory in Healthy Older adults and in Adults with Dementia of the Alzheimer type. Neuropsychology 11(3): 382-391 (1997).

[73] Tendolkar I, Schoenfeld A, Golz G, Fernandez G *et al.* Neural correlates of recognition memory with and without recollection in patients with Alzheimer's disease and healthy controls. Neuroscience Letters 263: 45-48 (1999).

[74] Koriat A, Levy-Sadot R, Edry E, de Marcas S. What do we know about what we cannot remember? Accessing the semantic attributes of words that cannot be recalled. Journal of Experimental Psychology: Learning, Memory and cognition 29: 1095-105 (2003).

[75] Metcalfe J, Schwartz B, Joaquim S. the Cue-Familiarity Heuristic in Metacognition, Journal of Experimental Psychology: Learning, Memory, and Cognition 19(4): 851-861 (1993).

[76] Hicks JL, Marsh RL. On predicting the future states of awareness for recognition of unrecallable items. Memory and cognition 30: 60-66 (2002).

[77] Brown AS. A review of the tip-of-the-tongue experience. Psychological Bulletin, 109(2): 204-223 (1991).

[78] Koriat A. How do we know that we know? The accessibility model of the feeling of knowing. Psychological Review 100: 609-639 (1993).

[79] Eysenck M. The Feeling Of Knowing a Word's meaning, British Journal Of Psychology 70: 243-251 (1979).

[80] Schacter DL, Worling J. attribute information and the feeling of knowing, Canadian Journal of Psychology 39(3): 467-475 (1985).

[81] Price JL, Morris JC. Tangles and plaques in nondemented aging and "preclinical" Alzheimer's disease. Annals of Neurology 45(3) (1999).

[82] Sperling R, Chua E, Cocchiarella A *et al.* Putting names to faces: Successful encoding of associative memories activates the anterior hippocampal formation. Neuroimage 20:1400-1410 (2003).

[83] Janowsky JS, Shimamura AP, Squire L.R. Memory and metamemory: Comparisons between patients with frontal lobe lesions and amnesic patients. Psychobiology, 17: 3-11 (1989).

[84] Levine B, Black S, Cabeza R, Sinden M, McIntosh A, Toth J, Tulving E, Stuss D. Episodic memory and the self in a case of isolated retrograde amnesia. Brain 121(10):1951-1973 (1998)

[85] Levine B, Freedman M, Dawson D, Black S, Stuss D. Ventral Frontal contribution to self-regulations: Convergence of episodic memory and inhibition. Neurocase 5(3):263-275 (1999).

[86] Parkin A, Bindschaedler C, Harsent L and Metzler C. Pathological false alarm rates following damage to the left frontal cortex. Brain and Cognition 32(1):14-27 (1996).

[87] Pannu JK and Kaszniak A. Metamemory Experiments in Neurological Populations: A review. Neuropsychology Review 15: 105-130 (2005).

[88] Conway MA. Memory and the Self, Journal of memory and Language 53: 594-628 (2005).

[89] Schnyer D, Verfaelli M, Alexander M, LaFleche G, Nicholls L, Kaszniak A. A role of right medial prefrontal cortex in accurate feeling-of-knowing judgments: evidence from patients with lesions to frontal cortex, Neuropsychologia 42: 957-966 (2004).

[90] Pinon K, Allain P, Zied Kefi M, Dubas F and Le Gall D. Monitoring processes and metamemory experience in patients with dysexecutive syndrome. Brain and Cognition, 57: 185-188 (2005).

[91] Kikyo H and Miyashita Y. Temporal lobe activations of "feeling-of-knowing" induced by face-name associations. Neuroimage 23:1348-57 (2004).
[92] Kikyo H, Ohki K and Miyashita Y. Neural correlates for feeling-of-knowing: an fMRI parametric analysis. Neurone,36:177-86 (2002).
[93] Maril A, Simons J, Mitchell J, Schwartz B and Schacter D. Feeling-of-knowing in episodic memory: and event-related fMRI study. Neuroimage 18: 827-836 (2003).
[94] Schnyer DM, Nicholls L and Verfaellie M. The role of VMPC in metamemorial judgments of content retrievability, Journal of Cognitive Neurosciences, 17:832-46 (2005).
[95] Vilkki J, Servo A and Surma-Aho O. Word list Learning and Prediction of recall after frontal lobe lesions. Neuropsychology 12: 268-277 (1998).
[96] Vilkki J, Virtanen S, Surma-Aho O and Servo A. Dual task performance after focal cerebral lesions and closed head injuries. Neuropsychologia, 34:, 1051-1056 (1996).
[97] Modirrousta M and Fellows L. Medial prefrontal cortex plays a critical and selective role in 'feeling of knowing' meta-memory judgments. Neuropsychologia, 46(12): 2958-65 (2008).
[98] Grady CL, Furey ML, Pietrini P, Horwitz B, Rappoport SI Altered brain functional connectivity and impaired short-term memory in Alzheimer's disease. Brain 124: 739-756 (2001).
[99] Wang L, Zang Y, He Y, Liang M, Zhang X, Tian L, Wu T, Jiang T, Li K. Changes in hippocampal connectivity in the early stages of Alzheimer's disease: Evidence from resting state fMRI. NeuroImage, in press.
[100] Chua E, Schacter D, Rand-Giovannetti E and Sperling R. Understanding metamemory: Neural correlates of the cognitive process and subjective level of confidence in recognition memory. NeuroImage 29: 1150-1160 (2006).
[101] Moscovitch M and Winocur G. The frontal cortex and working with memory. In D.T. Stuss & R.T. Knight (Eds.), Principles of frontal lobe function New York: Oxford University Press 188-209 (2002).
[102] Algarabel S, Escudero J, Mazón JF, Pitarque A, Fuentes M, Peset V and Lacruz L. Familiarity-based recognition in the young, healthy elderly, mild cognitive impaired and Alzheimer's patients. Neuropsychologia 47: 2056–64 (2009).
[103] Ally B, Gold C and Budson AE. An evaluation of recollection and familiarity in Alzheimer's disease and mild cognitive impairment using receiver operating characteristics. Brain and cognition 69: 504–13 (2009).
[104] Bastin C, Willems S, Genon S and Salmon E. Enhancing the salience of fluency improves recognition memory performance in mild Alzheimer's disease. Journal of Alzheimer's disease□: JAD 33, 1033–9 (2013).
[105] Genon S, *et al.* Verbal learning in Alzheimer's disease and mild cognitive impairment: fine-grained acquisition and short-delay consolidation performance and neural correlates. Neurobiology of aging 34, 361–73 (2013).
[106] Hudon C, Belleville S, and Gauthier S. The assessment of recognition memory using the Remember/Know procedure in amnestic Mild cognitive impairment and probable Alzheimer's disease. Brain and Cognition, 70(1), 171-179 (2009).
[107] van der Meulen M, Lederrey C, Rieger SW *et al.* Associative and Semantic Memory Deficits in Amnestic Mild Cognitive Impairment as Revealed by Functional Magnetic Resonance Imaging. Cognitive and behavioural neurology, 25: 195-215 (2012)
[108] Wolk D, Dunfee KL, Dickerson B, Aizenstein HJ, & DeKosky S. A medial temporal lobe division of labor: insights from memory in aging and early Alzheimer disease. Hippocampus 21: 461–6 (2011).

[109] Didic M. *et al.* Which memory system is impaired first in Alzheimer's disease? Journal of Alzheimer's disease□: JAD 27, 11–22 (2011).

[110] Wolk D, Mancuso L, Kliot D, Arnold SE, & Dickerson BC. Familiarity-based memory as an early cognitive marker of preclinical and prodromal AD. Neuropsychologia (in press).

[111] Tse, C., Balota, D. A., Moynan, S. C., Duchek, J. M. & Jacoby, L. L. The Utility of Placing Recollection in Opposition to Familiarity in Early Discrimination of Healthy Aging and Very Mild Dementia of the Alzheimer ' s Type. 24, 49–67 (2010).

[112] Abe, N. *et al.* False item recognition in patients with Alzheimer's disease. Neuropsychologia 49, 1897–902 (2011).

[113] Plancher, G., Guyard, A., Nicolas, S. & Piolino, P. Mechanisms underlying the production of false memories for famous people's names in aging and Alzheimer's disease. Neuropsychologia 47, 2527–36 (2009).

[114] Guerdoux E, Dressaire D, Martin S, Adam S, and Brouillet D. Habit and recollection in healthy aging, mild cognitive impairment, and Alzheimer's disease. Neuropsychology, 26: 517-33 (2012)

[115] Morris RG, and Mograbi DC. Anosognosia, autobiographical memory and self knowledge in Alzheimer's disease. Cortex (in press)

[116] Dodson CS, Spaniol M, O'Connor MK, Deason RG, Ally GA, Budson AE. Alzheimer's disease and memory-monitoring impairment: Alzheimer's patients show a monitoring deficit that is greater than their accuracy deficit. Neuropsychologia, 49: 2609 – 2618 (2011)

[117] Gallo DA, Cramer SJ, Wong JT, Bennett DA. Alzheimer's disease can spare local metacognition despite global anosognosia: Revisiting the confidence–accuracy relationship in episodic memory. Neuropsychologia 50: 2356–2364 (2012)

[118] Stewart G, McGeown WJ, Shanks MF, Venneri A. Anosognosia for memory impairment in Alzheimer's disease. Acta Neuropsychiatrica, 22: 180–187. (2010)

[119] Mograbi DC, Brown RG, Morris RG. Anosognosia in Alzheimer's disease--the petrified self. Conscious Cogn. 18: 989-1003 (2009)

[120] Mograbi DC, Brown RG, Salas C, Morris RG. Emotional reactivity and awareness of task performance in Alzheimer's disease. Neuropsychologia, 50: 2075-2084 (2012)

[121] Moulin CJA. Disordered recognition memory: Recollective confabulation. Cortex (in press)

[122] Clare L and Woods RT. Cognitive training and cognitive rehabilitation for people with early-stage Alzheimer's disease: a review. Neuropsychological Rehabilitation 14: 385-401 (2004).

[123] Souchay C, Moulin CJA, Isingrini M and Conway MA. Rehearsal strategy use in Alzheimer's disease. Cognitive Neuropsychology 25: 783-97 (2008).

[124] Boller B, Jennings JM, Dieudonné B, Verny M, Ergis AM. Recollection training and transfer effects in Alzheimer's disease: effectiveness of the repetition-lag procedure. Brain Cogn. 78:169-77 (2012).

[125] Jennings J and Jacoby L. Improving memory in older adults: Training recollection. Neuropsychological Rehabilitation 13: 417-440 (2003).

[126] Petersen R. C, Smith G E, Waring S. C, Ivnik R. J, Tangalos E. G and Kokmen E. Mild cognitive impairment: clinical characterization and outcome. Archives of Neurology 56: 303-308 (1999).

[127] Akhtar S, Moulin CJA, Bowie PCW. Are people with Mild Cognitive Impairment Aware of the benefits of Errorless Learning? Neuropsychological Rehabilitation 16: 329-346 (2006).

[128] Winstein CJ, Bentzen KR, Boyd L, Schneider LS. Does the cholinesterase inhibitor, donepezi, benefit both declarative and non-declarative processes in mild to moderate Alzheimer's disease? Current Alzheimer Research 4(3): 273-276 (2007).

CHAPTER 2

Common Biological Mechanisms in Alzheimer's Disease and Cancer

Maria I. Behrens[1,2,4,*], Daniela P. Ponce[2], Catherine M. Roe[3] and Felipe Salech[2]

[1]Departamento de Neurología y Neurocirugía, Hospital Clínico Universidad de Chile, Chile; [2]Instituto de Ciencias Biomédicas, Facultad de Medicina, Universidad de Chile, Chile; [3]Department of Neurology and the Charles F. and Joanne Knight Alzheimer Disease Center, Washington, University School of Medicine in St Louis and [4]Clínica Alemana de Santiago, Chile

Abstract: Epidemiological studies show an inverse association between Alzheimer's disease (AD) and cancer, such that the risk of developing cancer is significantly lower in patients with AD, while participants with a history of cancer in the past have a lower risk of developing AD. In cancer, cell regulation mechanisms are disrupted with augmentation of cell survival and/or proliferation, whereas conversely, AD is associated with increased neuronal death. Here we discuss the possibility that perturbations of mechanisms involved in cell survival/death regulation could be involved in both disorders. Mechanisms that induce changes in the activity of molecules with key roles in determining the decision to "repair and live"- or "die" could play a role in the pathogenesis of the two disorders. As examples, the roles of p53, PARP-1, the Wnt signaling pathway, and the process of adult neurogenesis are discussed as potential candidates that, speculatively, may explain an inverse association between AD and cancer.

Keywords: Alzheimer, cancer, neurogenesis, p53, PARP-1, Wnt signaling pathway.

AN INVERSE ASSOCIATION BETWEEN CANCER AND AD

Alzheimer's disease (AD) and cancer are two common disorders of the elderly. Age is the most important risk factor for AD and also for most cancers; therefore the increase in life expectancy is likely to increase the prevalence of these two disorders. However, there is data suggesting that these two disorders convey

***Corresponding author María Isabel Behrens:** Departamento de Neurología y Neurocirugía, Hospital Clínico Universidad de Chile, Santos Dumont 999, Clínica Alemana de Santiago, Chile; Tel: 56 2 2978 8260; Fax: 56 2 2737 8542; E-mail: behrensl@u.uchile.cl

D.K. Lahiri (Ed)

mutual protection. It intrigued us that residents in nursing homes, most of them suffering from some type of dementia, did not have a history of cancer, whereas many of those who were cognitively normal had had cancer in the past. This observation was followed by two longitudinal prospective studies in which we found an inverse association between cancer and AD [1, 2].

The first study, used archival data from 594 participants enrolled in longitudinal studies of memory and aging at the Knight Alzheimer's disease Research Center in Washington University School of Medicine in St Louis, where participants are cognitively evaluated annually with the Clinical Dementia Rating CDR [3], and a thorough medical history is obtained including a history of cancer, its type, treatment and date of diagnosis. The results showed an inverse association between AD and cancer; specifically, the rate of receiving a cancer diagnosis was significantly slower in the group of participants with dementia of the Alzheimer type, ($p < 0.001$, hazard ratio (HR) 0.391, 95% confidence interval (CI) 0.207-0.739), and conversely, participants with a history of any type of cancer in the past showed a slower rate of receiving a diagnosis of dementia of Alzheimer type with time. This last result did not reach statistical significance ($p = 0.06$, HR 0.400, CI 0.122-1.132), probably because of the small number of participants with a history of cancer in the past (N=50 patients). The inverse relationship was not accounted for by demographic factors such as age, sex, and education, as indicated by adjusted Cox proportional hazard models [1].

The incident cancers in the study groups were similar to those in the general US population [4], with skin cancers accounting for 57% of all neoplasias, most of them benign, ~80% basal or squamous cell carcinomas. We repeated the analysis in the skin cancer group specifically and found that, as with all cancers, the rate of skin cancer diagnosis was slower for participants with dementia of the Alzheimer type compared to non-demented individuals in both the log-rank test ($p <0.001$) and the Cox proportional hazard models ($p < 0.005$; hazard ratios (HR) between 0.22-0.26). Other cancer types were too infrequent in our sample to be analyzed separately. When combining all non-skin cancers into a single group, the rate of cancer diagnosis was slower with time for the dementia of Alzheimer type group, although the difference did not reach statistical significance (all $p>0.05$; HR between 0.65-0.83) [5].

The second analysis used data from the Cognition Substudy of the Cardiovascular Health Study (CHS) [6] to address the limitations of a selected population in our previous study. Cancer incidence was defined by hospitalization records to account for the limitation of self-report of cancer diagnosis [2]. The results analyzing 3020 participants confirmed those in our previous study; prevalent AD was associated with a reduced the risk of cancer (HR 0.31, 95% CI 0.12-0.86) after adjustment for demographic factors, smoking, obesity, and physical activity. Conversely, prevalent cancer was associated with a reduced risk of AD (HR 0.57, 95% CI 0.36-0.90) after adjustment for demographics, number of APOE4 alleles, hypertension, diabetes, and coronary heart disease. Furthermore, this study showed that the inverse association was present only for Alzheimer type dementia and not for vascular dementia or mixed -vascular plus Alzheimer- dementia. Vascular dementia is due to brain damage secondary to vascular pathology and not to a degenerative process as in dementia of the Alzheimer type.

Prior to our research in this area other studies, using cross-sectional and case-control designs, had reported a reduced prevalence of cancer among individuals with AD [7-12]. Recently, three additional longitudinal studies have found an inverse correlation between the risk of developing cancer and the risk of developing dementia. Driver *et al.,* [13] in a report using data from the Framingham Heart Study, evaluated 1278 participants older than 65 years of age with and without a history of cancer and free of dementia at baseline. Over a mean follow-up of 10 years they found that cancer survivors had a lower risk of probable AD (HR 0.67, CI 0.47-0.97), which was even lower for smoking related cancers (HR 0.26, CI 0.08-0.82). In a nested case-control analysis they found that the presence of AD was associated with a lower risk of subsequent cancer (HR 0.39, CI 0.26-0.58). In a population based registery study in Sweden with 19.756 cases and 147.324 age- and sex-matched controls Attner *et al.,* [14] reported lower rates of cancer diagnosis among patients with dementia (risk ratio = 0.60; 95% CI = 0.52-0.69). In accordance with our results in the skin cancer only group, White *et al.,* [15] recently followed 1,102 community-residing volunteers with a mean age of 79 years at enrollment and found that prevalent nonmelanoma skin cancer was associated with reduced risk of AD (HR 0.21; 95% CI 0.05-0.87; p =0.031) after adjustment for demographics, diabetes, hypertension, and coronary heart disease. In another study, in a large population-based incidence study in Northern Italy, Musicco *et al.,* [16] showed that the risk of cancer in AD patients was 50% reduced, and the risk of AD in patients with cancer was 35%

reduced. They also did separate subgroup analysis to indicate that the lower diagnosis was not due to underdiagnosis, for example, a lesser tendency to report a diagnosis of dementia in a patient with cancer, or to search for a cancer if the patient is demented [16].

Finally, in a retrospective national cohort of 3,499,378 veterans, Frain *et al.* communicated a reduced risk of Alzheimer's disease associated the majority of cancers. (Frain L, Swanson D, Betensky R, Cho K, Gagnon D, Kowall N, Lu KP, Gaziano M, Driver JA. A reduced risk of Alzheimer's disease is associated with the majority of cancers in a national cohort of veterans. Alzheimers Dement. 9(4):Suppl P617).

The relationship of dementia to the different types of cancers individually remains to be studied in more depth [17], as well as the role of environmental factors. However, there is an interesting possibility that one or more biological mechanisms may link AD and cancer. If such a mechanism can be identified, it might lead to better understanding of the pathology of these two disorders, as well as strategies to treatment development. The purpose of this review is to describe some potential biological links between the development of cancer and AD.

A COMMON BIOLOGICAL MECHANISM WITH OPPOSING EFFECTS

The neuropathological hallmarks of Alzheimer's disease include senile plaques composed of the beta amyloid (Aβ) peptide, and neurofibrillary tangles, consisting of intracellular deposits of an abnormally hyperphosphorylated tau protein. In addition, AD is characterized by extensive neuritic and synaptic degeneration and neuronal cell death. The leading explanation for the pathologic changes associated with AD is the "amyloid hypothesis" which states that the full manifestations of Alzheimer pathology are initiated by Aβ deposition [18].

Normal tissue function requires a match between the rate of cell loss and the rate of renewal. The maintenance of tissue homeostasis is achieved by efficient mechanisms that control genomic stability to prevent aberrant proliferation [9-21]. Intracellular stress pathways are able to recognize damage to the cell, and either induce DNA repair to mend the damage, or induce apoptosis or senescence [22]. In cancer this reparative process is defective, leading to excessive cell growth. Cancer is a disorder typified by uncontrolled, excessive cell growth, whereas conversely, AD and other neurodegenerative disorders are characterized by progressive dysfunction and neuronal loss.

One possible explanation for an inverse association between AD and cancer is that both diseases arise *via* malfunction of an underlying common mechanism that regulates cell survival. This mechanism could regulate the capability of cells to switch the cell machinery from a prone-to-death state (AD phenotype) to a prone-to-survive/grow state (cancer phenotype). In a prone-to die state, neurons would be more susceptible to cell death under stressors such as Aβ, tau hyperphosphorylation, oxidation, inflammation, or other unknown risk factors (the AD phenotype). At the same time, cells would respond to initiating cancer stimuli (UV radiation, for example) by death, reducing cancer susceptibility. Conversely, if cells are shifted to a survival/growth state, neurons would have a greater likelihood of surviving if subjected to stressors, while concomitantly becoming more susceptible to cancer development. Genetic polymorphisms in several key molecules that determine changes in their activity or variance in their DNA methylation could explain such opposing effects [23]. Here we discuss the possible involvement of the tumor suppressor p53, of PARP-1 and the Wnt signaling pathway as well as the role of adult neurogenesis in the pathophysiology of both cancer and AD.

The inverse association between cancer and AD described in the epidemiological studies was present in cancers of different organs, combining a cerebral disorder, such as AD, with tumors that are distributed in different organs outside the nervous system. This implies that a common biological mechanism would be applicable to all cells in the organism. In favor of a systemic deregulation of cell survival mechanisms, we recently showed that lymphocytes from AD patients had an increased vulnerability to oxidative stress-induced death, whereas cancer patients had an increased resistance to this type of death, compared to lymphocytes from healthy controls [24]. Instead, lymphocytes from aged healthy controls showed similar levels of overall survival than young donors when exposed to oxidative damage induce by H_2O_2, however the aged donors had increased apoptosis/necrosis ratios [25]. A greater susceptibility to death caused by apoptosis-inducing factors has also been reported in lymphocytes from AD patients [26]. In addition, lymphocytes and fibroblasts from AD patients show increased levels of p53 compared to healthy controls of comparable age [27-29]. Furthermore, fibroblasts derived from p53-mutated mice with enhanced p53 activity were more resistant to transformation by activated ras plus myc oncogene [30]. DNA microarrays studies of peripheral blood cells, have found similar patterns of gene differential expression as those encountered in studies of brain tissue -including aberrant gene expression of neuroinflammation and intracellular signalling proteins- supporting the suitability of peripheral cells for the study of AD pathogenesis [31].

The inverse association between cancer and AD might be extended to other neurodegenerative disorders, such as Parkinson's disease (PD), frontotemporal dementia and other tauopathies. Overall cancer mortality risk and tumor frequency are reduced in individuals with PD, for both smoking-related and non-smoking related cancers [32-34]. Of note, several genes known to be associated with PD were studied in cancer research before their involvement in PD was documented [35, 36]. Loss-of-function mutation in progranulin, a multifunctional protein involved in wound healing and inflammation has been reported in frontotemporal dementia [37-40]. Interestingly, overexpression of progranulin contributes to tumorigenesis in diverse cancers, including ovarian, breast, clear cell renal carcinoma and glioblastoma [41]. Not just neuronal cells but cells in other tissues could be more susceptible to degeneration. It is conceivable to speculate that other degenerative systemic disorders, such as osteoarthritis or osteoporosis, could also be associated with a reduced risk of cancer, and *vice versa*, patients with a history of cancer could have a reduced risk of systemic degenerative disorders.

TUMOR SUPPRESSORS IN CANCER AND AGING

In tissues with renewal capability, cell regeneration or reparation has evolved as an advantage in increased longevity compared to postmitotic tissues which lack this capability. However, this versatility to regenerate has the inherent risk of hyperproliferation and cancer. Thus, together with the renewal capacity that poses increased longevity there evolved mechanisms to suppress tumor formation [42]. Tumor suppressors are the main actors of the surveillance mechanism to avoid aberrant proliferation under normal conditions. Tumor suppressors regulate cell cycle checkpoint responses, detection and repair of DNA damage, mitogenic signaling, cell specification, protein ubiquitination and degradation, differentiation and migration, and angiogenesis [19]. Tumor suppressors can either eliminate potential cancer cells by inducing programmed cell death (apoptosis), or alternatively, they can induce permanent withdrawal from the cell cycle (cellular senescence). Apoptosis could give rise to a depletion of irreplaceable postmitotic cells in nonrenewable tissues; and, in the same way, to a depletion of proliferating or stem cell pools in renewable tissues. Similarly, senescence could deplete tissues of proliferating or stem cell pools, resulting in the accumulation of senescent cells. Thus, tumor suppressor mechanisms may be an example of evolutionary antagonistic pleiotropy [42-44], that is, they promote early-life survival by preventing the development of cancer, but eventually limiting longevity.

p53

The p53 gene is the prototypical tumor suppressor and its pathway is inactivated in most human cancers [21]. p53 is at the hub of numerous signaling pathways and can be described as a stress response gene; its product (the p53 protein) acts to induce apoptosis or cell-cycle arrest in response to DNA damage, thereby maintaining genetic stability in the organism by transcriptional and nontranscriptional mechanisms [21]. p53 deficient mice are developmentally normal, but susceptible to spontaneous tumors [45], and knocked-out p53 mice ($p53^{-/-}$) have a significantly higher number of proliferating cells than wild-type littermates in the lateral ventricle wall, as assessed by the incorporation of the nucleotide analogue bromodeoxyuridine [46].

As already mentioned the anticancer roles of p53 may come at the cost of proliferative reserve and thereby promote the aging phenotype [30, 42, 47, 48]. Tyner *et al.,* [30] created a transgenic mouse with a p53-mutation that confers an activated form of p53. They showed that these mice developed very few cancers, but showed several features of aging and had reduced longevity (26). Further support for the role of p53 in accelerating aging comes from data on transgenic mice that overexpress p44, a protein that enhances p53 activity, and showed shortened lifespan, accelerated aging, and an extraordinary low incidence of cancer compared to wild-type mice [49]. Furthermore, mice deficient in Zmpste24, a metallopeptidase involved in the processing of lamin A, show a senescence phenotype at the cellular level and accelerated aging at the organism level, together with a marked upregulation of p53 target genes [48]. As p53 enhancement leads to aging and reduced longevity, the opposite should be expected in p53 knockout mice. Mice genetically manipulated to activate the Arf/p53 pathway but conserving p53 normal regulation, show both cancer resistance and decreased aging [50], which is what would be expected if cancer is prevented [51, 52]. Therefore, the regulation of p53 activity is crucial to determine the role that p53 will assume. The same acetylation of the Lys amino acid at position 320 can promote neurite outgrowth in neuronal cells [53] or cell cycle arrest in other tissues [54]. In human population studies, the Arg 72 allele of the codon 72 Pro/Arg polymorphism of the p53 gene, resulting in a reduction in p53 activity, is associated with an increased longevity but also an enhanced cancer risk [55].

Therefore, the inactivation of p53 is known to be implicated in cancer development, and deregulation of p53 activation might play a role in promoting aging. Elevated p53 levels have been detected in the central nervous system of patients diagnosed with neurodegenerative diseases, such as Huntington's disease and Amyotrophic Lateral Sclerosis [56-58] and in the brains of AD [59-61] and Parkinson's disease patients [62, 63], and also in mouse models of several neurodegenerative diseases [64, 65].

The intracellular expression of the Aβ protein under a neuron-specific promoter led progressively to degeneration and death of neurons in the brains of transgenic mice and Aβ accumulation was correlated with activation of p53 [66]. In neuroblastoma cell lines, intracellular Aβ42 and Aβ40 directly activated the p53 promoter, resulting in p53-dependent apoptosis [59].

Mutations in the presenilins (PS1 and PS2), which form part of the gamma secretase complex that cleaves the amyloid precursor protein (APP) to generate Aβ, cause familial forms of AD and have also been shown to trigger p53-dependent cell death [67-69]. The intracellular C-terminal fragments of the gamma secretase cleavage of APP (AICD) trigger the activation of caspase-3 and an increase in p53 mRNA levels and activity [68]. A critical role for a presenilin/AICD-promyelocytic leukemia protein/p53 pathway has been proposed in AD pathogenesis [70]. Furthermore, it has been reported that inhibition of p53 in microglia attenuates the damage induced by Alzheimer peptides [71].

Taken together these results show that p53 regulation is extremely important to determine the fate of cells or tissues. It is conceivable that small deregulations towards one or the other side could favor survival/regeneration or death/senescence of the cells and explain the opposing results we found with regard to the development of cancer and DAT (Fig. **1**). Slight alterations in tumor suppressor activity, due for example to polymorphisms or differences in DNA methylation, could confer differential risks to AD or cancer across the lifespan. Patients with slight increases in the activity of tumor suppressor proteins would have lower risks of developing cancers, but instead would be at higher risk of developing AD. Augmented levels of tumor suppressors could also limit the renewal capacity of stem cells, and favor AD by preventing, in the long run, the reparation of dendrites and spines in damaged neurons and the replenishment of apoptotic cells. Similarly, the low incidence of AD in the cancer group could be explained by the presence of an inactivated form of a tumor suppressor, which in addition to assisting development of a cancer, could also favor a decreased susceptibility to neuronal death, conferring protection against AD. Microarray studies in the CA1 region of incipient AD patients showed upregulation of apparent glial transcription factor/epigenetic/tumor suppressor genes [72, 73].

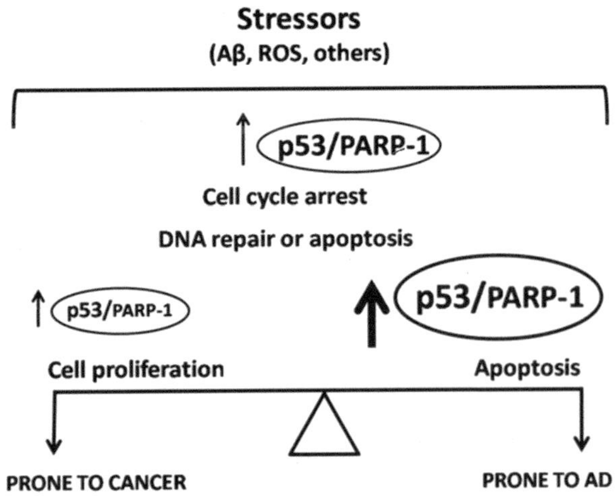

Figure 1: Proposed role of p53/PARP-1 in cancer and AD. In response to toxic or stress signals, p53 is activated through a number of post-translational modifications and induces cell cycle arrest among other functions. The decision is made whether to induce DNA repair or apoptosis of damaged cells to maintain genomic stability. If the cell machinery in the organism is shifted to higher p53 levels in response to stressors, the cells would be more prone to cell death and AD could develop. If, on the contrary, the cell machinery is shifted to low or no p53, the cells would be more prone to develop a cancer. PARP-1 and p53 have been recently proposed to regulate each other [99, 100]. ROS, reactive oxygen species. PARP-1, Poly (ADP-ribose) polymerase 1.

POLY (ADP-RIBOSE) POLYMERASE 1 (PARP-1)

Since the first report of a NAD-dependent protein modification now known as poly(ADP-ribosyl)ation, fifty years ago [74], several new biological functions have been described for the activity of PARP, the enzyme that catalyzes the reaction. PARP-1 is the best characterized of the 17 PARP sequences described in the human genome. It is a 116 kDa nuclear enzyme that catalyzes the transfer of the ADP-ribose moiety of nicotinamide adenine dinucleotide (NAD+) to nuclear proteins, such as transcription factors, histones and to PARP-1 itself, leading to the subsequent elongation of the polyADP ribose (PAR) polymer [75]. The first biological function described for PARP-1 was DNA repair. Upon DNA nicks, PARP-1 is activated and rapidly consumes nicotinamide adenine dinucleotide (NAD) to polymerize adenosine diphosphate (ADP)-ribose and covalently modify target proteins promoting chromatin relaxation and the recruitment of base-excision repair proteins to orchestrate DNA repair. Therefore, at low levels of activation PARP-1 has a protective role. However, following extensive DNA damage, such as those induced by excessive reactive oxygen species, PARP-1 is hyperactivated consuming large amounts of NAD+ and ATP and depriving the cell of energy, thereby promoting cell death by caspase-independent pathways, a form of necrotic cell death named parthanatos [76-78].

In this type of cell death, an apoptosis-inducing factor translocates to the nucleus from the intermembrane space of mitochondria and triggers chromatin condensation and DNA fragmentation, in a not yet well understood process [79-81]. PARP-1 has also been implicated in many physiological processes such as gene expression, maintenance of genomic stability and cell differentiation [75, 82, 83]. In addition, overactivation of PARP-1 is related to the development and progression of several chronic diseases such as diabetes, cancer, viral infections and neurodegenerative diseases [75]. In particular, parkinsonian neurotoxins lead to selective loss of dopaminergic neurons involving activation of PARP-1 [77, 84]. Increased poly (ADP-ribosyl) ation of nuclear proteins has been reported in the brains of AD patients [85], and an enhancement of PARP-1 activity is induced by amyloid beta in cells transfected with amyloid precursor protein, and in the brains of transgenic animals overproducing amyloid peptide [86, 87]. Nicotinamide, a PARP-1 inhibitor reduced the levels of oxidative stress, apoptosis and PARP-1 activity in an Aβ (1-42) induced rat model of AD [88]. To emphasize the PARP connection, significant differences in the distributions of PARP haplotype were observed in a case-control study between AD patients and controls (27). A PARP-1 dependent recruitment of the amyotrophic lateral sclerosis-associated protein FUS/TLS was recently described [89].

On the other hand, the inhibition of PARP-1 is being extensively studied in cancer research as a treatment for cancer. Inhibition of PARP-1 and PARP-2 activity is used to induce the death of tumor cells associated with genetic mutations in BRCA1 and BRCA2, or other tumors with non-functional homologous recombination repair [90]. PARP-1 functions by repairing single strand breaks which if unrepaired are converted into double strand breaks during DNA replication for cell division (increased in cancer cells). In this situation, cells with mutations in the double strand break repairing mechanisms, such as BRCA1 and BRCA2, generate genomic instability and are forced to death due to the rapid development of non-viable genetic errors [90]. PARP-1 and PARP-2 knockout mice show important deficiencies in DNA repair, and increased sensitivity to ionizing radiation and alkylating agents [91], so PARP inhibitors are also used as chemotherapy and radiation sensitizers in a other types of tumors [90, 92]. Several clinical studies with PARP inhibitors, mostly for breast and ovarian cancer, are currently been conducted [90]. PARP inhibitors have the advantage of not being toxic to healthy cells. Increased levels of PARP-1 expression and activity have been reported in prostate cancer cells [93], and PARP-1 hyperactivation is associated with cisplatin-resistance in human cancer cells [94]. The activation of PARP-1 seems to be a protective mechanism to trigger apoptosis of defective cells.

Finally, a relationship between PARP-1 activity and lifespan has been proposed. PARP-1 activity measured in permeabilized lymphocytes of 13 mammalian species strongly correlated with their lifespan [95]. Additionally, $PARP^{-/-}$ mice age prematurely [96], and poly(ADP-ribosyl)ation capacity declines with age in rodents as well as several cell types in humans, while centenarians have significantly higher poly(ADP-ribosyl)ation capacities than individuals of the average elder population [97, 98]. Our results showing that aging is associated with an increase in the apoptosis/necrosis ratio of H_2O_2-induced death of lymphocytes obtained from healthy control donors ranging from 24 to 95 years of age is in agreement with these results. Higher necrosis in young donors is in accordance with higher poly(ADP-ribosyl) ation capacity in this age category [25].

Interestingly, a recent report shows a link between p53 and PARP-mediated non-apoptotic cell death [99]. Montero *et al.,* 2013 showed that loss of p53 function promoted resistance to necrotic, PARP-mediated cell death in mouse embryonic fibroblasts, human colorectal, and human breast cancer cell lines, indicating that p53 is able to regulate not only apoptotic cell death, but also non-apoptotic, PARP dependent death. It was previously known that caspases are able to cleave PARP-1 and therefore interrupt NAD+ and ATP consumption needed for apoptotic death [100]. On the other hand, p53 is one of the targets of PARP-1, promoting its poly(ADP- ribosyl)ation and accumulation in the nucleus [101]. Therefore, p53 is a key protein orchestrating the different forms of cellular death pathways, whereby PARP-1 and p53 regulate each other, in a delicately regulated fashion.

In our studies of lymphocyte death induced by H_2O_2 oxidative stress we observed that inhibition of PARP-1 by preincubation with 3-Aminobenzamide significantly protected from cell death in all three groups of patients; healthy controls, patients with a previous skin cancer and AD patients. A significantly lower protection was obtained in AD lymphocytes [24] (Ponce *et al.,* in preparation). Interestingly, an increase in p53 has been reported in AD patients [29]. It is conceivable that in AD cells have increased levels of p53 that renders them more vulnerable to death, both by apoptosis and non-apoptotic, PARP-dependent death. The mechanism of PARP-1 regulation by p53 is unknown, but the action of sirt1 and Cathepsyn D has been suggested [100, 102, 103].

WNT SIGNALING PATHWAY

The Wnt (wingless-type murine-mammary tumour virus integration site) signaling pathway has an important role in many developmental and adult processes, such as gastrulation, axis formation, cell polarity, organ development and maintenance of stem cell pluripotency [104]. In the canonical pathway, wnt proteins bind to a complex cell-surface receptor that associates with a large cytoplasmic protein complex that ultimately stabilizes cytoplasmic β-catenin which translocates to the nucleus and promotes the expression of cell survival and proliferation promoting genes. In the absence of Wnt binding, GSK-3β which is part of the cytoplasmic complex phosphorylates β-catenin molecules which are then degradated through the ubiquitin-mediated degradation pathway, thus preventing their survival-promoting action.

The Wnt signaling pathway has been linked to neurodegeneration and cancer [104-107]. Perturbations of the Wnt signaling pathway are involved in colorectal cancer [108, 109] and several other cancers including prostate, lung and breast [108-112]. An upregulation of the Wnt signalling pathway has been described in skin cancers, both for melanomas and basal and squamous cell carcinomas [113-118].

A role for the Wnt signaling pathway has also been described in AD [107, 119-124]. Inestrosa and collaborators demonstrated a relationship between a loss of the wnt signaling pathway activity, with decreased cytoplasmic levels of β-catenin and Aβ-induced neurotoxicity. They found that inhibition of GSK-3β, a central modulator of the Wnt pathway, by lithium protected rat hippocampal neurons from Aβ-induced damage [125] and pre-treatment of neurons with wnt3a-conditioned media preserved neurons from Aβ neurotoxicity [126-128]. Wnt ligands were able to prevent the decrease in the number of neurites induced by Aβ in hippocampal primary cultures [106, 129-131]. Phosphorylation of tau stabilizes β catenin, antagonizing apoptosis, and the knock down of β-catenin produces an increase in the number of apoptotic cells reinforcing the action of β-catenin as a survival element in AD [132].

A study among bipolar patients reported a lower incidence of AD in patients who had been on lithium therapy [133], suggesting that GSK3 inhibition might have clinical benefits. Lithium treatment induced a reduction of GSK3β expression in hippocampal cells in culture and in the brain and leucocytes of rats treated with lithium [134]. β-catenin levels are markedly reduced in AD patients carrying presenilin-1 (PS-1) inherited mutations [135]. Furthermore, an association between a highly conserved LRP6 polymorphism and the risk of developing late-ons*et Al*zheimer's disease in ApoE 4 allele carriers was found in a case-control and a large family-based study of AD patients [136].

A subtle deregulation favoring Wnt activation could explain a greater tendency to tumor development, while at the same time favor neuronal survival and protect against degeneration. A small change towards suppression of Wnt signaling could explain a greater susceptibility to neuronal death or loss of dendritic spines, and protect against the development of cancer. Polymorphisms or epigenomic changes [23] in key molecules that might favor or un-favor the activity of the pathway could resolve the chances of developing a cancer, thus avoiding neurodegeneration, or developing AD, and avoiding hyperproliferation.

NEUROGENESIS

Another aproach to exploring a biological mechanism that may explain an inverse relationship between cancer and Alzheimer is through the study of changes in cellular proliferation in tissues, in this case in the adult brain. In the last decades, the generation of new neurons and subsequent differentiation of neural progenitor cells (NPC) has been consistently stated in the subventricular region of the lateral ventricles (SLV) and in the subgranular zone (SGZ) of the dentate gyrus in the hippocampus of adult brain throughout life [137]. In the dentate gyrus new neurons are integrated into existing circuits and shown to be important for learning and memory [137, 138]. Since this neurogenic niche is located in the hippocampus, and is related to the memory process it has been conjectured that it could participate in the pathogenesis of AD [139, 140].

Multiple animal models of AD have shown that alterations in the hippocampal neurogenesis is an early event in AD, and the progression of the pathological injury in the brain is associated with a decrease of neurogenesis in the SGZ of the hippocampus, although this finding depends on the animal model used and the set-up of the neurogenesis quantification method [139, 141]. Studies from autopsy brains of AD patients have also shown changes in hippocampal markers of neurogenesis [142]. The amyloid machinery participates in the regulation of adult neurogenesis. For example, the APP intracellular domain (AICD) has been shown to regulate hippocampal NPC proliferation and diferentiation [143], and sAPPα regulates the proliferation of NPC in the SVZ [144]. Recent studies have shown that overexpression of PS1 appears to modulate adult hippocampal progenitor proliferation and diferentiation in response to an enriched environment [145]. Nevertheless, the extent of neurogenesis can either increase or decrease during the progression of symptoms as a response to the neurodegenerative process [140].

Adult hippocampal neurogenesis is a highly regulated phenomenon. Interestingly, many of the signal transduction pathways important in regulating proliferation and differentiation of neural progenitors are the same pathways involved in cancer development [146]. We previously described the importance of p53 and wnt in cancer development. Studies in mice KO for p53 expression show an increase in cell proliferation in the hippocampus after gamma irradiation [147, 148]. Canonical Wnt signaling hyperactivation has been associated with the development of cancer in several niches such as skin, colon, and blood [149]. It has been shown that an increase in the activity of the canonical Wnt pathway is an important inducer of adult hippocampal neurogenesis increasing proliferation and subsequent differentiation of NPC into neurons by the expresión of neuroD1 and Prox1 gene [150-152] and that the inhibition of hippocampal canonical wnt signaling produces a decrease in hipocampal neurogenesis [150]. Recent studies have shown that changes in the expression of dickkopf, an inhibitor of the canonical wnt pathway, would be partly responsible for the reduced hippocampal neurogenesis associated with age and cognitive performance in older mice [153].

Taken together, these data show that increasing the activity of signaling pathways that produce cancer also cause an increase in hippocampal neurogenesis and conversely, a higher activity of suppressing tumor signaling pathways inhibits adult hippocampal neurogenesis. Therefore, a deregulation of neurogenesis may explain the inverse relationship between cancer and Alzheimer disease, and should be explored in the future.

CONCLUDING REMARKS

An inverse association between cancer and AD opens up numerous opportunities of investigation to explore the causes of both AD and cancer. A common biological mechanism inversely operating in the two disorders, leading to increased cell survival, or higher risk of cell death, could explain these results. Understanding the nature of the relationship between AD and cancer is crucial considering that treatments to prevent and treat one of the disorders might to a greater risk of developing the other. The identification of a common biological mechanism may provide insight into therapeutic strategies that could eventually aid in preventing both disorders.

Note added in proof. While this manuscript was in revision a study was published showing deregulation in opposite directions of molecular processes common to CNS disorders and Cancers that might explain the inverse comorbidity of these two disorder.[1] The authors performed a transcriptomic meta-analyses of three neurodegenerative disorders (Alzheimer's disease, Parkinson'sdisease and Schizophrenia) and three cancer types (Lung, Prostate, Colorectal) and found several genes and pathways that were deregulated in opposite directions. Interestingly, p53, wnt and Pin1 were among the pathways involved (1).

ACKNOWLEDGEMENTS

Supported by grants Fondecyt # 1080569, 1110189 (MIB) and grants P50-AG05681, P01-AG03991, P01 AG026276 from the National Institute on Aging, The Farrell Family Research Fund the Charles and Joanne Knight Alzheimer Research Initiative of the Washington University Knight Alzheimer Disease Research Center (CR), and the generous support of Fred Simmons and Olga Mohan.

CONFLICT OF INTEREST

The authors confirm that this chapter content has no conflict of interest.

DISCLOSURE

This chapter is an update of our previous publication in CAR "A Common Biological Mechanism in Cancer and Alzheimer's Disease?" published in 'CAR', Volume 6, Number 3, June, pp. 196 to 204.

REFERENCES

[1] Roe CM, Behrens MI, Xiong C, Miller JP, Morris JC. Alzheimer disease and cancer. Neurology. 2005;64(5):895-8.

[2] Roe CM, Fitzpatrick AL, Xiong C, Sieh W, Kuller L, Miller JP, *et al.,* Cancer linked to Alzheimer disease but not vascular dementia. Neurology. 2010;74(2):106-12.

---

[1]Ibanez K, Boullosa C, Tabares-Seisdedos R, Baudot A, Valencia A. Molecular Evidence for the Inverse Comorbidity between Central Nervous System Disorders and Cancers Detected by Transcriptomic Meta-analyses. PloS Genetics. 2014;10(2):e1004173.

[3] Morris JC. The Clinical Dementia Rating (CDR): current version and scoring rules. Neurology. 1993;43(11):2412-4.

[4] Parker SL, Tong T, Bolden S, Wingo PA. Cancer statistics, 1996. CA Cancer J Clin. 1996;46(1):5-27.

[5] Behrens MI, Roe CM, Morris JC. Inverse association between cancer and dementia of the Alzheimers type. In (Eds: von Bernhardy R, Inestrosa NC). Neurodegenerative diseases: From Molecular Concepts to Therapeutic Targets. Inc New York: Nova Science Publishers; 2008. p. PP. 111-20

[6] Fitzpatrick AL, Kuller LH, Ives DG, Lopez OL, Jagust W, Breitner JCS, *et al.,* Incidence and Prevalence of Dementia in the Cardiovascular Health Study. Journal of the American Geriatrics Society. 2004;52(2):195-204.

[7] JAN C. Mental Illness and Ageing Brain. London: Oxford University Press1962.

[8] Tirumalasetti F, Han L, Birkett DP. The relationship between cancer and Alzheimer's disease. J Am Geriatr Soc. 1991;39(8):840.

[9] DeSouky AL. The relationship between cancer and Alzheimer's disease. J Am Geriatr Soc. 1992;40(10):1075.

[10] Yamada M, Sasaki H, Mimori Y, Kasagi F, Sudoh S, Ikeda J, *et al.,* Prevalence and risks of dementia in the Japanese population: RERF's adult health study Hiroshima subjects. Radiation Effects Research Foundation. J Am Geriatr Soc. 1999;47(2):189-95.

[11] Beard CM, Kokmen E, Sigler C, Smith GE, Petterson T, O'Brien PC. Cause of death in Alzheimer's disease. Ann Epidemiol. 1996;6(3):195-200.

[12] Ganguli M, Dodge HH, Shen C, Pandav RS, DeKosky ST. Alzheimer disease and mortality: a 15-year epidemiological study. Arch Neurol. 2005;62(5):779-84.

[13] Driver JA, Beiser A, Au R, Kreger BE, Splansky GL, Kurth T, *et al.,* Inverse association between cancer and Alzheimer's disease: results from the Framingham Heart Study. BMJ. 2012;344:e1442.

[14] Attner B, Lithman T, Noreen D, Olsson H. Low cancer rates among patients with dementia in a population-based register study in Sweden. Dement Geriatr Cogn Disord. 2010;30(1):39-42.

[15] White RS, Lipton RB, Hall CB, Steinerman JR. Nonmelanoma skin cancer is associated with reduced Alzheimer disease risk. Neurology. 2013;80(21):1966-72.

[16] Musicco M, Adorni F, Di Santo S, Prinelli F, Pettenati C, Caltagirone C, *et al.,* Inverse occurrence of cancer and Alzheimer disease: a population-based incidence study. Neurology. 2013;81(4):322-8.

[17] Frain L, Swanson D, Betensky R, Cho K, Gagnon D, Kowall N, *et al.,* A reduced risk of Alzheimer's disease is associated with the majority of cancers in a national cohort of veterans In: AAIC, editor. Alzheimer's Association International Conference; Boston2013. p. P617.

[18] Hardy J. Alzheimer's disease: the amyloid cascade hypothesis: an update and reappraisal. J Alzheimers Dis. 2006;9(3 Suppl):151-3.

[19] Sherr CJ. Principles of tumor suppression. Cell. 2004;116(2):235-46.

[20] Riley T, Sontag E, Chen P, Levine A. Transcriptional control of human p53-regulated genes. Nat Rev Mol Cell Biol. 2008;9(5):402-12.

[21] Murray-Zmijewski F, Slee EA, Lu X. A complex barcode underlies the heterogeneous response of p53 to stress. Nat Rev Mol Cell Biol. 2008;9(9):702-12.

[22] Sharpless NE, DePinho RA. How stem cells age and why this makes us grow old. Nat Rev Mol Cell Biol. 2007;8(9):703-13.

[23] Tremolizzo L, Rodriguez-Menendez V, Brighina L, Ferrarese C. Is the inverse association between Alzheimer's disease and cancer the result of a different propensity to methylate DNA? Med Hypotheses. 2006;66(6):1251-2.

[24] Behrens MI, Silva M, Salech F, Ponce DP, Merino D, Sinning M, *et al.,* Inverse susceptibility to oxidative death of lymphocytes obtained from Alzheimer's patients and skin cancer survivors: increased apoptosis in Alzheimer's and reduced necrosis in cancer. J Gerontol A Biol Sci Med Sci. 2012;67(10):1036-40.

[25] Behrens MI, Silva M, Schmied A, Salech F, Manzur H, Rebolledo R, *et al.,* Age-dependent increases in apoptosis/necrosis ratios in human lymphocytes exposed to oxidative stress. J Gerontol A Biol Sci Med Sci. 2011;66(7):732-40.

[26] Lombardi VR, García M, Rey L, Cacabelos R. Characterization of cytokine production, screening of lymphocyte subset patterns and in vitro apoptosis in healthy and Alzheimer's Disease (AD) individuals. J Neuroimmunol. 1999;97(1-2):163-71.

[27] Uberti D, Lanni C, Racchi M, Govoni S, Memo M. Conformationally altered p53: a putative peripheral marker for Alzheimer's disease. Neurodegener Dis. 2008;5(3-4):209-11.

[28] Zhou X, Jia J. P53-mediated G(1)/S checkpoint dysfunction in lymphocytes from Alzheimer's disease patients. Neurosci Lett. 2010;468(3):320-5.

[29] Tan M, Wang S, Song J, Jia J. Combination of p53(ser15) and p21/p21(thr145) in peripheral blood lymphocytes as potential Alzheimer's disease biomarkers. Neurosci Lett. 2012;516(2):226-31.

[30] Tyner SD, Venkatachalam S, Choi J, Jones S, Ghebranious N, Igelmann H, *et al.,* p53 mutant mice that display early ageing-associated phenotypes. Nature. 2002;415(6867):45-53.

[31] Cooper-Knock J, Kirby J, Ferraiuolo L, Heath PR, Rattray M, Shaw PJ. Gene expression profiling in human neurodegenerative disease. Nat Rev Neurol. 2012;8(9):518-30.

[32] Vanacore N, Spila-Alegiani S, Raschetti R, Meco G. Mortality cancer risk in parkinsonian patients: a population-based study. Neurology. 1999;52(2):395-8.

[33] D'Amelio M, Ragonese P, Morgante L, Epifanio A, Callari G, Salemi G, *et al.,* Tumor diagnosis preceding Parkinson's disease: a case-control study. Mov Disord. 2004;19(7):807-11.

[34] Olsen JH, Friis S, Frederiksen K, McLaughlin JK, Mellemkjaer L, Møller H. Atypical cancer pattern in patients with Parkinson's disease. Br J Cancer. 2005;92(1):201-5.

[35] West AB, Dawson VL, Dawson TM. To die or grow: Parkinson's disease and cancer. Trends Neurosci. 2005;28(7):348-52.

[36] Staropoli JF. Tumorigenesis and neurodegeneration: two sides of the same coin? Bioessays. 2008;30(8):719-27.

[37] Pickering-Brown SM, Baker M, Gass J, Boeve BF, Loy CT, Brooks WS, *et al.,* Mutations in progranulin explain atypical phenotypes with variants in MAPT. Brain. 2006;129(Pt 11):3124-6.

[38] Mukherjee O, Pastor P, Cairns NJ, Chakraverty S, Kauwe JS, Shears S, *et al.,* HDDD2 is a familial frontotemporal lobar degeneration with ubiquitin-positive, tau-negative inclusions caused by a missense mutation in the signal peptide of progranulin. Ann Neurol. 2006;60(3):314-22.

[39] Behrens MI, Mukherjee O, Tu PH, Liscic RM, Grinberg LT, Carter D, *et al.*, Neuropathologic heterogeneity in HDDD1: a familial frontotemporal lobar degeneration with ubiquitin-positive inclusions and progranulin mutation. Alzheimer Dis Assoc Disord. 2007;21(1):1-7.

[40] Skoglund L, Brundin R, Olofsson T, Kalimo H, Ingvast S, Blom ES, *et al.*, Frontotemporal dementia in a large Swedish family is caused by a progranulin null mutation. Neurogenetics. 2009;10(1):27-34.

[41] Ong CH, Bateman A. Progranulin (granulin-epithelin precursor, PC-cell derived growth factor, acrogranin) in proliferation and tumorigenesis. Histol Histopathol. 2003;18(4):1275-88.

[42] Campisi J. Aging, tumor suppression and cancer: high wire-act! Mech Ageing Dev. 2005;126(1):51-8.

[43] Campisi J. Aging and cancer cell biology, 2008. Aging Cell. 2008;7(3):281-4.

[44] Papazoglu C, Mills AA. p53: at the crossroad between cancer and ageing. J Pathol. 2007;211(2):124-33.

[45] Donehower LA, Harvey M, Slagle BL, McArthur MJ, Montgomery CA, Butel JS, *et al.*, Mice deficient for p53 are developmentally normal but susceptible to spontaneous tumours. Nature. 1992;356(6366):215-21.

[46] Meletis K, Wirta V, Hede SM, Nistér M, Lundeberg J, Frisén J. p53 suppresses the self-renewal of adult neural stem cells. Development. 2006;133(2):363-9.

[47] Sharpless NE, DePinho RA. Telomeres, stem cells, senescence, and cancer. J Clin Invest. 2004;113(2):160-8.

[48] Varela I, Cadiñanos J, Pendás AM, Gutiérrez-Fernández A, Folgueras AR, Sánchez LM, *et al.*, Accelerated ageing in mice deficient in Zmpste24 protease is linked to p53 signalling activation. Nature. 2005;437(7058):564-8.

[49] Maier B, Gluba W, Bernier B, Turner T, Mohammad K, Guise T, *et al.*, Modulation of mammalian life span by the short isoform of p53. Genes Dev. 2004;18(3):306-19.

[50] Matheu A, Maraver A, Klatt P, Flores I, Garcia-Cao I, Borras C, *et al.*, Delayed ageing through damage protection by the Arf/p53 pathway. Nature. 2007;448(7151):375-9.

[51] García-Cao I, García-Cao M, Martín-Caballero J, Criado LM, Klatt P, Flores JM, *et al.*, "Super p53" mice exhibit enhanced DNA damage response, are tumor resistant and age normally. EMBO J. 2002;21(22):6225-35.

[52] Mendrysa SM, O'Leary KA, McElwee MK, Michalowski J, Eisenman RN, Powell DA, *et al.*, Tumor suppression and normal aging in mice with constitutively high p53 activity. Genes Dev. 2006;20(1):16-21.

[53] Di Giovanni S, Knights CD, Rao M, Yakovlev A, Beers J, Catania J, *et al.*, The tumor suppressor protein p53 is required for neurite outgrowth and axon regeneration. EMBO J. 2006;25(17):4084-96.

[54] Knights CD, Catania J, Di Giovanni S, Muratoglu S, Perez R, Swartzbeck A, *et al.*, Distinct p53 acetylation cassettes differentially influence gene-expression patterns and cell fate. J Cell Biol. 2006;173(4):533-44.

[55] van Heemst D, Mooijaart SP, Beekman M, Schreuder J, de Craen AJ, Brandt BW, *et al.*, Variation in the human TP53 gene affects old age survival and cancer mortality. Exp Gerontol. 2005;40(1-2):11-5.

[56] Bae BI, Xu H, Igarashi S, Fujimuro M, Agrawal N, Taya Y, *et al.*, p53 mediates cellular dysfunction and behavioral abnormalities in Huntington's disease. Neuron. 2005;47(1):29-41.

[57] Martin LJ. p53 is abnormally elevated and active in the CNS of patients with amyotrophic lateral sclerosis. Neurobiol Dis. 2000;7(6 Pt B):613-22.

[58] Ranganathan S, Bowser R. p53 and Cell Cycle Proteins Participate in Spinal Motor Neuron Cell Death in ALS. Open Pathol J. 2010;4:11-22.

[59] Ohyagi Y, Asahara H, Chui DH, Tsuruta Y, Sakae N, Miyoshi K, *et al.,* Intracellular Abeta42 activates p53 promoter: a pathway to neurodegeneration in Alzheimer's disease. FASEB J. 2005;19(2):255-7.

[60] Cenini G, Sultana R, Memo M, Butterfield DA. Elevated levels of pro-apoptotic p53 and its oxidative modification by the lipid peroxidation product, HNE, in brain from subjects with amnestic mild cognitive impairment and Alzheimer's disease. J Cell Mol Med. 2008;12(3):987-94.

[61] Hooper C, Meimaridou E, Tavassoli M, Melino G, Lovestone S, Killick R. p53 is upregulated in Alzheimer's disease and induces tau phosphorylation in HEK293a cells. Neurosci Lett. 2007;418(1):34-7.

[62] Mogi M, Kondo T, Mizuno Y, Nagatsu T. p53 protein, interferon-gamma, and NF-kappaB levels are elevated in the parkinsonian brain. Neurosci Lett. 2007;414(1):94-7.

[63] Alves da Costa C, Checler F. Apoptosis in Parkinson's disease: is p53 the missing link between genetic and sporadic Parkinsonism? Cell Signal. 2011;23(6):963-8.

[64] Martin LJ. Transgenic mice with human mutant genes causing Parkinson's disease and amyotrophic lateral sclerosis provide common insight into mechanisms of motor neuron selective vulnerability to degeneration. Rev Neurosci. 2007;18(2):115-36.

[65] Chou AH, Lin AC, Hong KY, Hu SH, Chen YL, Chen JY, *et al.,* p53 activation mediates polyglutamine-expanded ataxin-3 upregulation of Bax expression in cerebellar and pontine nuclei neurons. Neurochem Int. 2011;58(2):145-52.

[66] LaFerla FM, Hall CK, Ngo L, Jay G. Extracellular deposition of beta-amyloid upon p53-dependent neuronal cell death in transgenic mice. J Clin Invest. 1996;98(7):1626-32.

[67] Nguyen HN, Lee MS, Hwang DY, Kim YK, Yoon dY, Lee JW, *et al.,* Mutant presenilin 2 increased oxidative stress and p53 expression in neuronal cells. Biochem Biophys Res Commun. 2007;357(1):174-80.

[68] Alves da Costa C, Sunyach C, Pardossi-Piquard R, Sévalle J, Vincent B, Boyer N, *et al.,* Presenilin-dependent gamma-secretase-mediated control of p53-associated cell death in Alzheimer's disease. J Neurosci. 2006;26(23):6377-85.

[69] Checler F, Dunys J. p53, a pivotal effector of a functional cross-talk linking presenilins and Pen-2. Neurodegener Dis. 2012;10(1-4):52-5.

[70] Song H, Boo JH, Kim KH, Kim C, Kim YE, Ahn JH, *et al.,* Critical role of presenilin-dependent γ-secretase activity in DNA damage-induced promyelocytic leukemia protein expression and apoptosis. Cell Death Differ. 2013;20(4):639-48.

[71] Davenport CM, Sevastou IG, Hooper C, Pocock JM. Inhibiting p53 pathways in microglia attenuates microglial-evoked neurotoxicity following exposure to Alzheimer peptides. J Neurochem. 2010;112(2):552-63.

[72] Blalock EM, Geddes JW, Chen KC, Porter NM, Markesbery WR, Landfield PW. Incipient Alzheimer's disease: microarray correlation analyses reveal major transcriptional and tumor suppressor responses. Proc Natl Acad Sci U S A. 2004;101(7):2173-8.

[73] Blalock EM, Buechel HM, Popovic J, Geddes JW, Landfield PW. Microarray analyses of laser-captured hippocampus reveal distinct gray and white matter signatures associated with incipient Alzheimer's disease. J Chem Neuroanat. 2011;42(2):118-26.

[74] Chambon P, Weill JD, Mandel P. Nicotinamide mononucleotide activation of new DNA-dependent polyadenylic acid synthesizing nuclear enzyme. Biochem Biophys Res Commun. 1963;11:39-43.
[75] Virág L. 50Years of poly(ADP-ribosyl)ation. Mol Aspects Med. 2013;34(6):1043-5.
[76] Virág L, Robaszkiewicz A, Rodriguez-Vargas JM, Oliver FJ. Poly(ADP-ribose) signaling in cell death. Mol Aspects Med. 2013;34(6):1153-67.
[77] Lee Y, Karuppagounder SS, Shin JH, Lee YI, Ko HS, Swing D, *et al.,* Parthanatos mediates AIMP2-activated age-dependent dopaminergic neuronal loss. Nat Neurosci. 2013;16(10):1392-400.
[78] David KK, Andrabi SA, Dawson TM, Dawson VL. Parthanatos, a messenger of death. Front Biosci (Landmark Ed). 2009;14:1116-28.
[79] Moubarak RS, Yuste VJ, Artus C, Bouharrour A, Greer PA, Menissier-de Murcia J, *et al.,* Sequential activation of poly(ADP-ribose) polymerase 1, calpains, and Bax is essential in apoptosis-inducing factor-mediated programmed necrosis. Mol Cell Biol. 2007;27(13):4844-62.
[80] Yu SW, Wang H, Poitras MF, Coombs C, Bowers WJ, Federoff HJ, *et al.,* Mediation of poly(ADP-ribose) polymerase-1-dependent cell death by apoptosis-inducing factor. Science. 2002;297(5579):259-63.
[81] Baek SH, Bae ON, Kim EK, Yu SW. Induction of mitochondrial dysfunction by poly(ADP-ribose) polymer: implication for neuronal cell death. Mol Cells. 2013;36(3):258-66.
[82] Thomas C, Tulin AV. Poly-ADP-ribose polymerase: machinery for nuclear processes. Mol Aspects Med. 2013;34(6):1124-37.
[83] Kraus WL, Hottiger MO. PARP-1 and gene regulation: progress and puzzles. Mol Aspects Med. 2013;34(6):1109-23.
[84] Mandir AS, Przedborski S, Jackson-Lewis V, Wang ZQ, Simbulan-Rosenthal CM, Smulson ME, *et al.,* Poly(ADP-ribose) polymerase activation mediates 1-methyl-4-phenyl-1, 2,3,6-tetrahydropyridine (MPTP)-induced parkinsonism. Proc Natl Acad Sci U S A. 1999;96(10):5774-9.
[85] Love S, Barber R, Wilcock GK. Increased poly(ADP-ribosyl)ation of nuclear proteins in Alzheimer's disease. Brain. 1999;122(Pt 2):247-53.
[86] Abeti R, Abramov AY, Duchen MR. Beta-amyloid activates PARP causing astrocytic metabolic failure and neuronal death. Brain. 2011;134(Pt 6):1658-72.
[87] Martire S, Fuso A, Rotili D, Tempera I, Giordano C, De Zottis I, *et al.,* PARP-1 Modulates Amyloid Beta Peptide-Induced Neuronal Damage. PLoS One. 2013;8(9):e72169.
[88] Turunc Bayrakdar E, Uyanikgil Y, Kanit L, Koylu E, Yalcin A. Nicotinamide treatment reduces the levels of oxidative stress, apoptosis, and PARP-1 activity in Aβ(1-42)-induced rat model of Alzheimer's disease. Free Radic Res. 2014;48(2):146-58.
[89] Rulten SL, Rotheray A, Green RL, Grundy GJ, Moore DA, Gómez-Herreros F, *et al.,* PARP-1 dependent recruitment of the amyotrophic lateral sclerosis-associated protein FUS/TLS to sites of oxidative DNA damage. Nucleic Acids Res. 2014;42(1):307-14.
[90] Hilton JF, Hadfield MJ, Tran MT, Shapiro GI. Poly(ADP-ribose) polymerase inhibitors as cancer therapy. Front Biosci. 2013;18:1392-406.
[91] Bürkle A, Brabeck C, Diefenbach J, Beneke S. The emerging role of poly(ADP-ribose) polymerase-1 in longevity. Int J Biochem Cell Biol. 2005;37(5):1043-53.

[92] Guillot C, Hall J, Herceg Z, Merle P, Chemin I. Update on hepatocellular carcinoma breakthroughs: Poly(ADP-ribose) polymerase inhibitors as a promising therapeutic strategy. Clin Res Hepatol Gastroenterol. 2013.

[93] Salemi M, Galia A, Fraggetta F, La Corte C, Pepe P, La Vignera S, *et al.,* Poly (ADP-ribose) polymerase 1 protein expression in normal and neoplastic prostatic tissue. Eur J Histochem. 2013;57(2):e13.

[94] Michels J, Vitale I, Galluzzi L, Adam J, Olaussen KA, Kepp O, *et al.,* Cisplatin resistance associated with PARP hyperactivation. Cancer Res. 2013;73(7):2271-80.

[95] Grube K, Bürkle A. Poly(ADP-ribose) polymerase activity in mononuclear leukocytes of 13 mammalian species correlates with species-specific life span. Proc Natl Acad Sci U S A. 1992;89(24):11759-63.

[96] Piskunova TS, Yurova MN, Ovsyannikov AI, Semenchenko AV, Zabezhinski MA, Popovich IG, *et al.,* Deficiency in Poly(ADP-ribose) Polymerase-1 (PARP-1) Accelerates Aging and Spontaneous Carcinogenesis in Mice. Curr Gerontol Geriatr Res. 2008:754190.

[97] Chevanne M, Calia C, Zampieri M, Cecchinelli B, Caldini R, Monti D, *et al.,* Oxidative DNA damage repair and parp 1 and parp 2 expression in Epstein-Barr virus-immortalized B lymphocyte cells from young subjects, old subjects, and centenarians. Rejuvenation Res. 2007;10(2):191-204.

[98] Malanga M, Romano M, Ferone A, Petrella A, Monti G, Jones R, *et al.,* Misregulation of poly(ADP-ribose) polymerase-1 activity and cell type-specific loss of poly(ADP-ribose) synthesis in the cerebellum of aged rats. J Neurochem. 2005;93(4):1000-9.

[99] Montero J, Dutta C, van Bodegom D, Weinstock D, Letai A. p53 regulates a non-apoptotic death induced by ROS. Cell Death Differ. 2013;20(11):1465-74.

[100] Elkholi R, Chipuk JE. How do I kill thee? Let me count the ways: p53 regulates PARP-1 dependent necrosis. Bioessays. 2014;36(1):46-51.

[101] Valenzuela MT, Guerrero R, Núñez MI, Ruiz De Almodóvar JM, Sarker M, de Murcia G, *et al.,* PARP-1 modifies the effectiveness of p53-mediated DNA damage response. Oncogene. 2002;21(7):1108-16.

[102] Rajamohan SB, Pillai VB, Gupta M, Sundaresan NR, Birukov KG, Samant S, *et al.,* SIRT1 promotes cell survival under stress by deacetylation-dependent deactivation of poly(ADP-ribose) polymerase 1. Mol Cell Biol. 2009;29(15):4116-29.

[103] Tu HC, Ren D, Wang GX, Chen DY, Westergard TD, Kim H, *et al.,* The p53-cathepsin axis cooperates with ROS to activate programmed necrotic death upon DNA damage. Proc Natl Acad Sci U S A. 2009;106(4):1093-8.

[104] Coombs GS, Covey TM, Virshup DM. Wnt signaling in development, disease and translational medicine. Curr Drug Targets. 2008;9(7):513-31.

[105] Maiese K, Li F, Chong ZZ, Shang YC. The Wnt signaling pathway: aging gracefully as a protectionist? Pharmacol Ther. 2008;118(1):58-81.

[106] Caricasole A, Bakker A, Copani A, Nicoletti F, Gaviraghi G, Terstappen GC. Two sides of the same coin: Wnt signaling in neurodegeneration and neuro-oncology. Biosci Rep. 2005;25(5-6):309-27.

[107] Inestrosa NC, Toledo EM. The role of Wnt signaling in neuronal dysfunction in Alzheimer's Disease. Mol Neurodegener. 2008;3:9.

[108] Buongiorno P, Pethe VV, Charames GS, Esufali S, Bapat B. Rac1 GTPase and the Rac1 exchange factor Tiam1 associate with Wnt-responsive promoters to enhance beta-catenin/TCF-dependent transcription in colorectal cancer cells. Mol Cancer. 2008;7:73.

[109] Firestein R, Bass AJ, Kim SY, Dunn IF, Silver SJ, Guney I, *et al.,* CDK8 is a colorectal cancer oncogene that regulates beta-catenin activity. Nature. 2008;455(7212):547-51.

[110] Karim R, Tse G, Putti T, Scolyer R, Lee S. The significance of the Wnt pathway in the pathology of human cancers. Pathology. 2004;36(2):120-8.

[111] Fiorentino M, Zadra G, Palescandolo E, Fedele G, Bailey D, Fiore C, *et al.,* Overexpression of fatty acid synthase is associated with palmitoylation of Wnt1 and cytoplasmic stabilization of beta-catenin in prostate cancer. Lab Invest. 2008;88(12):1340-8.

[112] Veeck J, Bektas N, Hartmann A, Kristiansen G, Heindrichs U, Knüchel R, *et al.,* Wnt signalling in human breast cancer: expression of the putative Wnt inhibitor Dickkopf-3 (DKK3) is frequently suppressed by promoter hypermethylation in mammary tumours. Breast Cancer Res. 2008;10(5):R82.

[113] Coe BP, Lockwood WW, Girard L, Chari R, Macaulay C, Lam S, *et al.,* Differential disruption of cell cycle pathways in small cell and non-small cell lung cancer. Br J Cancer. 2006;94(12):1927-35.

[114] Da Forno PD, Pringle JH, Hutchinson P, Osborn J, Huang Q, Potter L, *et al.,* WNT5A expression increases during melanoma progression and correlates with outcome. Clin Cancer Res. 2008;14(18):5825-32.

[115] Liu ZL, Li Y, Kong QY, Zhan C, Wang Q, Chen XY, *et al.,* Immunohistochemical profiling of Wnt, NF-kappaB, Stat3 and Notch signaling in human epidermal tumors. J Dermatol Sci. 2008;52(2):133-6.

[116] Yang SH, Andl T, Grachtchouk V, Wang A, Liu J, Syu LJ, *et al.,* Pathological responses to oncogenic Hedgehog signaling in skin are dependent on canonical Wnt/beta3-catenin signaling. Nat Genet. 2008;40(9):1130-5.

[117] Malanchi I, Peinado H, Kassen D, Hussenet T, Metzger D, Chambon P, *et al.,* Cutaneous cancer stem cell maintenance is dependent on beta-catenin signalling. Nature. 2008;452(7187):650-3.

[118] Asplund A, Gry Björklund M, Sundquist C, Strömberg S, Edlund K, Ostman A, *et al.,* Expression profiling of microdissected cell populations selected from basal cells in normal epidermis and basal cell carcinoma. Br J Dermatol. 2008;158(3):527-38.

[119] Adams PD, Enders GH. Wnt-signaling and senescence: A tug of war in early neoplasia? Cancer Biol Ther. 2008;7(11):1706-11.

[120] Toledo EM, Colombres M, Inestrosa NC. Wnt signaling in neuroprotection and stem cell differentiation. Prog Neurobiol. 2008;86(3):281-96.

[121] De Ferrari GV, Moon RT. The ups and downs of Wnt signaling in prevalent neurological disorders. Oncogene. 2006;25(57):7545-53.

[122] Magdesian MH, Carvalho MM, Mendes FA, Saraiva LM, Juliano MA, Juliano L, *et al.,* Amyloid-beta binds to the extracellular cysteine-rich domain of Frizzled and inhibits Wnt/beta-catenin signaling. J Biol Chem. 2008;283(14):9359-68.

[123] Caricasole A, Copani A, Caraci F, Aronica E, Rozemuller AJ, Caruso A, *et al.,* Induction of Dickkopf-1, a negative modulator of the Wnt pathway, is associated with neuronal degeneration in Alzheimer's brain. J Neurosci. 2004;24(26):6021-7.

[124] Ghanevati M, Miller CA. Phospho-beta-catenin accumulation in Alzheimer's disease and in aggresomes attributable to proteasome dysfunction. J Mol Neurosci. 2005;25(1):79-94.

[125] De Ferrari GV, Chacón MA, Barría MI, Garrido JL, Godoy JA, Olivares G, *et al.,* Activation of Wnt signaling rescues neurodegeneration and behavioral impairments induced by beta-amyloid fibrils. Mol Psychiatry. 2003;8(2):195-208.

[126] Alvarez AR, Godoy JA, Mullendorff K, Olivares GH, Bronfman M, Inestrosa NC. Wnt-3a overcomes beta-amyloid toxicity in rat hippocampal neurons. Exp Cell Res. 2004;297(1):186-96.

[127] Busciglio J, Lorenzo A, Yeh J, Yankner BA. beta-amyloid fibrils induce tau phosphorylation and loss of microtubule binding. Neuron. 1995;14(4):879-88.

[128] Takashima A, Honda T, Yasutake K, Michel G, Murayama O, Murayama M, *et al.,* Activation of tau protein kinase I/glycogen synthase kinase-3beta by amyloid beta peptide (25-35) enhances phosphorylation of tau in hippocampal neurons. Neurosci Res. 1998;31(4):317-23.

[129] Inestrosa NC, Varela-Nallar L, Grabowski CP, Colombres M. Synaptotoxicity in Alzheimer's disease: the Wnt signaling pathway as a molecular target. IUBMB Life. 2007;59(4-5):316-21.

[130] De Ferrari GV, Inestrosa NC. Wnt signaling function in Alzheimer's disease. Brain Res Brain Res Rev. 2000;33(1):1-12.

[131] Mudher A, Lovestone S. Alzheimer's disease-do tauists and baptists finally shake hands? Trends Neurosci. 2002;25(1):22-6.

[132] Li HL, Wang HH, Liu SJ, Deng YQ, Zhang YJ, Tian Q, *et al.,* Phosphorylation of tau antagonizes apoptosis by stabilizing beta-catenin, a mechanism involved in Alzheimer's neurodegeneration. Proc Natl Acad Sci U S A. 2007;104(9):3591-6.

[133] Nunes PV, Forlenza OV, Gattaz WF. Lithium and risk for Alzheimer's disease in elderly patients with bipolar disorder. Br J Psychiatry. 2007;190:359-60.

[134] Mendes CT, Mury FB, de Sá Moreira E, Alberto FL, Forlenza OV, Dias-Neto E, *et al.,* Lithium reduces Gsk3b mRNA levels: implications for Alzheimer Disease. Eur Arch Psychiatry Clin Neurosci. 2009;259(1):16-22.

[135] Zhang Z, Hartmann H, Do VM, Abramowski D, Sturchler-Pierrat C, Staufenbiel M, *et al.,* Destabilization of beta-catenin by mutations in presenilin-1 potentiates neuronal apoptosis. Nature. 1998;395(6703):698-702.

[136] De Ferrari GV, Papassotiropoulos A, Biechele T, Wavrant De-Vrieze F, Avila ME, Major MB, *et al.,* Common genetic variation within the low-density lipoprotein receptor-related protein 6 and late-ons*et Al*zheimer's disease. Proc Natl Acad Sci U S A. 2007;104(22):9434-9.

[137] Lazarov O, Mattson MP, Peterson DA, Pimplikar SW, van Praag H. When neurogenesis encounters aging and disease. Trends Neurosci. 2010;33(12):569-79.

[138] Deng W, Aimone JB, Gage FH. New neurons and new memories: how does adult hippocampal neurogenesis affect learning and memory? Nat Rev Neurosci. 2010;11(5):339-50.

[139] Mu Y, Gage FH. Adult hippocampal neurogenesis and its role in Alzheimer's disease. Mol Neurodegener. 2011;6:85.

[140] Lazarov O, Marr RA. Neurogenesis and Alzheimer's disease: at the crossroads. Exp Neurol. 2010;223(2):267-81.

[141] Varela-Nallar L, Aranguiz FC, Abbott AC, Slater PG, Inestrosa NC. Adult hippocampal neurogenesis in aging and Alzheimer's disease. Birth Defects Res C Embryo Today. 2010;90(4):284-96.

[142] Jin K, Peel AL, Mao XO, Xie L, Cottrell BA, Henshall DC, *et al.,* Increased hippocampal neurogenesis in Alzheimer's disease. Proc Natl Acad Sci U S A. 2004;101(1):343-7.

[143] Ghosal K, Stathopoulos A, Pimplikar SW. APP intracellular domain impairs adult neurogenesis in transgenic mice by inducing neuroinflammation. PLoS One. 2010;5(7):e11866.

[144] Caillé I, Allinquant B, Dupont E, Bouillot C, Langer A, Müller U, *et al.,* Soluble form of amyloid precursor protein regulates proliferation of progenitors in the adult subventricular zone. Development. 2004;131(9):2173-81.

[145] Veeraraghavalu K, Sisodia SS. Mutant presenilin 1 expression in excitatory neurons impairs enrichment-mediated phenotypes of adult hippocampal progenitor cells. Proc Natl Acad Sci U S A. 2013;110(22):9148-53.

[146] Gage FH. Molecular and cellular mechanisms contributing to the regulation, proliferation and differentiation of neural stem cells in the adult dentate gyrus. Keio J Med. 2010;59(3):79-83.

[147] Uberti D, Piccioni L, Cadei M, Grigolato P, Rotter V, Memo M. p53 is dispensable for apoptosis but controls neurogenesis of mouse dentate gyrus cells following gamma-irradiation. Brain Res Mol Brain Res. 2001;93(1):81-9.

[148] Medrano S, Scrable H. Maintaining appearances--the role of p53 in adult neurogenesis. Biochem Biophys Res Commun. 2005;331(3):828-33.

[149] Reya T, Clevers H. Wnt signalling in stem cells and cancer. Nature. 2005;434(7035):843-50.

[150] Lie DC, Colamarino SA, Song HJ, Désiré L, Mira H, Consiglio A, *et al.,* Wnt signalling regulates adult hippocampal neurogenesis. Nature. 2005;437(7063):1370-5.

[151] Kuwabara T, Hsieh J, Muotri A, Yeo G, Warashina M, Lie DC, *et al.,* Wnt-mediated activation of NeuroD1 and retro-elements during adult neurogenesis. Nat Neurosci. 2009;12(9):1097-105.

[152] Karalay O, Doberauer K, Vadodaria KC, Knobloch M, Berti L, Miquelajauregui A, *et al.,* Prospero-related homeobox 1 gene (Prox1) is regulated by canonical Wnt signaling and has a stage-specific role in adult hippocampal neurogenesis. Proc Natl Acad Sci U S A. 2011;108(14):5807-12.

[153] Seib DR, Corsini NS, Ellwanger K, Plaas C, Mateos A, Pitzer C, *et al.,* Loss of Dickkopf-1 restores neurogenesis in old age and counteracts cognitive decline. Cell Stem Cell. 2013;12(2):204-14.

CHAPTER 3

Cholesterol in Alzheimer's Disease: Unresolved Questions

Massimo Stefani* **and Gianfranco Liguri**

Department of Biochemical Sciences and Research Centre on Neurodegeneration (CIMN), University of Florence, Florence, Italy

Abstract: The role of cholesterol as a susceptibility factor or a protective agent in neurodegeneration and, more generally, in amyloid-induced cytotoxicity is still controversial. Epidemiological studies on the hypercholesterolemia-AD risk relation and some reports indicating a beneficial effect of statin therapy suggest cholesterol as a susceptibility factor in AD. The ApoE4 genotype as a prevalent genetic risk factor for AD and the function of ApoE as main cholesterol carrier in the brain also underlie a close cholesterol load-AD risk relation. Finally, cell biology evidences support a critical involvement of lipid raft cholesterol in the modulation of β- and γ-cleavage of APP with altered Aβ production.

However, little exchange does exist between circulating and brain cholesterol, the latter arising from endogenous synthesis. In addition, increasing evidence supports the idea that amyloid cytotoxicity in most cases is initiated by oligomer recruitment at the cell membrane with oligomer nucleation, loss of membrane integrity, Ca^{2+} ingress into the cell, oxidative stress and apoptosis. In such a scenario, increased membrane cholesterol seems to be protective by disfavouring aggregate binding to the membrane. Recent findings also point at a key role performed by lipid rafts and their proteins and indicate that a reduction of cellular cholesterol favours co-localization of BACE1 and APP in non-raft membrane domains and hinders generation of plasmin, an Aβ-degrading enzyme. Finally, recent researches on Seladin-1, involved in cholesterol biosynthesis, show that modulation of membrane cholesterol affects Aβ generation and cell resistance against Aβ oligomer toxicity. These data confirm previous findings indicating a reduction of the cholesterol/phospholipid ratio in aged and AD brains.

The aim of this review is to critically discuss some of the main results reported in the recent years in this field supporting a role of cholesterol either as a susceptibility factor or as a protective agent in AD.

Keywords: Alzheimer's disease, Aβ peptides, APP, neurodegeneration, amyloid, cholesterol.

***Corresponding author Massimo Stefani:** Department of Biochemical sciences, University of Florence, Viale Morgagni m50, 50134 Florence, Italy; Tel: +39.0554598307; Fax: +39.0554598905; E-mail:stefani@scibio.unifi.it

D.K. Lahiri (Ed)

INTRODUCTION

Around one century ago, on November 3rd, 1906, the German physician Alois Alzheimer in a scientific meeting at the Tubingen University discussed an unusual case of dementia in one of his patients, Auguste D. Since then, and particularly in the past few decades, the incidence in the developed countries of the Alzheimer's disease (AD), the most prevalent form of senile dementia, and other neurodegenerative diseases has dramatically increased. Such a rise, thought to depend mainly on the extended life expectancy in the population, results in severe social and health problems that are expected to worsen in the near future.

Presently, in the developed countries, AD affects around 10% of the people over age 60 years and 45% of the people over age 85 years [1]; an increasing number of cases of sporadic AD in young people (early-onset sporadic AD) have also been described. Finally, the NIH estimates indicate that, at the present time, the number of AD-affected people in the world is over 15 millions (4.7 in the USA) and this number is expected to reach 50 millions (13.8 in the USA) by 2050, with total estimated worldwide costs of US$ 604 billion in 2010 [2]. These numbers are significantly higher when including people with mild cognitive impairment or other pre-dementia conditions likely evolving to overt AD. These data account for the intense efforts spent by researchers to investigate the molecular and cellular features underlying the clinical signs of AD as well as the genetic [3] and environmental risk factors (including diabetes mellitus, diet, physical and mental activity, cardiovascular disease and hypercholesterolemia) involved in its pathogenesis in addition to ageing. A large amount of knowledge as been gained in the past decade on these issues mainly thanks to epidemiological studies, to genetic studies of the familial forms of AD and to the increasing use of animal models. However, in spite of such dramatic increase of information, much must still be learnt on the molecular, cellular and environmental factors that are really involved in the onset of the much more prevalent sporadic forms of AD and the ways these factors affect each other. The substantial absence of resolutive therapies for AD is largely due to such a lack of knowledge.

AD is characterized by the presence of proteinaceous deposits (senile and diffuse plaques) in the cerebral vessels and in the parenchyma of the affected brain regions; these, include the prefrontal and entorhinal cortex and the hippocampus, where the plaques are surrounded by dead and dystrophic neurons (reviewed in [4]). The major components of the plaques are fibrillar aggregates of the Aβ peptides, mainly Aβ40, Aβ42 and their 3-40 or 3-42 pyroglutamate derivatives (the longer Aβ42 isoform and its 3-42 pyroglutamate derivative being much more pathogenic than Aβ40). Aβ peptides arise from proteolytic processing of the extracellular and transmembrane regions of the amyloid precursor protein (APP), a membrane protein with still unknown function (reviewed in [4]). Extensive research has highlighted a link between AD and vascular injury in the brain; accordingly, AD and vascular dementia are now recognized as distinct, yet coexisting processes, both contributing to the clinical signs of dementia [5]. It is now established that Aβ42 and its 3-42 pyroglutamate derivative are the main components of the fibrillar material in the plaques, whereas both Aβ40 and Aβ42 are found in the cerebral vessel deposits. In addition, fibrillar aggregates of the microtubule-associated protein tau in a hyperphosphorylated form are found as paired helical filaments and neurofibrillary tangles in neuronal cells of most AD patients [6]. These data have led to propose the amyloid cascade hypothesis of AD whereby Aβ deposits in the brain parenchyma are the main cause, rather than an epiphenomenon, of the disease [7].

Presently, the overproduction and/or the reduced clearance of Aβ peptides are considered key factors underlying their fibrillar polymerization, a key event in AD pathogenesis. Actually, many *in vitro* studies have shown that synthetic Aβ peptides readily polymerize into amyloid oligomers and fibrils very similar to those found in *in vivo* deposits; moreover, the neuritic dystrophy and synaptic failure elicited in cultured neuronal cells by those aggregates and resulting in cell degeneration seem to arise from the interaction of the latter with the cell membrane [8,9].

During the past decade, the awareness has grown that, contrary to what it was believed previously, at least in most cases mature amyloid fibrils are substantially devoid of direct toxicity to cells whereas their unstable precursors in the fibrillization path, oligomers or prefibrillar aggregates of Aβ peptides (or other proteins in different amyloid diseases), are endowed with the highest cytotoxicity [10] (see later). At least in most cases, protein/peptide oligomer cytotoxicity seems to arise from the ability of these unstable immature aggregation forms and their monomeric unstable precursors to inappropriately interact with cellular components including cell membranes; the consequent disruption of membrane integrity and non-specific permeabilization, alteration of ion (particularly free Ca^{2+}) distribution, ER, mitochondrial and oxidative stress, and derangement of specific signalling pathways, would eventually lead to cell death (reviewed in [11]). Actually, many recent reports have convincingly shown that Aβ oligomers do form *in vivo* and that their presence is directly associated with synaptic dysfunction and cell impairment [12-17]. Considerable evidence also supports the idea that Aβ (and other protein/peptide) oligomerization can be accelerated by the interaction with synthetic and cell membranes depending on environmental conditions and membrane lipid composition.

Token together, all these data support the concept of a central role of Aβ peptides in AD pathogenesis at the molecular and functional level and of the interaction between peptide oligomers and the cell membrane as a key event in the path of peptide polymerization and oligomer cytotoxicity, even though recently the significance of the amyloid cascade hypothesis has been revisited [18].

These considerations account for the great interest of studying the molecular and physicochemical features of the interaction between peptide/proteins and surfaces as well as the effect of the chemical composition of the latter. The present review is aimed at providing information on the research in this field, particularly for what the role of cholesterol in AD pathogenesis is concerned.

BRAIN CHOLESTEROL METABOLISM

Cholesterol is an essential component of the plasma membrane of all cells, where it increases membrane rigidity reducing lipid disorder; it is found mainly in the cytofacial leaflet, where, together with sphingolipids and gangliosides, is concentrated in detergent-resistant membrane fractions (lipid rafts) and plays key roles in neuronal development as well as in the maintenance of neuronal plasticity and function (reviewed in [19]). Lipid rafts are rigid and dynamic assemblies of membrane proteins and lipids that float freely within the liquid-disordered phase of the cell membrane bilayer (reviewed in [20]). In lipid rafts, cholesterol is thought to act as a spacer between the hydrocarbon chains of the sphingolipids and as a dynamic glue that holds together rafts upon assembly. Cholesterol removal results in raft disassembly with dissociation, deregulation and/or inactivation of most raft proteins.

The brain synthesizes essentially all of its cholesterol and does not appear to depend on the circulating pool of the steroid; actually, the plasma lipoproteins do not cross the blood-brain barrier (BBB) and do not deliver significant amounts of cholesterol to the CNS [21]. Neuronal cells appear to synthesize cholesterol during development, whereas mature neurons progressively lose such ability, getting cholesterol from glial cells, particularly astrocytes [22,23].

The rate-limiting step of cholesterol synthesis is the reaction catalyzed by 3-hydroxy-3-methylglutarylCoA reductase (HMGCoAR), whose activity is controlled by the levels of cholesterol itself "Fig. (**1**)". Thus HMGCoAR has been a good candidate for pharmacological treatment of hypercholesterolemia using statins, chemical analogues of cholesterol. However, reducing cholesterol synthesis at one of its earliest steps by HMGCoAR inhibition can also hinder the synthesis of downstream intermediates with important physiological functions; the latter include farnesylpyrophosphate, a precursor of molecules involved in cell signalling and inflammation, and ubiquinone, an antioxidant molecule participating as an electron carrier to the mitochondrial respiratory chain.

Another important reaction of cholesterol synthesis is the reduction of desmosterol to cholesterol, the last step of the pathway. The reaction is catalyzed by the product of *Dhcr24*, an evolutionarily conserved gene on chromosome 1 with homologies to a family of FAD-dependent oxidoreductases and marked sequence homology to the *Diminuto/Dwarf1* gene described in *A. thaliana* and *C. elegans* [24,25]. The *Dhcr24* gene product, also known as Seladin-1 (SELective Alzheimer's Disease INdicator-1) is found in the CNS and other organs and tissues including lung, adrenal gland, testis, ovary, prostate, stomach and liver. Seladin-1 levels appear to be down-regulated following cell differentiation [26] and in AD brains, thus establishing a possible link between this protein and AD [27] (see later). In humans, functional deficiencies of Seladin-1 result in desmosterolosis, a disorder characterized by elevated plasma levels of desmosterol and by developmental anomalies [25]. Besides contributing to cholesterol synthesis, Seladin-1 possesses other less characterized activities, including anti-apoptotic effects, possibly through caspase-3 inhibition, modulation of cell responses to oxidative and oncogenic stimuli, and regulation of Ras-induced senescence [28].

In the adult brain, the astrocytes not only synthesize, but also internalize and recycle the cholesterol released from degenerating nerve terminals to deliver it back to neurons [29]; this activity requires cholesterol binding to one of the variants of apolipoprotein E (ApoE), a major lipoprotein in the CNS [30]. ApoE is the main carrier of cholesterol in brain and a ligand for cell surface lipoprotein receptors such as the LDLR and the LDLR-related proteins (LRP); ApoE also regulates lipid transport to neurons and clears cholesterol from the extracellular space [31]. The fusion with lysosomes of the internalized endosomes containing ApoE-cholesterol-phospholipid complexes results in the intracellular release of cholesterol, with reduction of endogenous synthesis by HMGCoAR inhibition and storage upon fatty acid esterification by acylCoA:cholesterol acyltransferase (ACAT) [31]. The main product of brain cholesterol metabolism is the 24-hydroxy derivative that is translocated to the circulating blood through the BBB (see next section).

That ApoE plays a pivotal role in AD pathogenesis (reviewed in [32]) is confirmed by the recognised role of its ε4 variant as the main genetic risk factor for sporadic AD [33].

Although the mechanisms underlying the pathogenic effects of the ApoE4 phenotype are still poorly understood, recently a possible molecular basis for such a behaviour has been proposed and supported by *in vitro* and *in vivo* studies. In fact, it has been shown that ApoE4 promotes Aβ production [34], aggregation, and amyloid plaque formation by displaying weaker affinity for Aβ peptides than the other, less or non pathogenic ApoE variants [35]. As a consequence, the ApoE4 variant displays reduced ability to clear Aβ peptides from the cells *via* ApoE receptors expressed in neurons and in the BBB, with increase of the load of intracellular Aβ and its oligomerization [35]. ApoE4 can also be toxic to neurons in a way independent of Aβ aggregation and clearance [36], for example by undergoing enhanced proteolytic degradation with production of toxic fragments (reviewed in [37, 38]), thus raising the possibility that multiple pathways are involved in its pathogenic effects. ApoE4 also displays reduced uptake by LDLR with a possible further decrease of Aβ clearance (reviewed in [39]). The importance of ApoE4 as a prominent risk factor for AD has prompted intense research aimed at developing new therapeutics targeted at this ApoE variant (reviewed in [40]).

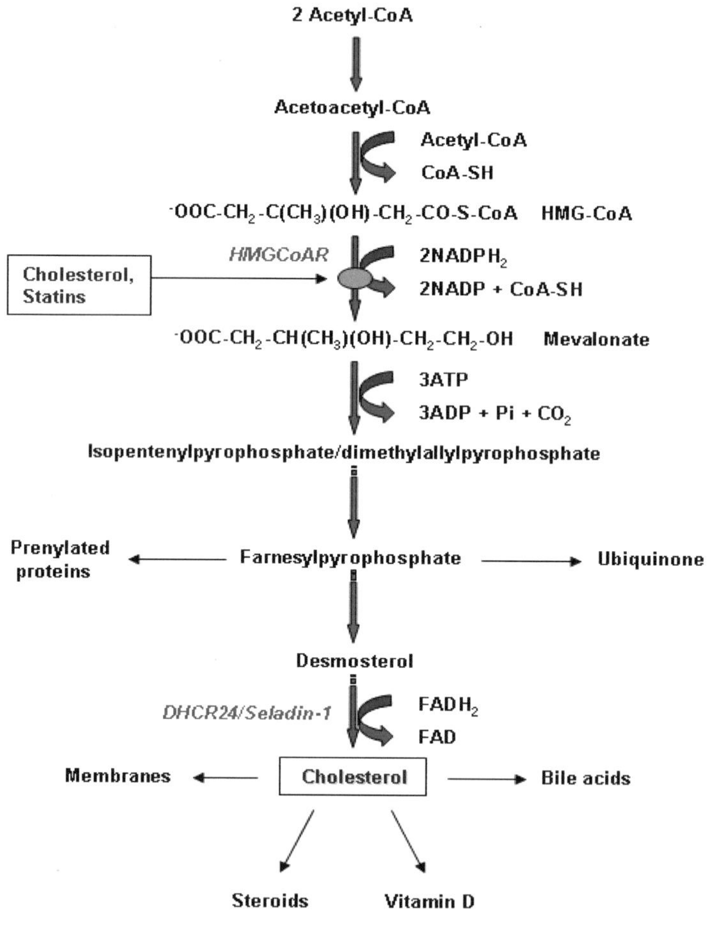

Figure 1: Cholesterol biosynthesis. The pathway is controlled at the level of the 3-hydroxy-3-methylCoA (HMGCoA) reductase-catalyzed reaction by cholesterol inhibition. The pharmacological effect of statins, structural analogues of cholesterol, mimics the inhibitory effect of cholesterol on HMGCoA. The last step of cholesterol synthesis is catalyzed by a desmosterol reductase also known as Seladin-1, that has been shown to affect cell sensitivity to Aβ peptides by modulating the cellular levels of cholesterol. For detail see under the text.

Finally, recent findings suggest that the lipoprotein receptor LRP1, a neuronal receptor essential for proper ApoE endocytosis and catabolism, affects the CNS levels of ApoE (decrease) and cholesterol (increase); in addition, LRP1 expression appears to be under negative transcriptional control of the APP and/or its intracellular domain (AICD) resulting from α/β- and γ-secretase sequential cleavage of the APP itself [35]. The APP ligand, F-spondin, is also apparently able to regulate APP cleavage by inhibiting β-secretase (BACE1) and, consequently, the AICD-dependent transactivation in cultured cells [41]. Although the exact role of the AICD in the transcriptional regulation of target genes must still be assessed, these data support the idea that cholesterol metabolism and transport in the CNS are, at least in part, under the control of the products of APP processing [42]. It has been speculated that decreased LRP1 levels in AD are directly responsible for cholesterol loss and related synaptic dysfunction [35] and that treatment with γ-secretase inhibitors could increase LRP1 expression and function in cholesterol metabolism and clearance, thus resulting beneficial.

CHOLESTEROL TRAFFICKING BETWEEN THE BLOOD AND THE CNS

Cholesterol exchanges between the CNS and the circulating blood imply the participation of the BBB, that hinders the direct passage to the CNS of the blood cholesterol and limits the reverse passage of cholesterol from the CNS to the venous circulation; the latter restriction appears to be reduced in AD, where an increased transport of cholesterol coming from degenerating neurons and the impaired transport by the ApoE4 variant have been reported [43,44].

In addition to the transport by ApoE4, most of the brain cholesterol is translocated to the circulation across the BBB in the form of the oxidized derivative 24S-hydroxycholesterol (24SOH-Chol) produced by a cholesterol 24-hydroxylase [45] responsible for the catabolism of around 40% of the cholesterol turned of in the brain. Since most of the circulating 24SOH-Chol arises from brain cholesterol, its plasma levels can be considered a measure of cholesterol turnover in the CNS [46] resulting from the balance between cerebral production and hepatic elimination and related to the number of metabolically active neurons in the brain.

Accordingly, the study of plasma 24SOH-Chol is likely to offer an insight about brain cholesterol turnover with a limited diagnostic power [47]. Finally, a fraction of brain cholesterol could be translocated to the blood by transport systems involving ATP-binding cassette membrane transport proteins such as ABCA1. Recently, it has been reported that ABCA1 is required to maintain normal CNS levels of either ApoE and ApoE-containing lipoproteins [48,49]. Conversely, dietary and pharmacological modulation of the levels of cholesterol appear to affect ApoE expression [50].

The intact BBB normally prevents cholesterol import into the CNS from the peripheral circulation; however, vascular injury can affect the translocation inside the CNS of cholesterol-carrying lipoproteins, with possible increase of membrane cholesterol and consequences for the regulation of secretase activity and the generation of Aβ peptides (see later). Data reported using Tg2576 APP transgenic mice as AD models indicate that impaired BBB results in Aβ deposition [51], a possible link between vascular injury and AD risk.

In addition to 24SOH-Chol, another cholesterol oxidized derivative, 27-hydroxycholesterol (27OH-Chol), found in the circulating blood and mainly originating from extra-CNS sources, can cross the BBB. Hence, any vascular damage can decrease the levels of 24SOH-Chol and increase those of 27OH-Chol in the CNS. Recent studies indicate that, in early AD, 24SOH-Chol increases in both the CSF and the peripheral circulation, possibly reflecting increased brain cholesterol turnover, whereas in late AD the 24SOH-Chol concentration in the CSF falls, indicating reduced cholesterol metabolism or transport as disease progresses [46,52]. These data suggest monitoring the 24SOH-Chol:27OH-Chol ratio in the CSF as a possible indicator of AD progression.

IS HIGH CHOLESTEROL A RISK FACTOR AND STATIN TREATMENT BENEFICIAL IN AD PATHOGENESIS?

In spite of the intense research carried out in recent times, the role of cholesterol as a risk factor for AD remains controversial (reviewed in [53, 54-57]). In the past 15 years, several epidemiological studies have stressed an association between high plasma cholesterol, mainly in mid age, and increased susceptibility to sporadic late-onset AD (reviewed in [53]). More recently, early mild hypercholesterolemia has been associated with increased risk for AD [58]. Moreover, increased consumption of polyunsaturated fatty acids (notably the omega-3 family) associated with a low intake of hydrogenated fats seems to reduce the risk of developing AD and other dementias, particularly those associated with vascular alterations (reviewed in [53]). However, these studies do not assess whether high circulating cholesterol in directly associated with AD or, rather, it increases brain vessel atherosclerosis with reduction of blood circulation and oxygen supply to the CNS resulting in cerebral parenchyma stress and increased susceptibility to AD damage [59,60]. The latter view is supported by the findings that cerebral and circulating cholesterol belong to distinct pools (see above). In addition, recent data indicate that Aβ peptides enhance vasoconstriction, reduce cerebral blood flow [61] and increase ROS production by NADPH oxidase, with further cerebrovascular alterations [62]. Such effects could worsen vascular endothelial damage and reduce brain parenchyma perfusion in the presence of atheromatous plaques. When added to the effect of age in reducing cerebral blood flow responses *via* Nox-derived ROS in mice [63], and to the findings indicating that Nox2-dependent ROS production is the final common pathway for the vascular alterations induced by both aging and Aβ [64], these data could provide a rationale explaining, at least in part, age and high blood cholesterol as main risk factors for sporadic AD.

The lack of a direct effect of circulating cholesterol on AD risk is further supported by the notion that there is very little exchange between circulating and brain cholesterol (see above) thus questioning the importance of those statins able to cross the BBB (including atorvastatin, simvastatin and lovastatin) as possible drugs for AD therapy (reviewed in [59]). The use of statins as possible pharmacological agents in the treatment of AD stems from retrospective clinical studies indicating that individuals chronically treated with these drugs display lower risk of developing late-onset AD [64]. The idea was supported by findings indicating that treating with statins cultured human hippocampal neurons and neuroblastoma cells expressing the amyloidogenic Swedish mutation of APP resulted in reduced Aβ production, increased α-secretase activity [65,66] and lowered inflammatory response to Aβ aggregates [67]. Moreover, inhibition by statins of the synthesis of geranylgeranyl isoprenoids, previously shown to be involved in the regulation of Aβ production plays an important role in statin-mediated reduction of Aβ secretion [68]. Statin treatment also contributes to maintain cholesterol distribution in the cell membrane and normal function of membrane proteins while hindering APP cleavage and Aβ production [69]. Decreased Aβ production has also been shown in guinea pigs treated with high doses of statins [65,70]. However, recent studies do not support these conclusions (reviewed in [53]), [59] and other prospective studies failed to show a beneficial effect of statins in AD treatment [71], though in a very recent clinical trial the use of statins resulted in significant reduction of the risk for AD [72]. The reported anti-inflammatory activity of statins could provide a rationale for their possible beneficial effects in AD [73].

Several unresolved questions raise doubts on the beneficial effects of statins in neurodegeneration and on the notion that high brain cholesterol is associated with brain dysfunction. These include (i.) the absence of solid data that high neuronal cholesterol increases Aβ production; (ii.) the findings indicating Seladin-1 down-regulation and cholesterol decrease in AD brains [24]; (iii.) the reduction of the Aβ degrading enzyme plasmin in AD brains resulting from raft disassembly (see later); (iv.); the increase of amyloid production and neurodegeneration in female mice treated with brain permeant statins [74]; and (v.) the evidence that defective cholesterol metabolism and trafficking are present in the familial forms of a number of neurodegenerative diseases [75]; on this aspect, a recent study has indicated that in human AD cases a significant increase of the content of cholesterol in specific layers of the cortex does exist, even though the density of neurofibrillary tangles and of senile plaques was not statistically associated to cholesterol abundance, leading to propose that cholesterol overload can be a new independent alteration in AD cortex [76].

Altogether, a substantial lack of effects of statins as AD drugs has became evident (reviewed in [53]). This view is supported by the very few retrospective analyses and randomized double blinded studies pointing toward an AD risk-reducing effect of statins [77], in front of the substantial lack of positive indications by all the prospective epidemiological studies and short or long term clinical trials with simvastatin and atorvastatin in mild to moderate AD patients [78]. Presently, other randomized trials are being carried out on cognitive outcomes in mild to moderate AD [79]. These and other trials, together with safety studies, are expected to definitively answer the question of the possible efficacy and safety of the statin treatment in AD (reviewed in [80]).

SURFACES ARE INDUCTORS OF PROTEIN/PEPTIDE AGGREGATION

In spite of the conflicting data on the effect of circulating and brain cholesterol on AD, undoubtedly a cholesterol-AD link must exist. As pointed out above, cell cholesterol in mainly located at the cell plasma membrane, and membrane environment is of fundamental importance in regulating membrane protein degradation and in modulating protein/peptide fibrillization. Actually, membranes and their lipid domains can contribute to protein/peptide fibrillization, particularly to the nucleation of the most toxic early amyloid oligomers, as either the primary sources of the aggregating peptide monomers and/or as enhancers of protein aggregation. In addition to the Aβ peptides, other examples of amyloidogenic peptides arising from membrane protein processing include the ABri/ADan peptides resulting from BRI protein processing and the peptides medin and gelsolin produced from the partial proteolysis of lactadherin and wild-type gelsolin, respectively [81,82]. Accordingly, it is not surprising that any modification in the membrane lipid composition and membrane environment can result in modification of processing of membrane proteins with possible enhancement of amyloidogenic peptide production (see later).

The surface or the hydrophobic interior of the plasma membrane can also induce structural changes in proteins and peptides, with exposure of hydrophobic core residues and the peptide backbone, often favouring aggregation-prone conformational states that lead to aggregation variants with different structural features [83]; these in some way are comparable to prion strains and can be endowed with different toxicities [84], as it has been shown for the prion protein, Aβ and other peptides [85-89]. The two-dimensional environment of synthetic or biological surfaces may favour protein/peptide aggregation in various ways. It can enhance aggregate nucleation by recruiting protein/peptide monomers increasing their local concentration and proximity and altering their structural features [90-92]; such effect can considerably accelerate aggregate nucleation and fibril growth

[88-90] favouring lipid extraction and disruption of membrane integrity [85,93]. It is also believed that surfaces can catalyze the formation of amyloid aggregates by a mechanism substantially different from that occurring in the three-dimensional environment of the bulk solution [90] and that depends on the membrane lipid content [85]. Conversely, the interaction of several proteins/peptides, including Aβ, with the cell, notably neuronal, membranes depend on, and can modify, membrane physicochemical properties such as charge, hydrophobicity, density of lipid packing, curvature, fluidity or lipid dynamics, that are in relation with the membrane lipid composition; consequently, the structural integrity of the membrane can be altered [86,93] and the activity of several membrane proteins and signalling pathways modified [94-97]. The above effects depend on the physicochemical features of either the surface and the monomer, the folded or unfolded state of the latter and the way it interacts with the surface (see later). This holds true also for early oligomeric assemblies, that have been shown to interact with phospholipid bilayers modifying their structure and permeability (see later) and impairing the function of membrane-bound proteins (reviewed in [11]).

The relation among membrane lipid composition, peptide/protein monomer recruitment, early aggregate nucleation and the ability of the aggregates to grow on, or to bind to, and to disassemble, the cell membrane is supported by several lines of evidence. It has been reported repeatedly that anionic surfaces, membranes rich in anionic phospholipids and even anionic macromolecules are potent inductors of beta-sheet structures by acting as conformational catalysts for amyloids [98] and stimulating protein aggregation [11,90,99-101]. Anionic phospholipid- and ganglioside-rich membranes, such as the neuronal membranes of AD people [102], have also been proposed to interact with amyloid aggregates by recognizing a shared fold [99]. These data also provide clues to explain the different vulnerability of neuronal populations to the toxic insult given by protein folding variants and their early aggregates.

The role of membrane cholesterol and gangliosides in modulating protein aggregation at the membrane and aggregate interaction with the cell membranes has also been investigated in detail (see later). However, even in this case conflicting data on the effect of cholesterol on Aβ peptide production, aggregation and toxicity have been reported [55,56].

Aβ OLIGOMERS ARE POTENT NEUROTOXINS

The amyloid cascade hypothesis is supported by a large number of data on many *in vivo* and *in vitro* amyloidogenic proteins indicating a direct cytotoxic effect of amyloid aggregates (reviewed in [10]). Until recently, mature amyloid fibrils, the main protein component found in pathological amyloid deposits, were considered the true cytotoxic agents. Therefore, it appeared likely that the pathogenic features underlying AD and other amyloid diseases were a consequence of the interaction with cells of extracellular or intracellular deposits of the fibrillar material. Besides providing a theoretical frame to understand the molecular basis of these diseases, such a scenario stimulated the exploration of therapeutic approaches to amyloidoses that were mainly focused at searching molecules able to hinder the growth and deposition of amyloid fibrils.

However, increasing evidence indicates that, at least in most cases, the early oligomeric pre-fibrillar aggregates preceding the appearance of the mature fibrils are the most highly cytotoxic species. This finding has been extended practically to all proteins and peptides associated with amyloid diseases, including Aβ peptides, α synuclein, amylin, beta2-microglobulin, transthyretin and others [13,15,103-109] and to proteins and peptides not associated with disease [110]. If we accept the idea that pre-fibrillar aggregates are the most highly cytotoxic species, mature fibrils could be considered as inert, harmless deposits of the latter and hence their growth could be interpreted as a cell defense mechanism rather than a pathological feature. However, mature fibrils can be cytotoxic indirectly, in tissue, notably by activating an inflammatory response with activation of macrophages and, in the CNS, glial cells resulting in the production of cell damaging cytokines. Fibril toxicity can also result from any leakage of toxic oligomeric species from fibril ends which, in turn, can depend on fibril conformational features and stability [111-113]. The high cytotoxicity of the early oligomeric aggregates and the possible, yet variable, indirect toxicity of mature fibrils can also explain the lack of direct correlation between density of fibrillar plaques in the brains of AD victims and severity of their clinical symptoms. Actually, experimental imaging techniques show the presence of severe burden of amyloid in most asymptomatic elderly people [114,115].

The growing awareness that the early oligomeric species in the fibrillization path are the most potent toxins to cells stems in particular from a large number of studies on Aβ aggregation both *in vitro* and *in vivo* and Aβ aggregate neurotoxicity (reviewed in [116]). The idea that Aβ oligomers are produced inside neuronal cells and are responsible for neuronal impairment was proposed over ten years ago by the William Klein group [117]. However, one of the first evidences that Aβ oligomers are really produced in cultured cells and impair neuronal cell physiology and viability came in 2002, when the Dennis Selkoe group showed that Aβ oligomers are formed and secreted soon after peptide generation in model cultured cells overexpressing APP containing the V717F AD mutation; they also showed that cerebral microinjection of the cell medium containing these oligomers, but not Aβ monomers nor fibrils, potently inhibited hippocampal long-term potentiation in rats [13]. Since then, many studies have confirmed the Selkoe results progressively leading to assess the nature of those Aβ oligomers as spherical trimer-hexamer to 24mer aggregates (ADDLs, amylospheroids) [15,16,118,119], their presence inside AD brains [14,17], their formation within neuronal cells [12,120,121], their ability to impair memory and cognitive function [15,17], and their involvement in physical degeneration of synapses [122].

The cell membranes, and their physicochemical features and biological activities appear to play key roles in Aβ (and other aggregating neuropeptide) generation, oligomerization and clearance as well as in their interaction with the oligomers and in the cytotoxicity of the latter. The growing awareness of the importance of these themes accounts for the large number of studies aimed at assessing the nature of these relationships. Particular emphasis has been given to the role performed by membrane cholesterol in all these aspects.

CELL CHOLESTEROL AFFECTS Aβ PRODUCTION, AGGREGATION AND TOXICITY

As reminded above, a number of *in vitro* and *in vivo* studies using cultured cells and animal models have investigated the link between cell cholesterol levels, Aβ peptide generation and aggregation and cell viability. Since Aβ peptide production and aggregation is considered the key event in neuronal dysfunction, mainly at the synaptic level, and in early tissue impairment in AD, any factor modulating APP processing can be of the outmost importance in AD pathogenesis. Many factors have been reported to modulate APP processing at the neuronal membrane; among these, membrane cholesterol appears to play a direct or indirect pivotal role.

The content of membrane cholesterol can modulate Aβ peptide production, aggregation and clearance in various ways, particularly by affecting the stability of lipid rafts and other membrane domains where APP and some APP processing secretases are located, as well as the activity of raft-associated proteins. In particular, the following effects/actions have been highlighted: (i.) membrane cholesterol can affect the cellular localization and the activity of the APP and the secretases modulating APP processing through the amyloidogenic or the non-amyloidogenic pathway; (ii.) membrane cholesterol can modulate the production of plasmin, a major protease involved in Aβ clearance; (iii.) membrane cholesterol and Aβ production can be affected by sphingolipid processing; (iv.) membrane cholesterol can affect the way Aβ peptides interact with the plasma membrane favouring or disfavouring aggregate nucleation; (v.) membrane cholesterol can hinder the interaction of Aβ oligomers with the cell membrane thus avoiding their cytotoxic effects; (vi.) membrane cholesterol can affect the extent and the way amyloid monomers or oligomers interact with raft-associated membrane proteins; (vii.) membrane cholesterol interacts with adjacent ganglioside molecules, particularly GM1, modulating their conformation and exposure of the negatively charged region.

MEMBRANE CHOLESTEROL MODULATES THE AMYLOIDOGENIC AND THE NON-AMYLOIDOGENIC PATHWAYS

Lipid rafts harbour many membrane proteins including APP and some secretases [123-125]. They also appear to be involved in many membrane processes, including APP (as well as other membrane protein) processing, thus providing a possible rationale for the cholesterol-AD link and the observed increased risk for AD in hypercholesterolemic people (see above). In particular, the content of membrane cholesterol and the functional organization of lipid rafts appear to markedly affect the way APP is processed by the α-, β-, and γ-secretases thus favouring the non-amyloidogenic or the amyloidogenic pathway, with increased or reduced Aβ40/42 production [126-128].

The raft dependence of the generation of amyloidogenic derivatives of proteins and peptides does not appear to be limited to APP and Aβ peptides. Actually, several lines of evidence support the idea that the pathological conversion of the cellular (PrP^c) to the infectious scrapie (PrP^{sc}) form of the prion protein occurs at the lipid rafts [129,130] and that sphingolipid depletion increases PrP^{sc} production in neuroblastoma cells infected with prions [131]. Finally, the PrP^c conformation can be stabilized upon association with lipid rafts in the secretory pathway [132] favoring its interaction with Aβ oligomers [132a]. Accordingly, it has been proposed that the aggregation of the soluble Aβ peptides and the prion protein can be a raft-associated process [125] and that any alteration of cholesterol (as well as sphingolipid) homeostasis can be a shared primary cause of a number of neurodegenerative diseases [125].

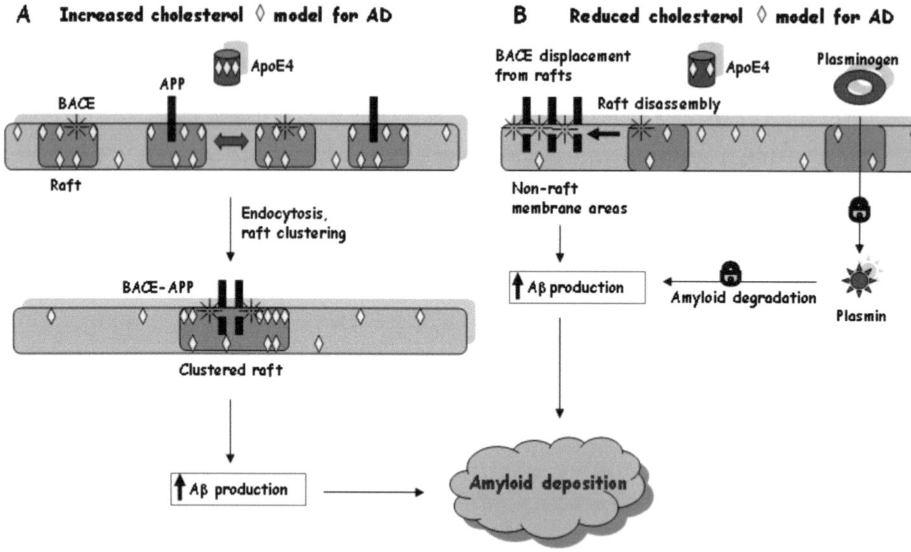

Figure 2: The high (A) and low (B) neuronal membrane cholesterol models of AD pathogenesis. The high cholesterol model assumes that low neuronal membrane cholesterol is protective against AD. In fact, high membrane cholesterol would result in increased lipid raft co-clustering and APP-BACE1 co-localization thus favouring the amyloidogenic pathway of APP processing with increased Aβ production. On the contrary, the low membrane cholesterol model envisages a protective role of relatively high amounts of membrane cholesterol assuming that APP is located in non-raft membrane domains. High membrane cholesterol would maintain APP and BACE1 separated into different membrane domains thus reducing Aβ generation. Under low cholesterol

conditions, following lipid raft disassembly BACE1 would translocate to non raft domains thus favouring its association with APP and starting the amyloidogenic pathway of APP processing. Under these conditions, the production of Aβ peptides would be further increased by the reduced activation of plasminogen to plasmin, a raft-associated event. For details see under the text.

Several reports indicate that α-secretase and BACE1 compete for APP and that such competition depends on APP compartmentalization in the cell membrane [133]; in addition, recent findings support the idea that the way APP is processed by the cell depends on the membrane localization of the APP itself and the various secretases. However, conflicting data have been reported on the effect of membrane cholesterol on APP processing. Several findings indicate that in peripheral and neuronal cell lines low membrane cholesterol and increased membrane fluidity stimulate the non-amyloidogenic pathway (α/γ-secretase cleavage); this could result from reduced activity of BACE1 (β-secretase), the enzyme starting the amyloidogenic pathway, and from increased α-secretase activity and APP content in the cell membrane, where it can undergo α-secretase cleavage [126]. The latter data have been confirmed by more recent findings showing increased levels of BACE1, Aβ and phosphorylated tau in the hippocampus of rats fed with a long-term diet enriched in cholesterol. However, most of these data were obtained in cells heavily perturbed by chemical treatment with methyl-β-cyclodextrin or lovastatin. The former extracts cholesterol from the plasma membrane, thus heavily affecting lipid rafts, and is a general endocytosis inhibitor, whereas statins have been shown to alter APP processing by modifying cell cholesterol distribution, rather than total levels, with its increase in the exofacial membrane leaflet, [134].

As it has been reported that Aβ production depends on the expression of endocytic molecules, a model of APP processing has been proposed in which BACE1 and APP are segregated into different rafts thus hindering β-cleavage [135]. The model postulates that two pools of APP do exist in the cells, one associated with membrane rafts and another out of rafts, where α-cleavage occurs, suggesting that only the raft-localized APP processing results in Aβ generation [124]. According to this model, lipid raft clustering in endocytic vesicles would bring into close contact APP and BACE1, with increased β-cleavage in the amyloidogenic pathway. Such a scenario would be favoured by high levels of brain cholesterol possibly associated with the ApoE4 phenotype "Fig. (**2A**)".

The beneficial effects of low brain cholesterol resulting from this model are strongly questioned by several studies carried out on experimental systems close to the physiological and pathological situations. Actually, many data suggest that cholesterol loss in neuronal membranes enhances amyloid peptide generation [59,136], thus agreeing with a beneficial effect of brain cholesterol against AD and questioning the experimental and clinical retrospective studies supporting the view that reducing brain cholesterol is protective against AD. Moreover, in the hippocampus of both humans and transgenic mice only a very moderate amount of APP and BACE1 is found in the same membrane environment; these co-localized APP and BACE1 fractions increase markedly in AD patients and in rodents with a moderate reduction of brain cholesterol [127]. Similarly, altered lipid composition with ganglioside increase, cholesterol decrease and lipid raft alterations have been found in temporal cortex samples from AD brains [137]. Finally, a recent study has investigated the regulation of α-secretase and BACE1 activities by the cholesterol metabolites 24SOH-Chol and 27OH-Chol. In cultured SH-SY5Y neuroblastoma cells, 24SOH-Chol, the main cholesterol metabolite in the brain (see above), was shown to exert a unique modulatory role on APP processing by reducing BACE1 activity, increasing α-secretase activity and the α/β-secretase activity ratio [138]. Such study confirmed preceding data showing a selective up regulation of the cholesterol-24 hydroxylase around neuritic plaques and the potent inhibition of APP processing by 24SOH-Chol [139].

The protective effect of cell cholesterol against Aβ production and cytotoxicity is convincingly confirmed by more recent investigations on the relation between Seladin-1, cholesterol levels and Aβ generation in neuronal cells. Seladin-1-deficient mice show reduced brain cholesterol and disorganized lipid rafts with impaired plasmin activation and BACE1 displacement to APP-containing membrane fractions, resulting in increased Aβ production through the amyloidogenic pathway. The opposite effects were found in Seladin-1-overexpressing mice [128]. Finally, the beneficial effect of increased cholesterol following Seladin-1 over expression has recently been confirmed in a study showing that cultured cells enriched in membrane cholesterol by Seladin-1 over expression display reduced ability to bind externally supplied Aβ oligomers with increased resistance to their cytotoxic effects, whereas the opposite was seen in the same cells made poor in cholesterol following treatment with the Seladin-1 inhibitor desmosterol [140]. Finally, a related study has recently shown that seladin-1 is directly involved in estrogen-mediated neuroprotection; the investigation reported that silencing of the *seladin-1* gene determined the loss of the protective effect of 17βE2 against β-amyloid toxicity and caspase-3 activation. through the estrogen responsive elements found in the coding region of the gene encoding Seladin-1 [141].

These data, together with those indicating a specific down-regulation of Seladin-1 [24] and a reduced level of cholesterol in the brains of AD patients [142], establish a role of this enzyme in lipid raft formation, modulation of APP processing, Aβ generation and clearance, and cell resistance to Aβ oligomer cytotoxicity. However, recent data question the significance of the seladin-1 gene as a selective AD indicator [143]. On the basis of these and other findings, a different scenario has been proposed, in which BACE1, but not APP, is localized to lipid rafts [127]. As a consequence, a moderate loss of membrane cholesterol would result in raft disassembly and increased BACE1-APP co-localization in non-raft membrane domains, with increased β-cleavage. Under these conditions, a lack of activation of the Aβ-degrading enzyme plasmin, a raft-associated event, would also occur [144] further reinforcing the load of Aβ peptides. According to this model, membrane cholesterol would act in keeping separated APP and BACE1 by distributing the latter in membrane compartments (rafts) distinct from those occupied by APP, with reduced β-cleavage of the latter; any loss of membrane cholesterol would thus result in raft disassembly favouring the escape of BACE1 to APP-enriched non raft domains and hindering plasminogen activation (see later), thus enhancing the amyloidogenic pathway and the build-up of Aβ peptides "Fig. (**2B**)".

THE CERAMIDE-CHOLESTEROL RELATION CAN AFFECT MEMBRANE PROPERTIES AND Aβ GENERATION

Sphingolipids are also key lipid raft components and, as such, important in affecting APP processing as well as Aβ binding to, insertion into, and aggregation onto the plasma membrane; The importance of sphingolipids has been highlighted in the case of solid-supported lipid bilayers by plasmon waveguide resonance experiments demonstrating that Aβ aggregation requires a sphingomyelin (SM)-rich environment and occurs at the bilayer surface in the absence of cholesterol [145]. Actually, several reports support the notion that lipid metabolism controls APP processing [146], that Aβ production is affected by cholesterol levels and lipid trafficking (see above) and, conversely, that APP processing affects cholesterol and SM metabolism [147] thus providing a consistent mechanism of cross-regulation of the two processes.

These and other studies have led to propose a model of Aβ-regulated cholesterol and SM metabolism whereby the γ-secretase activity controls the activity of various enzymes involved in lipid metabolism, thus affecting lipid levels. The model predicts that the combined effects of the cellular levels of cholesterol and SM controls γ-secretase activity and hence APP cleavage with different consequences on lipid metabolism regulation by Aβ peptides. By activating the neutral sphingomyelinase (SMase), the latter would down regulate SM levels, whereas Aβ40 would lower cholesterol levels by reducing its *de novo* synthesis following inhibition of HMGCoA reductase. On turn, the modification of membrane lipid composition (reduction of cholesterol and SM levels) produced by Aβ40/42 would affect γ-secretase activity thus providing a feed-back mechanism [147].

One of the products of the neutral SMase activity at the cell surface is ceramide. The latter is important as signalling molecule involved in many biochemical (regulation of sphingolipid and glycolipid levels, production of bioactive sphingolipids), biological (cell growth, proliferation and lifespan, apoptosis, vesicular trafficking and neuronal differentiation) and pathological (inflammation, tumorigenesis, diabetes and neurodegenerative diseases) processes (reviewed in [148]); in addition, a critical role of ceramide in cell membrane and/or membrane raft re-organization has been supported by many recent studies (reviewed in [149]). Actually, ceramide molecules modify the membrane properties following their tendency to spontaneously self-associate into ceramide-enriched membrane microdomains displaying the tendency to fuse into large macrodomains [150]. Moreover, ceramide molecules strongly stabilize rafts due to their close packing and tend to displace cholesterol from rafts in artificial membranes [151] thus potentially affecting APP processing (see preceding section). The activation of the acid SMase by stress stimuli such as oxidative stress, γ- and UV-irradiation, bacterial and viral infections results in ceramide release with the formation of ceramide-enriched platforms and the activation of death receptors, an event associated with the ceramide pro-apoptotic effect (reviewed in [149]) (see later). A possible role of ceramide in APP processing and Aβ generation due to its ability to stabilize BACE1 is also emerging [152]. However, whether ceramide regulates one or more molecular events associated to AD pathogenesis must still be assessed.

MEMBRANE CHOLESTEROL AFFECTS PLASMINOGEN ACTIVATION

Aβ-degrading enzymes are involved in the physiological regulation of the levels of Aβ peptides and their early aggregates in the brain. Altered levels of these enzymes have been shown in AD and cerebral amyloid angiopathy (CAA) and could be influenced by the ApoE genotype. The Aβ-degrading enzymes include nephrylisin, the insulin-degrading enzyme (IDE), the endothelin-converting enzymes and plasmin, whereas conflicting results have been reported for the angiotensin-converting enzyme (reviewed in [153]). Aβ degradation by proteolysis is of great importance for its reflexes on Aβ turnover and biology and can represent a possible target for AD therapy [154]. Of particular importance in either aspect could be the role played by plasmin, although several recently performed association studies do not support the notion that common polymorphisms in the plasminogen genes influence the development of late-onset AD [155].

Plasmin is a raft-resident serine protease generated from the inactive precursor plasminogen, whose activation by tissue-type or urokinase-type plasminogen activator (tPA) is a raft-dependent event [144]. Plasmin cleaves Aβ peptides at multiple sites thus preventing their aggregation [156]. Significantly increased plasmin levels have been found in the frontal cortex and the hippocampus of AD people carrying the ApoE4 genotype respect to unaffected age-matched controls [144]. These data were complemented by *in vivo* studies on APP transgenic mouse models showing that reduced tPA activity correlated with Aβ accumulation [157]. Plasmin seems also to enhance APP α-cleavage, in addition to Aβ degradation, further underscoring its potential importance to AD pathogenesis [144]. Finally, the low neuronal membrane cholesterol model of AD pathogenesis proposes that any loss of membrane cholesterol resulting in lipid raft disorganization would hinder plasminogen activation, a raft-associated process, with loss of plasmin activity and increased levels of Aβ peptides and their oligomers (see above).

It is also worth mentioning previous data indicating that tPA is able to bind to, and to be stimulated by, not only fibrin but also other protein/peptide oligomers with cross-beta structure such as amyloids (reviewed in [158]). Therefore, Aβ peptides and their oligomers would directly favour plasmin formation and hence their own degradation thus highlighting a possible further regulatory negative feedback mechanism.

The multiplicity of Aβ-degrading enzymes within the brain, together with the existence of several possible ways to regulate the production and the clearance of Aβ peptides could probably limit the impact of the deficiency of any particular Aβ-degrading enzyme on AD pathogenesis. However, a declined capacity to degrade Aβ peptides, together with other age-related functional impairment could contribute to the accumulation of Aβ peptides and their oligomers in the brain parenchyma and vessels, with neuronal impairment and the progressive appearance of the signs of AD and CAA.

MEMBRANE CHOLESTEROL CAN MODULATE Aβ AGGREGATION

Aβ peptides are amphipathic molecules, containing a hydrophilic N-terminal stretch (residues 1-28) and a hydrophobic C-terminal domain (residues 29-40/42) partially spanning the APP transmembrane domain. In solution, Aβ peptides display a substantially unfolded conformation with reduced content of secondary structure; however, the latter increases considerably in phospholipid vesicles particularly when enriched in cholesterol and gangliosides [159,160] thus underscoring the role of membranes in modulating peptide structure and aggregation. Actually, structural perturbations may be expected to occur in proteins/peptides following their interaction with membranes thus enhancing their rate of fibrillization (reviewed in [161]). Therefore, it is not surprising that membrane lipid composition affects remarkably the effect of a membrane on a protein/peptide structure and aggregation propensity (see above). For example, Aβ40 oligomerization has been shown to occur during the isolation of lipid rafts [162]. Therefore, the role of cholesterol and gangliosides in modulating either protein aggregation at the membrane level and aggregate interaction with the cell membranes (see later) appears of great importance.

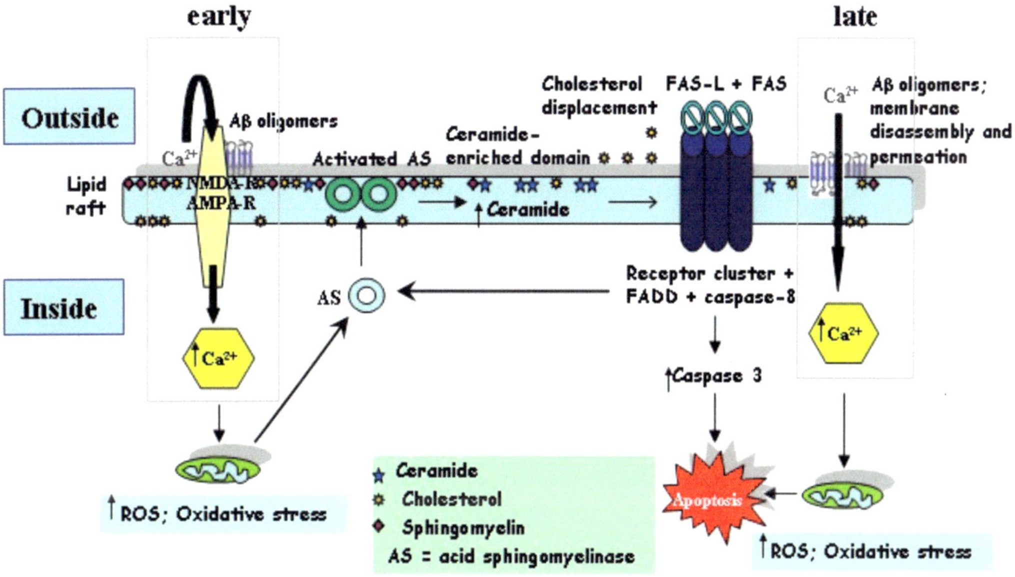

Figure 3: Sphingomyelin (SM) processing by neutral or acid sphingomyelinase (AS) can affect membrane lipid composition and amyloid cytotoxicity. The model proposes a two-step toxic effect of amyloid oligomers. Initially, the oligomers would interact with the neuronal membrane at specific sites, notably the AMPA and NMDA glutamatergic Ca^{2+} channels favouring uncontrolled Ca^{2+} ingress into the cell. The intracellular Ca^{2+} rise would elicit an oxidative stress condition with AS activation resulting in some increase of the content of membrane ceramide coming from SM hydrolysis and favouring the appearance of ceramide-enriched domains with pull-out of cholesterol molecules. These modifications would favour oligomerization and activation of different membrane receptors including death receptors triggering the apoptotic pathway. The second step would envisage a substantially non-specific interaction of the amyloid oligomers with the cell membrane; the latter would result in membrane disassembly and permeabilization with a second pulse of intracellular Ca^{2+} reinforcing the condition of oxidative stress and the impairment of mitochondrial activity. At the same time, or even at later times of exposure to Aβ oligomers, the glutamatergic Ca^{2+} channels can be internalized by endocytosis thus reducing Ca^{2+} influx by this route. For details see under the text.

The ability of Aβ peptides to insert into the membrane seems to depend on the membrane cholesterol:phospholipid ratio. In synthetic, low cholesterol DMPC vesicles, Aβ preferentially localizes at the membrane surface exhibiting an aggregation-prone β-structure; on the contrary, in the same vesicles containing 33% cholesterol the C-terminal tail of the peptide inserts into the membrane with an altered, α-helix-rich, structure that hinders peptide aggregation [159]. These data support the idea that the content in cholesterol affects the way Aβ peptides interact with the phospholipid bilayer and their ability to insert in the latter, modulating its aggregation into fibrillar assemblies. Increased Aβ40 retention onto, or into, acidic phospholipid membranes has also been reported, either way of interaction resulting in different outcomes. The peptide anchored *via* its C-terminal tail, presumably in its native, partially α-helical structure, remained monomeric; conversely, upon peptide interaction at the membrane surface, peptide aggregation was accelerated [87] indicating that a delicate balance between two different mechanisms of peptide-membrane interaction could possibly be involved in AD pathophysiology. Overall, when added to the fact that membrane cholesterol can also modulate Aβ production (see above) and Aβ cytotoxicity (see below), these data further support the AD-cholesterol link.

MEMBRANE CHOLESTEROL MODULATES Aβ CYTOTOXICITY

The biochemical effects of Aβ oligomers accounting for their toxicity are under investigation and must be added to the biological effects of monomeric Aβ peptides to complete the picture. The reported biological effects of monomeric Aβ peptides include interaction with TNFR1 and the p75 neurotrophin receptor, with induction of neuronal death [163,164], inflammation and cholinergic dysfunction in the rat brain through activation of the p38 MAPK pathway [165] and other signalling pathways [166,167]. Aβ40 has also been reported to up regulate APAF-1 expression and neuronal NF-κB translocation eventually leading to neuronal death [165]. Other effects related to AD pathology include the ability of Aβ peptides to disassemble microtubules [168] and to bind to soluble tau promoting its hyperphosphorylation by glycogen synthase kinase-3β [169]. Aβ can also interact with its homologue sequence in APP, inducing homo-oligomerization of the latter and its of BACE1-cleaved C-terminal fragment eventually leading to cell death [170]. Finally recent data demonstrate that, Aβ can be toxic to neurons by interacting with the PrP^c with resulting activation of the Fyn kinase pathway [171].

Aβ oligomer toxicity has been associated basically with the ability of these assemblies to interact with the cell membranes disrupting membrane integrity and altering specific membrane functions. Actually, it has repeatedly been reported that pre-fibrillar aggregates of many peptides and proteins either associated or not-associated with disease are able to interact with synthetic phospholipid bilayers [172-177] and with cell membranes [104,178-180]. Such an interaction results in loss of membrane integrity, derangement of selective ion permeability and impairment of specific membrane-bound protein function [94,95,181,182], and appears to be modulated by membrane biophysical features, and hence by the lipid (particularly cholesterol) and GM1 content in the membrane, increasing in cholesterol-poor or GM1-rich membranes and *vice versa* [8,9]. On this aspect, it has recently been reported that the GM1-Abeta complex favors subsequent aggregation behaving as an aggregation nucleus [182a]. Recent data also indicate that membrane-oligomer interaction also depends on oligomer biophysical features, depending on the conditions oligomers are grown, such that it has been proposed that oligomer cytotoxicity is not an intrinsic, but, rather, an emerging property of a more complex oligomer-membrane system [183,184] (Fig. **4**).

The cytotoxicity data agree with the notion that one of the earliest modifications in cells exposed to Aβ (and other protein) toxic oligomers is a significant increase of the intracellular free Ca^{2+} associated with oxidative stress. These biochemical modifications appear to be rather common to many types of cultured cells exposed to pre-fibrillar aggregates of many different peptides and proteins (reviewed in [11]). Actually, many data support the idea that Aβ oligomer cytotoxicity following association with the cell membrane depends on membrane physical features including fluidity, compactness, curvature and others, resulting from lipid composition. Since differing cell types display different average membrane lipid composition, for example in terms of cholesterol or ganglioside content, this could contribute to explain the variable susceptibility to the same toxic oligomeric species of varying cell types in culture and in tissue, or of the same cells in different differentiation stages or cell cycle phases [8,9].

If we consider that Aβ oligomer cytotoxicity appears to require oligomer interaction with the cell membrane, the question arises as to whether such an interaction is non-specific or it occurs at the level of specific membrane proteins or domains. Apart the most recently proposed Aβ interactors (APP, PrP^c, see above), in the past, several candidate cell surface proteins, including RAGE, have been considered as possible receptors of amyloids or their precursors, particularly in the case of Aβ peptides [185]. However, increasing evidence suggests that additional binding sites must be involved in the interaction of amyloids of different peptides and proteins with the neuronal plasma membrane [82,181,182]. This is confirmed by recent findings indicating that Aβ oligomers accumulate within dendritic arbors, attach selectively to dendrites in culture [14] and bind to the neuronal surface in small punctate clusters that co-localize with a subpopulation of synaptic terminals at undefined specific locations [186].

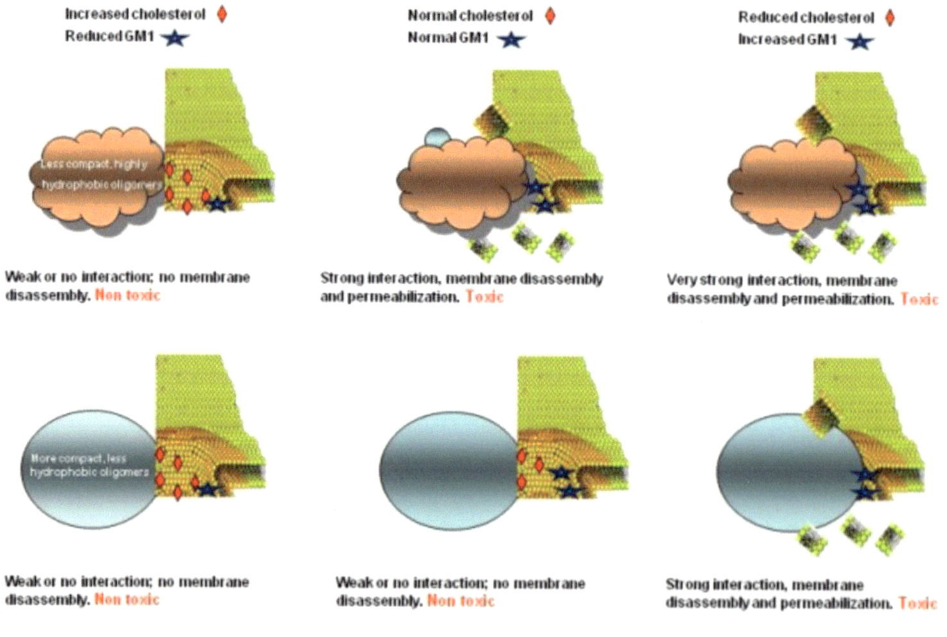

Figure 4: The idea that amyloid cytotoxicity stems from a complex interplay between oligomer and membrane biophysical properties has led to consider that amyloid-membrane interaction results in a system. The features of such a system depend on oligomer properties determined by the conditions of oligomer nucleation and growth, such as stability, compactness and hydrophobic exposure; they also depend on membrane properties resulting from lipid composition, such as rigidity/fluidity, lateral pressure, hydrophobicity and electrostatic potential. In particular, the

content of cholesterol and GM1, key components of lipid rafts, appears to modulate the ability of amyloid oligomers with different biophysical properties to interact with, disassemble and permeabilize the cell membrane. For details see in the text.

A number of reports also support the possibility that Aβ oligomers interact with glutamatergic calcium channels such as the AMPA and NMDA receptors. It is not clear whether such an interaction occurs directly with the receptor or with the lipid raft domain where the receptor itself is located, however the receptor is supposed to be initially activated following such an interaction thus accounting, at least in part, for the early free Ca^{2+} increase in the exposed cells [181,182]. At later times, the oligomer-receptor complexes could hinder NMDA receptor-mediated Ca^{2+} influx into active dendritic spines inducing spine loss and receptor internalization by endocytosis, thus reverting the initial activation effects [187,188]. Recently, a similar behaviour has been reported for amyloid aggregates of a protein not associated with amyloid diseases, suggesting that NMDA and AMPA receptors can be generic interaction sites for amyloids [189]. Membrane cholesterol can modulate aggregate-cell interaction by affecting the physical state of the rafts harbouring those receptors.

A model describing the final apoptotic outcome in Aβ oligomer-exposed cells could tentatively be proposed taking into account the data on cell permeabilization to Ca^{2+} by Aβ peptides and their oligomers together with the relation between Ca^{2+} increase, oxidative stress and stress-activated acid SMase resulting in ceramide increase and cholesterol displacement from the cell membrane (see above). On this aspect, a critical role of gangliosides and sphingolipids as critical player in senescence and in Alzheimer's disease has recently emerged [190] (see also above). As far as the effects on cell calcium are concerned, Aβ oligomers could affect free Ca^{2+} levels and cell viability by a two step mechanism "Fig. (**3**)". In the first, early, step the interaction of Aβ oligomers with the cell membrane would increase the intracellular Ca^{2+} by impairing AMPA and/or NMDA receptor regulation [181,182]. The resulting, initially reversible, increase of cytosolic Ca^{2+} would elicit rapid oxidative stress with acid SMase activation, ceramide increase, membrane cholesterol displacement and formation of ceramide-enriched domains. The latter would serve clustering and activation of receptors involved in several signalling pathways, including death receptors such as FAS [145], with further SMase activation, FADD recruitment and pro-caspase-8 activation, thus triggering the apoptotic pathway. This model does not exclude late effects of Aβ oligomers, including receptor endocytosis and non-specific membrane permeabilization due to physical disruption of the phospholipid bilayer, enhanced Ca^{2+} increase and activation of the intrinsic (mitochondrial) apoptotic pathway "Fig. (**3**)". The model could, in part, implement those previously reported to account for the effects of the reduction or the increase of membrane cholesterol (see above), contributing to a scenario that must necessarily be much more complex.

CONCLUDING REMARKS

The relation between membrane lipid composition (mainly in terms of cholesterol, ganglioside and sphingomyelin content), Aβ generation and aggregation as well as aggregate cytotoxicity and AD pathogenesis requires more extensive research to provide further knowledge and to reconcile some contradictory data. However, the data presently available support the idea that, in general, the presence of cholesterol in the cell membrane can modulate cell vulnerability to amyloids in several ways with opposite effects. Cholesterol can favour APP processing with increased production of Aβ peptides thus resulting amyloidogenic; altered content of membrane cholesterol can also induce conformational changes of specific protein/peptides; increased content of membrane cholesterol induces higher membrane rigidity that can be protective disfavouring aggregate interaction with cell membranes and reducing aggregate cytotoxicity following perturbation of membrane integrity. The relation between hypercholesterolemia and brain cholesterol levels is not ascertained, even taking into account that circulating and brain cholesterol are substantially separate pools. Although several epidemiological studies seem to prove that hypercholesterolemia is a risk factor for AD, conflicting data have emerged from clinical studies on statin efficacy as potential anti-AD drugs. New ideas are also emerging on the molecular basis of the ApoE4 genotype as the main recognised genetic risk factor for AD. Finally, alternative hypotheses based on conflicting data have been proposed on the relation between high brain cholesterol and AD risk involving APP, its processing enzymes, their lipid raft location and trafficking between the plasma membrane and the endosome compartments.

The presence of conflicting lines of evidences highlights the need of a more extensive information on the link between cholesterol and the molecular and cellular basis of AD suggesting new ideas and approaches for therapy.

ACKNOWLEDGEMENTS

The authors thank the Regione Toscana for financial support.

CONFLICT OF INTEREST

The authors confirm that this chapter content has no conflict of interest.

DISCLOSURE

This chapter is an update of our previous publication in CAR "Cholesterol in Alzheimer's Disease: Unresolved Questions"" published in 'CAR', Volume 6, Number 1, February, pp. 15 to 29.

ABBREVIATIONS

24SOH-Chol	=	24S-hydroxycholesterol
27OH-Chol	=	27-hydroxycholesterol
AD	=	Alzheimer's disease
AICD	=	APP intracellular domain
ApoE	=	Apolipoprotein E
APP	=	Amyloid precursor protein
BACE1	=	Beta-amyloid converting enzyme
BBB	=	Blood-brain barrier
CAA	=	Cerebral amyloid angiopathy
CNS	=	Central nervous system
CSF	=	Cerebrospinal fluid
HMGCoAR	=	3-hydroxy-3-methylglutarylCoA reductase

LRP = LDL-receptor-related proteins

RAGE = Receptor of advanced glycation end-products;

Seladin-1 = Selective Alzheimer's disease indicator-1

SM = Sphingomyelin

SMase = Sphingomyelinase

tPA = Tissue-type plasminogen activator

REFERENCES

[1] 1.Von Strauss E, Viitanen M, De Ronchi D, Winblad B, Fratiglioni L. Aging and the occurrence of dementia: findings from a population-based cohort with a large sample of nonagenarians. Arch Neurol 56: 587-592 (1999).

[2] Wimo A, Jönsson L, Bond J, Prince M and Winblad B. Alzheimer Disease International. The worldwide economic impact of dementia. Alzheimers Dement. 9: 1-11 (2013).

[3] Bettens K, Sleegers K and Van Broeckhoven C. Genetic insights in Alzheimer's disease. Lancet Neurol. 12: 92-104 (2013).

[4] Selkoe DJ. Alzheimer's disease: genes, proteins, and therapy. Physiol Rew 81: 741-766 (2001).

[5] De la Torre JC. Is Alzheimer's disease a neurodegenerative or a vascular disorder? Data, Dogma and Dialectics. Lancet Neurol 3: 184-190 (2004).

[6] Probst A, Langui D and Ulrich J. Alzheimer's disease: a description of the structural lesions. Brain Pathol 1: 229-239 (1991).

[7] Hardy J and Selkoe DJ. The amyloid hypothesis of Alzheimer's disease: progress and problems on the road to therapeutics. Science 297: 353-356 (2002).

[8] Cecchi C, Baglioni S, Fiorillo C, Pensalfini A, Liguri G, Nosi D, Rigacci S, Bucciantini M and Stefani M. Insights into the molecular basis of the differing susceptibility of varying cell types to the toxicity of amyloid aggregates J Cell Sci 118: 3459-3470 (2005).

[9] Cecchi C, Pensalfini A. Stefani M, Baglioni S, Fiorillo C, Cappadona S, Caporale R, Nosi D, Ruggiero M and Liguri G. Replicatine neuroblastoma cells in different cell cycle phases display different vulnerability to amyloid toxicity. J. Mol. Med. 86: 197-209 (2008).

[10] Selkoe DJ. Folding proteins in fatal ways. Nature 426: 900-904 (2003).

[11] Stefani M. Generic cell dysfunction in neurodegenerative disorders: role of surfaces in early protein misfolding, aggregation and aggregate cytotoxicity. The Neuroscientist 13: 519-531 (2007).

[12] Gouras GK, Tsai, J, Nasslund J, Vincent B, Edgar M, Checler F, Greefiels JP, Haroutunian V, Buxbaum JD, Xu H, Greengard P and Relkin NR. Intraneuronal Aβ accumulation in human brain. Am J Pathol 156: 15-20 (2000).

[13] Walsh DM, Klyubin I, Fadeeva JV, Cullen WK, Anwyl R, Wolfe MS, Rowan MJ and Selkoe DJ. Naturally secreted oligomers of amyloid β protein potently inhibit hippocampal long-term potentiation *in vivo*. Nature 416: 535-539 (2002).

[14] Gong Y, Chang I, Viola KI, Lacor PN, Lambert MP, Finch CE, Krafft GA and Klein WI. Alzheimer's disease-affected brain: presence of oligomeric Aβ ligands (ADDLs) suggests a molecular basis for reversible memory loss. Proc Natl Acad Sci USA 100: 10417-10422 (2003).

[15] Cleary JP, Walsh DM, Hofmeister JJ, Shankar GM, Kuskowski MA, Selkoe DJ and Ashe KH. Natural oligomers of the amyloid-β protein specifically disrupt cognitive function. Nat Neurosci 8: 79-84 (2005).

[16] Townsend M, Shankar GM, Mehta T, Walsh DM and Selkoe DJ. Effects of secreted oligomers on amyloid β-protein on hippocampal synaptic plasticity: a potent role for trimers. J Physiol 572.2: 477-492 (2006).

[17] Lesné S. Koh MT, Kotlinek L, Kayed R, Glabe CG, Yang A, Gallagher M and Ashe KH. Nature 440: 352-357 (2006).

[18] 18.Fjell AM and Walhovd KB. Neuroimaging results impose new views on Alzheimer's disease--the role of amyloid revised. Mol Neurobiol. 45: 153-72 (2012).

[19] Ledesma MD and Dotti CG. Amyloid excess in Alzheimer's disease: what is cholesterol to be blamed for? FEBS Lett 580: 5525-5532 (2006).

[20] Simons K and Ehehalt R. Cholesterol, lipid rafts, and disease. J Clin Invest 110: 597-603 (2002).

[21] Turley SD, Burns DK, Rosenfeld CR and Dietschy JM. Brain does not utilize low density lipoprotein-cholesterol during fetal and neonatal development in the sheep. J Lipid Res 37: 1953-1961 (1996).

[22] Poirier J, Baccichet A, Dea D and Gauthier S. Cholesterol synthesis and lipoprotein reuptake during synaptic remodelling in hippocampus in adult rats Neuroscience 55: 81-90 (1993).

[23] Pfrieger FW. Cholesterol homeostasis and function in neurons of the central nervous system. Cell Mol Life Sci 60:1158-11571 (2003).

[24] Greeve I, Hermans-Borgmeyer I, Brellinger C, Kasper D, Gomez-Isla T, Behl C, Levkau B and Nitsch RM. The human DIMINUTO/DWARF1 homolog seladin-1 confers resistance to Alzheimer's disease-associated neurodegeneration and oxidative stress. J Neurosci 20: 7345-7352 (2000).

[25] Waterham HR, Koster J, Romeijn GJ, Hennekam RC, Vreken P, Andersson HC, FizPatrick DR, Kelley RI and Wanders RJ. Mutations in the 3beta-hydroxysterol Delta24-reductase gene cause desmosterolosis, an autosomal recessive disorder of cholesterol biosynthesis. Am J Human Genet 69: 685-694 (2001).

[26] Benvenuti S, Saccordi R, Luciani P, Urbani S, Deledda C, Cellai I, Arancini F, Squecco R, Rosati F, Danza G, Gelmini S, Greve I, Rossi M, Maggi R, Serio M and Peri A. neuronal differentiation of human mesenchymal stem cells: changes in the expression of the Alzheimer's disease-related gene seladin-1. Exp Cell Res 312: 2592-2604 (2006).

[27] Iivonen S, Hiltunen M, Alafuzoff I, Mannermaa A, Kerokoski P, Puoliväli J, Salminen A, Helisalmi S and Soininen H. Seladin-1 transcription is linked to neuronal degeneration in Alzheimer's disease. Neuroscience 113: 301-310 (2002).

[28] Wu C, Miloslavskaya I, Demontis S, Maestro R and Galaktionov K. Regulation of cellular response to oncogenic and oxidative stress by Seladin-1. Nature 432: 640-645 (2004).

[29] Jurevics H and Morell P. Cholesterol for synthesis of myelin is made locally, not imported into brain. J Neurochem 64: 895-901 (1995).

[30] Mahley RW. Apolipoprotein E: cholesterol transport protein with expanding role in cell biology. Science 240: 622-630 (1988).

[31] Poirier J. Apolipoprotein E and cholesterol metabolism in the pathogenesis and treatment of Alzheimer's disease. Trends Mol Med 9: 94-101 (2003).

[32] Liu CC, Kanekiyo T, Xu H and Bu G. Apolipoprotein E and Alzheimer disease: risk, mechanisms and therapy. Nat Rev Neurol. 9: 106-118 (2013).

[33] Corder EH, Saunders AM, Strittmatter WJ, Schmechel DE, Gaskell PC, Small GW, Roses AD, Haines JL and Pericak-Vance MA Gene dose of apolipoprotein E type 4 allele and the risk of Alzheimer's disease in late-onset families. Science 261: 921-923 (1993).

[34] Ye S, Huang Y, Mullerdorff K, Dong I, Griedt G, Meng EC, Cohen FE, Kuntz ID, Weisgraber KH and Mahley RW. Apolipoprotein (apo) E4 enhances amyloid β peptide production in cultured neuronal cells: ApoE structure as a potential therapeutic target Proc Natl Acad Sci USA 102: 18700-18705 (2005).

[35] Liu Q, Zerbinatti CV, Zhang J, Hoe H-S, Wang B, Cole SL, Herz J, Muglia L and Bu G. Amyloid precursor protein regulates brain apolipoprotein A and cholesterol metabolism through lipoprotein receptor LRP1. Cell 56: 66-78 (2007).

[36] Huang Y. Molecular and cellular mechanisms of apolipoprotein E4 neurotoxicity and potential therapeutic strategies Curr Opin Drug Discover Dev 9: 627-641 (2006).

[37] Mahley RW, Huang Y and Weisgraber KH. Detrimental effects of apolipoprotein E4: potential therapeutic targets in Alzheimer's disease. Curr Alz Res 4: 537-540 (2007).

[38] Marques MA, Owens PA and Crutcher KA. Progress toward identification of protease activity involved in proteolysis of apolipoprotein E in human brain. J Mol Neurosci. 24: 73-80 (2004).

[39] Donahue JE and Johanson CE. Apolipoprotein E, Amyloid-beta, and blood-brain barrier permeability in Alzheimer disease. J Neuropathol Exp Neurol 67: 261-270 (2008).

[40] Refolo LM and Fillit HM. Apolipoprotein E4 as a target for developing new therapeutics for Alzheimer's disease. J Mol Neurosci 23: 151-155 (2004).

[41] Ho A and Sudhof TC. Binding of F-spondin to amyloid-β precursor protein: a candidate amyloid-β precursor protein ligand that modulates amyloid-β precursor protein cleavage. Proc Natl Acad Sci USA 101: 2548-2553 (2004).

[42] Grimm MO, Grimm HS, Pätzold AJ, Zinser EG, Halonen R, Duering M, Tschäpe JA, De Strooper B, Müller U, Shen J and Hartmann T. Regulation of cholesterol and sphingomyelin metabolism by amyloid-beta and presenilin. Nat Cell Biol. 7: 1118-1123 (2005).

[43] Heverin M, Meaney S, Lütjohann D, Diczfalusy U, Wahren J and Björkhem I. Changes in the levels of cerebral and extracerebral sterols in the brain of patients with Alzheimer's disease J Lipid Res 45: 186-193 (2004).

[44] Schönknecht P, Lütjohann D, Pantel J, Bardenheuer H, Hartmann T, von Bergmann K, Beyreuther K and Schröder J. Cerebrospinal fluid 24S-hydroxycholesterolis increased in patients with Alzheimer's disease compared to healthy controls. Neurosci Lett 324: 83-85 (2002).

[45] Combarros O, Infante J, Llorca J and Berciano J. Genetic association of CYP46 and risk for Alzheimer's disease. Dement Geriatr Cogn Disord 18: 257-260 (2004).

[46] Kölsch H, Heun R, Kerksiek A, Bergmann KV, Maier W and Lütjohann D. Altered levels of plasma 24S-hydroxycholesterol and 7-hydroxycholesterol in demented patients. Neurosci Lett 368: 303-308 (2004).

[47] Leoni V and Caccia C. 24S-hydroxycholesterol in plasma: A marker of cholesterol turnover in neurodegenerative diseases. Biochimie. 95: 595-612 (2013).

[48] Hirsch-Reinshagen V, Zhou S, Burgess BL, Bernier L, McIsaac SA, Chan JY, Tansley GH, Cohn JS, Hayden MR and Wellington CL. Deficiency of ABCA1 impairs Apolipoprotein E metabolism in brain. J Biol Chem 279: 41197-41207 (2004).

[49] Wahrle SE, Jiang H, Parsadanian M, Legleiter J, Han X, Fryer JD, Kowalewski T and Holtzman DM. ABCA1 is required for normal central nervous system ApoE levels and for lipidation of astrocyte-secreted ApoE. J Biol Chem 279: 40987-40993 (2004).

[50] Petanceska SS, DeRosa S, Sharma A, Diaz N, Duff K, Tint SG, Refolo LM and Pappolla M. Changes in apolipoprotein E expression in response to dietary and pharmacological modulation of cholesterol. J Mol Neurosci. 20: 395-406 (2003).

[51] Ujiie M, Dickstein DL, Carlow DA and Jefferies WA. Blood-brain barrier permeability precedes senile plaque formation in an Alzheimer's disease model. Microcirculation 10: 463-470 (2003).

[52] Locatelli S, Lütjohann D, Schmidt HH, Otto C, Beisiegel U and von Bergmann K. Reduction of plasma 24S-hydroxycholesterol (cerebrosterol) levels using high-dosage simvastatin in patients with hypercholesterolemia: evidence that simvastatin affects cholesterol metabolism in the human brain. Arch Neurol 59: 213-216 (2002).

[53] Shobab LA, Hsiung G-YR and Feldman HH. Cholesterol in Alzheimer's disease. The Lancet 5:841-852 (2004).

[54] Puglielli L, Tanzi RE and Kovacs DM. Alzheimer's disease: the cholesterol connection. Nat Neurosci 6: 7212-72121 (2003)

[55] Koudinov AR and Koudinova NV. Cholesterol homeostasis failure as a unifying cause of synaptic degeneration J Neurol Sci 229-230:233-240 (2005).

[56] Sjögren M, Mielke M, Gustafson D, Zandi P and Skoog I. Cholesterol and Alzheimer's disease – is there a relation? Mech Ageing Develop 127: 138-147 (2006).

[57] Reiss AB and Voloshyna I. Regulation of cerebral cholesterol metabolism in Alzheimer disease. J Investig Med. 60: 576-582 (2012).

[58] Pappolla MA, Bryant-Thomas TK, Herbert D, Pacheco J, Fabra Garcia M, Manjon M, Girones X, Henry TL, Matsubara E, Zambon D, Wolozin B, Sano M, Cruz-Sanchez FF, Thal LJ, Petanceska SS and Refolo LM. Mild hypercholesterolemia is an early risk factor for the development of Alzheimer amyloid pathology. Neurology. 61: 199-205 (2003).

[59] Ledesma, MD and Dotti CG. The conflicting role of brain cholesterol in Alzheimer's disease: lessons from the brain plasminogen system. Biochem Soc Symp 72: 129-138 (2005).

[60] Beach TG, Wilson JR, Sue LI, Newell A, Poston M, Cisneros R, Pandya Y, Esh C, Connor DJ, Sabbagh M, Walker DG and Roher AE. Circle of Willis atherosclerosis: association with Alzheimer's disease, neuritic plaques and neurofibrillary tangles. Acta Neuropathol. 113:13-21 (2007).

[61] Thomas T, Thomas G, McLendon C, Sutton T and Mullan M. β-amyloid-mediated vasoactivity and vascular endothelial damage. Nature 380: 168-171 (1996).

[62] Park L, Zhou P, Pitstick R, Capone C, Anrather J, Norris EH, Younkin L, Younkin S, Carlson G, McEwen BS and Iadecola C. Nox2-derived radicals contribute to neurovascular and behavioural dysfunction in mice overexpressing the amyloid precursor protein. Proc Natl Acad Sci USA 105: 1347-1352 (2008).

[63] Park L, Anrather J, Girouard H, Zhou P and Iadecola C. Nox-2-derived reactive oxygen species mediate neurovascular dysregulation in the aging mouse brain. J Cereb Blood Flow Metab. 27: 1908-1918 (2007).

[64] Zandi PP, Sparks DL, Khachaturian AS, Tschanz J, Norton M, Steinberg M, Welsh-Bohmer KA and Breitner JC. Cache County study investigators. Do statins reduce the risk of incident dementia and Alzheimer's disease? The Cache County study Arch. Gen Psychiatry 62: 217-224 (2005).

[65] Fassbender K, Simons M, Bergmann C, Stroick M, Lutjohann D, Keller P, Runz H, Kuhl S, Bertsch T, von Bergmann K, Hennerici M, Beyreuther K and Hartmann T. Simvastatin strongly reduces levels of Alzheimer's disease beta-amyloid peptides Abeta-42 and Abeta-40 *in vitro* and *in vivo*. Proc Natl Acad Sci USA 98: 5856-5861 (2001)

[66] Parvathy S, Ehrlich M, Pedrini S, Diaz N, Refolo L, Buxbaum JD, Bogush A, Petanceska S and Gandy S. Atorvastatin-induced activation of Alzheimer's alpha secretase is resistant to standard inhibitors of protein phosphorylation-regulated ectodomain shedding. J Neurochem 90: 1005-1010 (2004).

[67] Sun YX, Crisby M, Lindgreen S and Janciauskene S. Pravastatin inhibits pro-inflammatory effects of Alzheimer's peptide Abeta(1-42) in glioma cell culture. Pharmacol Res 47: 119-126 (2003).

[68] Zhou Y, Suram A, Venugopal C, Prakasam A, Lin S, Su Y, Li B, Paul SM and Sambamurti K. Geranylgeranyl pyrophosphate stimulates gamma-secretase to increase the generation of Abeta and APP-CTFgamma. FASEB J. 22: 47-54 (2008).

[69] Kirsch C, Eckert GP and Mueller WE. Statin effects on cholesterol micro-domains in brain plasma membranes. Biochem Pharmacol 65: 843-856 (2003).

[70] Lütjohann D, Stroick M, Bertsch T, Kühl S, Lindenthal B, Thelen K, Andersson U, Björkhem I, Bergmann Kv K and Fassbender K. High doses of simvastatin, pravastatin and cholesterol reduce brain cholesterol synthesis in guinea pigs. Steroids 69: 431-438 (2004).

[71] MRC/BHF Heart Protection Study of cholesterol lowering with simvastatin in 20, 536 high-risk individuals: a randomized placebo-controlled trial. Lancet 360: 7-22 (2002).

[72] Sparks DL, Kryscio RJ, Sabbagh MN, Connor DJ, Sparks LM and Liebsack C. Reduced risk of incident AD with elective statin use in a clinical trial cohort. Curr Alzheimer Res. 5: 416-421 (2008).

[73] Vaughan CJ and Gotto Jr AM. Update on statins: 2003. Circulation 110: 886-892 (2004).

[74] Park I-H, Hwang EM, Hong HS, Boo JH, Oh SS, Lee J, Jung MW, Bang OY, Kim SU and Mook-Jung I. Lovastatin enhances Abeta production and senile plaque deposition in female Tg2576 mice. Neurobiol Aging 24: 637-643 (2003).

[75] Vance JE, Hayashi H and Karten B. Cholesterol homeostasis and glial cells. Sem Cell Develop Biol 16: 193-212 (2005).

[76] Lazar AN, Bich C, Panchal M, Desbenoit N, Petit VW, Touboul D, Dauphinot L, Marquer C, Laprévote O, Brunelle A and Duyckaerts C. Time-of-flight secondary ion mass spectrometry (TOF-SIMS) imaging reveals cholesterol overload in the cerebral cortex of Alzheimer disease patients. Acta Neuropathol 125: 133-144 (2013).

[77] Sparks DL, Sabbagh NM, Connor DJ, Lopez J, Launer LJ, Browne P, Wasser D, Johnson-Traver S, Lochhead J and Ziolwolski C. Atorvastatin for the treatment of mild to moderate Alzheimer's disease: preliminary results. Arch Neurol 62: 753-757 (2005).

[78] Sparks DL, Lemieux SK, Haut MW, Baxter LC, Johnson SC, Sparks LM, Sampath H, Lopez JE, Sabbagh MH and Connor DJ. Hippocampal volume change in the Alzheimer disease cholesterol-lowering treatment trial. Cleve Clin J Med 75 Suppl 2: S87-93 (2008).

[79] Jones RW, Kivipelto M, Feldman H, Sparks L, Doody R, Waters DD, Hey-Hadavi J, Breazna A, Schindler RJ and Ramos H. LEADe investigators. The Atorvastatin/Donepezil in Alzheimer's Disease Study (LEADe): design and baseline characteristics. Alzheimers Dement. 4: 145-153 (2008).

[80] Burgos JS, Benavides J, Douillet P, Velasco J and Valdivieso F. How statins could be evaluated successfully in clinical trials for Alzheimer's disease? Am J Alzheimers Dis Other Demen. 27: 151-3 (2012).

[81] Peng S, Glennert J and Westermark P. Medin-amyloid: a recently characterized age-associated arterial amyloid form affects mainly arteries in the upper part of the body. Amyloid 12: 96-102 (2005).

[82] Huff ME, Balch WE and Kelly JW. Pathological and functional amyloid formation orchestrated by the secretory pathway. Curr Opin Struct Biol 13: 674-682 (2003).

[83] Kakio A, Yano Y, Takai D, Kuroda Y, Matsumoto O, Kozutsumi Y and Matsuzaki K. Interaction between amyloid beta-protein aggregates and membranes. J Pept Sci 10: 612-621 (2004).

[84] Meyer-Luhemann M, Coomaraswamy J, Bolmont T, Kaeser S, Schaefer C, Kilger E, Neuenscwander A, Abramowski D, Frey P, Jaton A, Vigouret J-M, Paganetti P, Walsh DM, Metthews PM, Ghiso J, Staufenbiel M, Walzer LC and Jucker M. Exogenous induction of cerebral β-amyloidogenesis is governed by agent and host. Science 313: 1781-1784 (2006).

[85] Yip CM, Elton EA, Darabie AA, Morrison MR and McLaurin J. Cholesterol, a modulator of membrane-associated Aβ-fibrillogenesis and neurotoxicity. J Mol Biol 311: 723-734 (2001).

[86] Kazlauskaite J, Senghera N, Sylvester I, Vénien-Bryan C and Pinheiro TJT. Structural changes of the prion protein in lipid membranes leading to aggregation and fibrillization. Biochemistry 42: 3295-3304 (2003).

[87] Bokvist M, Lindström F, Watts A and Gröbner G. Two types of Alzheimer's β-amyloid (1-40) peptide membrane interactions: aggregation preventing transmembrane anchoring *vs.* accelerated surface fibril formation. J Mol Biol 335: 1039-1049 (2004).

[88] Engel MFM, Yiggitop HA, Eigersma RC, Rijkers DTS, Liskamp RMJ, de Kruijff B, Höppener JWM and Killian A. Islet amyloid polypeptide inserts into phospholipid monolayers as monomer. J Mol Biol 356: 783-789 (2006).

[89] Lührs T, Zahn R and Wüthrich K. Amyloid formation by recombinant full-length prion proteins in phospholipid bicelle solutions. J Mol Biol 357: 833-841 (2006).

[90] Zhu M, Souillac PO, Ionesco-Zanetti C, Carter SA and Fink AL. Surface-catalyzed amyloid fibril formation. J Biol Chem 277: 50914-50922 (2002).

[91] Sethuraman A and Belfort G. Protein structural perturbation and aggregation on homogeneous surfaces. Biophys J 88: 1322-1333 (2005).

[92] Koppaka V and Axelsen PH Accelerated accumulation of amyloid beta proteins on oxidatively damaged lipid membranes. Biochemistry 39: 10011-10016 (2000).

[93] Porat Y, Kolusheva S, Jelinek R and Gazit E. The human islet amyloid polypeptide forms transient membrane-active prefibrillar assemblies. Biochemistry 42: 10971-10977 (2003).

[94] Mattson MP. Impairment of membrane transport and signal transduction systems by amyloidogenic proteins. Methods Enzymol 309: 733-768 (1999).

[95] Kourie JI and Henry CL. Ion channel formation and membrane-linked pathologies of misfolded hydrophobic proteins: the role of dangerous unchaperoned molecules. Clin Exp Pharmacol Physiol 29: 741-753 (2002).

[96] Hou X, Richardson SJ, Aguilar MI and Small DH. Binding of amyloidogenic transthyretin to the plasma membrane alters membrane fluidity and induces neurotoxicity. Biochemistry 44: 11618-11627 (2005).

[97] Um JW and Strittmatter SM. Amyloid-β induced signaling by cellular prion protein and Fyn kinase in Alzheimer disease. Prion 7: 37-41 (2013).

[98] Jayakumar R, Jayaraman M, Koteeswarl D and Gomath K. Cytotoxic and membrane perturbation effects of a novel amyloid forming model, peptide poly(leucine-glutamic acid). J Biochem (Tokyo) 136: 457-462 (2004).

[99] Zhao H, Tuominen EKJ and Kinnunen PKJ. Formation of amyloid fibers triggered by phosphatidylserine-containing membranes. Biochemistry 43: 10302-10307 (2004).

[100] Suk JY, Zhang F, Balch WE, Linhardt RJ and Kelly JW. Heparin accelerates gelsolin amyloidogenesis. Biochemistry 45: 2234-2242 (2006).

[101] Necula M, Chirita C and Kuret J. Rapid anionic micelle-mediated α-synuclein fibrillization *in vitro*. J Biol Chem 278: 46674-46680 (2002).

[102] Wells K, Farooqui AA, Liss L and Horrocks LA. Neural membrane phospholipids in Alzheimer disease. Neurochem. Res., 20: 1329-1333 (1995).

[103] Bhatia R, Lin H and Lal R. Fresh and nonfibrillar amyloid β protein(1-42) induces rapid cellular degeneration in aged human fibroblasts: evidence for AβP-channel-mediated cellular toxicity. FASEB J 14: 1233-1243 (2000).

[104] Conlon IJ, Dunn GA, Mudge AW and Raff MC. Extracellular control of cell size. Nat Cell Biol 3: 918-921 (2001).

[105] Conway KA, Lee S-J, Rochet JC, Ding TT, Williamson RE and Lansbury PT. Acceleration of oligomerization not fibrillization is a shared property of both alpha-synuclein mutations linked to early-onset Parkinson's disease. Implication for pathogenesis and therapy Proc Natl Acad Sci USA 97: 571-576 (2000).

[106] Nilsberth C, Westlind-Danielssnon A, Eckman CB, Condron MM, Axelman K, Forsell C, Stenh C, Luthman J, Teplow DB, Younkin SG, Naslund J and Lannfelt L. The "arctic" APP mutation. (E693G) causes Alzheimer's disease by enhanced Aβ protofibril formation. Nat Neurosci 4: 887-893 (2001).

[107] Sousa MM, Cardoso I, Fernandes R, Guimaraes A and Saraiva MJ. Deposition of transthyretin in early stages of familial amyloidotic polyneuropathy. Am J Pathol 159: 1993-2000 (2001).

[108] Poirier MA, Li H, Macosko J, Cail S, Amzel M and Ross CA. Huntingtin spheroids and protofibrils as precursors in polyglutamine fibrillization. J Biol Chem 277: 41032-41037 (2002).

[109] Chung J, Yang H, de Beus MD, Ryu CY, Cho K and Colòn W. Cu/Zn superoxide dismutase can form pore-like structures. Biochem Biophys Res Commun 312: 973-876 (2003).

[110] Bucciantini M, Giannoni E, Chiti F, Baroni F, Formigli L, Zurdo J, Taddei N, Ramponi G, Dobson CM and Stefani M. Inherent toxicity of aggregates implies a common mechanism for protein misfolding diseases Nature 416: 507-511 (2002).

[111] Koffie RM, Meyer-Luehmann M, Hashimoto T, Adams KW, Mielke ML, Garcia-Alloza M, Micheva KD, Smith SJ, Kim ML, Lee VM, Hyman BT and Spires-Jones TL. Oligomeric amyloid beta associates with postsynaptic densities and correlates with excitatory synapse loss near senile plaques. Proc Natl Acad Sci USA 106: 4012-4017 (2009).

[112] Xue W-F, Hellewell AL, Gosal WS, Homans SW, Hewitt EW and Radford SE. Fibril fragmentation enhances amyloid cytotoxicity. J Biol Chem 284: 34272-3482 (2009).
[113] Martins IC, Kuperstein I, Wilkinson H, Maes E, Vambrabant M, Jonckheere W, Van Gelder P, Hartmann D, D'Hooge R, De Strooper B, Schymkowitz J and Rousseau F. Lipids revert inert Abeta amyloid fibrils to neurotoxic protofibrils that affect learning in mice. EMBO J 27: 224-233 (2008).
[114] Mintun MA, Larossa GN, Sheline YI, Dence CS, Lee SY, Mach RH, Klunk WE, Mathis CA, DeKosky ST and Morris JC. [11C]PIB in a nondemented population: potential antecedent marker of Alzheimer disease. Neurology 67: 446-452 (2006).
[115] Dickson DW. Correlation of synaptic and pathological markers with cognition of the elderly. Neurobiol Aging 16: 285-298 (1995).
[116] Walsh DM and Selkoe DJ. Oligomers on the brain: the emerging role of soluble protein aggregates in neurodegeneration. Protein Peptide Lett 11: 1-16 (2004).
[117] Lambert MP, Barlow AK, Chromy BA, Edwards C, Freed R, Liosatos M, Morgan TE, Rozovsky I, Trommer B, Viola KL, Wals P, Zhang C, Finch CE, Krafft GA and Klein WL. Diffusible, nonfibrillar ligands derived from Abeta1-42 are potent central nervous system neurotoxins. Proc Natl Acad Sci U S A 95: 6448-53 (1998).
[118] Chromy BA, Nowak RJ, Lambert MP, Viola KI, Chang L, Velasco PT, Jones BW, Fernandez SJ, Lacor PN, Horowitz P, Finch CE, Krafft GA and Klein WL. Self-assembly of Aβ1-42 into globular neurotoxins. Biochemistry 42: 12749-12760 (2003).
[119] Hoshi M, Sato M, Matsumoto S, Noguchi A, Yasutake K, Yoshida N and Sato K. Spherical aggregates of β-amyloid (amylospheroid show high neurotoxicity and activate tau protein kinase I/glycogen synthase kinase-3β. Proc Natl Acad Sci USA 100: 6370-6375 (2003).
[120] Walsh DM, Tseng BP, Rydel RE, Podlisny MB and Selkoe DJ. The oligomerization of amyloid β-protein begins intracellularly in cell derived from human brain. Biochemistry 39: 10831-10839 (2000).
[121] Billings LM, Oddo S, Green KN, McGaugh JL and LaFerla F. Intraneuronal Aβ causes the onset of early Alzheimer's disease-related cognitive deficits in transgenic mice. Neuron 45: 675-688 (2005).
[122] Mucke L, Masliah E, Yu GQ, Mallory M, Rockenstein EM, Tatsuno G, Hu K, Kholodenko D, Johnson-Wood K and McConlogue L. High-level neuronal expression of abeta 1-42 in wild-type human amyloid protein precursor transgenic mice: synaptotoxicity without plaque formation. J Neurosci 20: 4050-4058 (2000).
[123] Lee SJ, Liyanage U, Bickel PE, Xia W, Lansbury PT and Kosik KS. A detergent-insoluble membrane compartment contains A beta *in vivo*. Nat Med 4: 730-734 (2003).
[124] Ehehalt R, Keller P, Haass C, Thiele C and Simons K. Amyloidogenic processing of the Alzheimer beta-amyloid precursor protein depends on lipid rafts. J Cell Biol 160: 113-123 (2003).
[125] Kakio A, Nishimoto S, Kozutsumi Y and Matsuzaki K. Formation of a membrane-active form of amyloid beta-protein in raft-like model membranes. Biochem Biophys Res Commun 303: 514-518 (2003).
[126] Kojro E, Gimpl G, Lammich S, März W and Fahrenholz F. Low cholesterol stimulates the nonamyloidogenic pathway by its effect on the α-secretase ADAM 10 Proc Natl Acad Sci USA, 98: 5815-5820 (2001).
[127] Abad-Rodriguez J, Ledesma MD, Craessaerts K, Perga S, Medina M, Delacourte A, Dingwall C, De Strooper B and Dotti CG. Neuronal membrane cholesterol loss enhances amyloid peptide generation. J Cell Biol 167: 953-960 (2004).

[128] Crameri A, Biondi E, Kuehnle K, Lütjohann D, Thelen KM, Perga S, Dotti CG, Nitsch RM, Ledesma MD and Mohajeri MH. The role of seladin-1/DHCR24 in cholesterol biosynthesis, APP processing and Abeta generation *in vivo*. EMBO J 25: 432-443 (2006).
[129] Prusiner SB, Scott MR, deArmond SJ and Cohen FE. Prion Protein Biology. Cell 93: 337-348 (1998).
[130] Harris DA. Cellular biology of prion diseases. Clin Microbiol Rev 12: 429-444 (1999).
[131] Naslavsky N, Shmeeda H, Friedlander G, Yanai A, Futerman AH, Barenholz Y and Taraboulosi A. Sphingolipid depletion increases formation of the scrapie prion protein in neuroblastoma cells infected with prions. J Biol Chem 274: 20763-20771 (1999).
[132] Laurén J, Gimbel DA, Nygaard HB, Gilbert JW and Strittmatter SM. Cellular prion protein mediates impairment of synaptic plasticity by amyloid-beta oligomers. Nature. 457: 1128-1132 (2009)
a) Sarnataro D, Campana V, Paladino S, Stornaiuolo M, Nitsch L and Zurzolo C. PrP^c association with lipid rafts in the early secretory pathway stabilizes its cellular conformation Mol Biol Cell 15: 4031-4042 (2004).
[133] Gandhi S, Refolo LM and Sambamurti K. Amyloid precursor protein compartmentalization restricts beta-amyloid production: therapeutic targets based on BACE compartmentalization. J Mol Neurosci. 24: 137-43 (2004).
[134] Burns MP, Igbavboa U, Wang L, Wood WG and Duff K. Cholesterol distribution, not total levels, correlate with altered amyloid precursor protein processing in statin-treated mice. Neuromol Med 8: 319-328 (2006).
[135] Reid PC, Urano Y, Kodama T and Hamakubo T. Alzheimer's disease: cholesterol, membrane rafts, isoprenoids and statins. J Cell Mol Med 11: 383-392 (2007).
[136] Arispe N and Doh M. Plasma membrane cholesterol controls the cytotoxicity of Alzheimer's disease Aβ(1-40) and (1-42) peptides. FASEB J 16: 1526-1536 (2002).
[137] Molander-Melin M, Blennow K, Bogdanovic N, Dellheden B, Månsson JE and Fredman P. Structural membrane alterations in Alzheimer brains found to be associated with regional disease development; increased density of gangliosides GM1 and GM2 and loss of cholesterol in detergent-resistant membrane domains. J Neurochem 92: 171-182 (2005).
[138] Famer D, Meaney S, Mousavi M, Nordberg A, Björkhem I and Crisby M. Regulation of alpha- and beta-secretase activity by oxysterols: cerebrosterol stimulates processing of APP *via* the alpha-secretase pathway. Biochem Biophys Res Commun 359: 46-50 (2007).
[139] Brown J III, Theisler C, Silberman S, Magnuson D, Gottardi-Littell N, Lee JM, Yager D, Crowley J, Sambamurti K, Rahman MM, Reiss AB, Eckman CB and Wolozin B. Differential expression of cholesterol hydroxylases in Alzheimer's disease J Biol Chem 279: 34674-34681 (2004).
[140] Cecchi C, Rosati F, Pensalfini A, Formigli L, Nosi D, Liguri G, Dichiara F, Morello M, Danza G, Pieraccini G, Peri A, Serio M and Stefani M. Seladin-1/DHCR24 protects neuroblastoma cells against abeta toxicity by increasing membrane cholesterol content. J Cell Mol Med 12: 1990-2002 (2008).
[141] Luciani P, Deledda C, Rosati F, Benvenuti S, Cellai I, Dichiara F, Morello M, Vannelli GB, Danza G, Serio M and Peri A. Seladin-1 is a fundamental mediator of the neuroprotective effects of estrogen in human neuroblast long-term cell cultures. Endocrinology 149: 4256-4266 (2008).
[142] Mason RP, Shoemaker WJ, Shajenko L, Chambers TE and Herbette LG. Evidence for changes in the Alzheimer's disease brain cortical membrane structure mediated by cholesterol. Neurobiol. Aging, 13: 413-419 (1992).

[143] Sharpe LJ, Wong J, Garner B, Halliday GM and Brown AJ. Is seladin-1 really a selective Alzheimer's disease indicator? J Alzheimers Dis 30: 35-39 (2012).

[144] Ledesma MD, Abad-Rodriguez J, Galvan C, Biondi E, Navarro P, Delacourte A, Dingwall C and Dotti CG. Raft disorganization leads to reduced plasmin activity in Alzheimer's disease brains. EMBO Rep 4: 1190-1196 (2003).

[145] Devanathan S, Salamon Z, Lindblom G, Gröbner G and Tollin G. Effects of sphingomyelin, cholesterol and zinc ions on the binding, insertion and aggregation of the amyloid Aβ1-40 peptide in solid-supported lipid bilayers. FEBS J 273: 1389-1402 (2006).

[146] Puglielli L, Tanzi R and Kovacs DM. Alzheimer's disease: the cholesterol connection Nature Neurosci 6: 345-351 (2003).

[147] Grimm MO, Grimm HS, Pätzold AJ, Zinser EG, Halonen R, Duering M, Tschäpe J.-A, De Strooper B, Müller U, Shen J and Hartmann T. Regulation of cholesterol and sphingomyelin metabolism by amyloid-β and presenilin. Nat Cell Biol 7: 1118-1123 (2005).

[148] Costantini C, Kolasani RMK and Puglielli L. Ceramide and cholesterol: possible connections between normal aging of the brain and Alzheimer's disease. Just hypotheses or molecular pathways to be identified? Alz Dem 1: 43-50 (2005).

[149] Grassmé H, Riethmüller J and Gulbins E. Biological aspects of ceramide-enriched membrane domains Progress Lipid Res 46: 161-170 (2007).

[150] Holopainen JM, Subramanian M and Kinnunen PK. Sphingomyelinase induces lipid microdomain formation in a fluid phosphatidylcholine/sphingomyelin membrane. Biochemistry 37: 17562-17570 (1998).

[151] London M and London E. Ceramide selectively displaces cholesterol from ordered lipid domains (rafts): implication for lipid raft structure and function. J Biol Chem 279: 9997-10004 (2004).

[152] Puglielli L, Ellis BC, Saunder's AJ and Kovacs DM. Ceramide stabilizes beta-site amyloid precursor protein degrading enzyme 1 and promotes amyloid beta peptide biogenesis. J Biol Chem 278: 19777-19783 (2003).

[153] Scott Miners J, Baig S, Palmer J, Palmer LE, Kehoe PG and Love S. Aβ-degrading enzymes in Alzheimer's disease. Brain Pathol 18: 240-252 (2008).

[154] Nalivaeva NN, Fisk LR, Belyaev ND and Turner AJ. Amyloid-degrading enzymes as therapeutic targets in Alzheimer's disease. Curr Alzheimer Res 5: 212-224 (2008).

[155] Shibata N, Kawarai T, Meng Y, Lee JH, Lee HS, Wakutani Y, Shibata E, Pathan N, Bi A, Sato C, Sorbi S, Bruni AC, Duara R, Mayeux R, Farrer LA, George-Hyslop PS and Rogaeva E. Association studies between the plasmin genes and late-onset Alzheimer's disease. Neurobiol Aging 28:1041-1043 (2007).

[156] Tucker HM, Kihiko-Ehmann M, Wright S. Rydel RE and Estus S. Tissue plasminogen activator requires plasminogen to modulate amyloid-beta neurotoxicity and deposition J Neurochem 75: 2172-2177 (2000).

[157] Cacquevel M, Launay S, Castel H, Benchename K, Cheenne S, Buee L. Moons L, Delacourte A, Carmeliet P and Vivien D. Ageing and amyloid-beta peptide deposition contribute to an impaired brain tissue plasminogen activator activity by different mechanisms. Neurobiol Dis 27: 164-173 (2007).

[158] Kranenburg O. Bouma B. Kroon-Batenburg LMJ. Reijerkerk A. Wu Y-P. Voest EE and Gebbink MFBG. Tissue-type plasminogen activator is a multiligand cross-β structure receptor. Curr Biol 12: 1833-1839 (2002).

[159] Ji S-R, Wu Y and Sui S-f. Cholesterol Is an Important Factor Affecting the Membrane Insertion of β-Amyloid Peptide (Aβ1-40), Which May Potentially Inhibit the Fibril Formation J Biol Chem 277: 6273-6279 (2002).
[160] Choo-Smith L, Garzon-Rodriguez W, Glabe CG and Surewicz WK. Acceleration of amyloid fibril formation by specific binding of Abeta-(1-40) peptide to ganglioside-containing membrane vesicles. J Biol Chem 272: 22987-22990 (1997).
[161] McLaurin J, Yang D, Yip CM and Fraser PE. Review: modulating factors in amyloid-beta fibril formation. J Struct Biol 130: 259-270 (2000).
[162] Yu W, Zou K, Gong JS, Ko M, Yanagisawa K and Michikawa M. Oligomerization of amyloid beta-protein occurs during the isolation of lipid rafts. J Neurosci Res. 80: 114-119 (2005).
[163] Li R, Yang L, Lindholm K, Konishi Y, Yue X, Hampel H, Zhang D and Shen Y. Tumor necrosis factor death receptor signalling cascade is required for amyloid-beta protein-induced neuron death. J Neurosci 24: 1760-1771 (2004).
[164] Sotthibundhu A, Sykes AM, Fox B, Underwood CK, Thangnipon W and Coulson EJ. Beta-amyloid(1-42) induces neuronal death through the p75 neurotrophin receptor. J Neurosci 28: 3941-3946 (2008).
[165] Giovannini MG, Scali C, Prosperi C, Bellucci A, Vannucchi MG, Rosi S, Pepeu G and Casamenti F. β-Amyloid-induced inflammation and cholinergic hypofunction in the rat brain *in vivo*: involvement of the p38MAPK pathway. Neurobiol Dis 11: 257-274 (2002).
[166] Combs CK, Johnson DE, Cannady SB, Lehman TM and Landreth GE. Identification of microglia signal transduction pathways mediating a neurotoxic response to amyloidogenic fragments of β-amyloid and prion protein. J Neurosci 19: 928-939 (1999).
[167] Bozyczko-Coyne D, Saporito MS and Hudkins RL. Targeting the JNK pathway for therapeutic benefit in CNS disease. Curr Drug Targets CNS Neurol Disord 1: 31-49 (2002).
[168] King ME, Kan HM, Baas PW, Elisir A, Glabe CG and Bloom GS. Tau-dependent microtubule disassembly initiated by prefibrillar beta-amyloid J Cell Biol 175: 541-546 (2006)
[169] Guo JP. Arai T, Miklossy J and McGeer PL. Abeta and tau form soluble complexes that may promote self aggregation og both into the insoluble forms observed in Alzheimer's disease. Proc Natl Acad Sci USA 103: 1953-1958 (2006).
[170] Shaked GM, Kummer MP, Lu DC, Galvan V, Bredesen DE and Koo EH. Aβ induces cell death by direct interaction with its cognate extracellular domain on APP (APP 597-624). FASEB J 20: 1254-1256 (2006).
[171] Um JW, Nygaard HB, Heiss JK, Kostylev MA, Stagi M, Vortmeyer A, Wisniewski T, Gunther EC and Strittmatter SM. Alzheimer amyloid-β oligomer bound to postsynaptic prion protein activates Fyn to impair neurons. Nature Neurosci 15: 1227-1235 (2012).
[172] Arispe N, Rojas E and Pollard HD. Alzheimer's disease amyloid beta protein forms calcium channels in bilayer membranes: blockade by tromethamine and aluminium. Proc Natl Acad Sci USA 89: 10940-10944 (1993).
[173] Mirzabekov TA, Lin MC and Kagan BL. Pore formation by the cytotoxic islet amyloid peptide amylin. J Biol Chem 271: 1988-1992 (1996).
[174] Lin MC, Mirzabekov T and Kagan BL. Channel formation by a neurotoxic prion protein fragment. J Biol Chem 272: 44-47 (1997).
[175] Kourie JI. Synthetic C-type mammalian natriuretic peptide forms large cation selective channels. FEBS Lett 445: 57-62 (1999).

[176] Hirakura Y and Kagan BL. Pore formation by beta-2-microglobulin: a mechanism for the pathogenesis of dialysis-associated amyloidosis. Amyloid 8: 94-100 (2001).

[177] Volles MJ and Lansbury PT. Vesicle permeabilization by protofibrillar α-synuclein: comparison of wild-type with Parkinson's disease linked mutants and insights in the mechanisms. Biochemistry 40: 7812-7819 (2001).

[178] Ding TT, Lee S-J, Rochet J-C and Lansbury PT. Annular α-synuclein protofibrils are produced when spherical protofibrils are incubated in solution or bound to brain-derived membranes. Biochemistry 41: 10209-10217 (2002).

[179] Hirakura Y, Carreras I, Sipe JD and Kagan BL. Channel formation by serum amyloid A: a potential mechanism for amyloid pathogenesis and host defense. Amyloid 9: 13-23 (2002).

[180] Kourie JI and Shorthouse AA. Properties of cytotoxic peptide-induced ion channels. Am J Physiol Cell Physiol 278: C1063-C1087 (2000).

[181] De Felice FG. Velasco PT. Lambert MP. Viola K. Fernandez SJ. Ferriera ST and Klein WL. Aβ oligomers induce neuronal oxidative stress through an N-methyl-D-aspartate receptor-dependent mechanism that is blocked by the Alzheimer drug memantine. J Biol Chem 282: 11590-11601 (2007).

[182] Okada T, Ikeda K, Wakabayashi M, Ogawa M and Matsuzaki K. Formation of toxic Abeta(1–40) fibrils on GM1 ganglioside-containing membranes mimicking lipid rafts: polymorphisms in Abeta(1–40) fibrils, J. Mol. Biol. 382: 1066–1074 (2008).
a) Resende R. Pereira C. Agostinho P. Vieira AP. Malva JO and Oliveira CR. Susceptibility of hippocampal neurons to Aβ peptide toxicity is associated with perturbations of Ca^{2+} homeostasis. Brain Res1143: 11-21 (2007).

[183] Evangelisti E, Cecchi C, Cascella R, Sgromo C, Liguri G, Dobson CM, Chiti F and Stefani M. Membrane lipid composition and its physicochemical properties define cell vulnerability to aberrant protein oligomers. J Cell Sci 125: 2416-2427 (2012).

[184] Campioni S, Mannini B, Pensalfini A, Zampagni M, Parrini C, Evangelisti E, Relini A, Stefani M, Dobson CM, Cecchi C and Chiti F. Aberrant protein oligomer structures are causatively linked to cellular dysfunction. Nat Chem Biol 6: 140-147 (2010).

[185] Yan SD, Stern D, Kane MD, Kuo YM, Lampert HC and Roher AE. RAGE-Abeta interactions in the pathophysiology of Alzheimer's disease. Resto Neurol Neurosci 12: 167-173 (1998).

[186] Lacor PN, Buniel MC, Chang L, Fernandez SJ, Gong Y, Viola KL, Lambert M, Velasco PT, Bigio EH, Finch CE, Krafft G and Klein WL. Synaptic targeting by Alzheimer's-related amyloid β oligomers. J Neurosci 24: 10191-10200 (2004).

[187] Shankar GM, Bloodgood BL, Townsend M, Walsh DM, Selkoe DJ and Sabatini BL. Natural oligomers of the Alzheimer amyloid-β protein induce reversible synapse loss by modulating an NMDA-type glutamate receptor-dependent signalling pathway. J Neurosci 271: 2866-2875 (2007).

[188] Snyder EM, Nong Y, Almeida CG, paul S, Moran T, Choi EY, Nairn AC, Salter MW, Lombroso PJ, Gouras GK and Greengard P. Regulation of NMDA receptor trafficking by amyloid β. Nature Neurosci 8: 1051-1058 (2005).

[189] Pellistri F, Bucciantini M, Relini A, Nosi D, Gliozzi A, Robello M and Stefani M. Non-specific interaction of prefibrillar amyloid aggregates with NMDA and AMPA receptors results in Ca^{2+} increase in primary neuronal cells. J Biol Chem 283: 29950-2960 (2008).

[190] van Echten-Deckert G and Walter J. Sphingolipids: critical players in Alzheimer's disease. Prog Lipid Res 51: 378-393 (2012).

CHAPTER 4

Metals in Alzheimer's Disease: A Combined Experimental and Numerical Approach

Silvia Morante* **and Giancarlo Rossi**

Dipartimento di Fisica, Università di Roma "Tor Vergata" and INFN, Sezione di Roma "Tor Vergata", Via della Ricerca Scientifica, 00133 Roma, Italy

Abstract: Alzheimer disease is a pathology causing severe problems with memory, thinking and behavior. It accounts for the majority of dementia cases and is the sixth leading cause of death in developed countries. Unfortunately a real cure is still missing and the drug treatments today available can only reduce symptoms. It belongs to a large class of diseases, called amyloidosis, in which endogenous proteins or peptides undergo a misfolding process switching from the physiological soluble configuration to a pathological fibrillar insoluble state. An important, but not yet fully elucidated, rôle appears to be played in these processes by transition metals (mainly copper and zinc) that have been observed to be present in fairly large amounts in patient's neurological plaques. In this review we will show that the challenging problem of understanding the physico-chemical basis of protein misfolding and aggregation can be successfully investigated with a combination of modern spectroscopic techniques and advanced *first principle* numerical simulations. In particular, it will be shown that different metals can rival in peptide binding thus adding support to the hypothesis that metal dyshomeostasis may be relevant in the Alzheimer disease development.

Keywords: Amyloidosis, Aβ-peptide, *ab initio* molecular dynamics, metal ions, X-ray Absorption Spectroscopy.

1. INTRODUCTION

Although the discovery of the presence of iron-containing compounds in blood can be traced back to the beginning of the 19th century, it is not more than fifty years that chemistry started a systematic study of rôle of metals in biology, that eventually led to the opening of a new branch of chemistry nowadays called "bioinorganic chemistry".

***Corresponding author Silvia Morante:** Dipartimento di Fisica, Università di Roma "*Tor Vergata*", INFN, Sezione di Roma "*Tor Vergata*", *Via* della Ricerca Scientifica, 00133 Roma, Italy; Tel: +390672594554; Fax: +39062023507; E-mail: silvia.morante@roma2.infn.it

D.K. Lahiri (Ed)

The 1950' renaissance of transition metal coordination chemistry was due to both the important new insights obtained from the application of ligand field theory [1] on the basic reaction mechanisms involving metal complexes, and to the increasing power of experimental and theoretical tools developed for the purpose of studying structural and kinetic properties of these biological systems at the molecular level.

Metals are electropositive elements characterized by ductility, malleability, brightness, and high conductance of heat and electricity. They can replace the hydrogen of an acid and form bases with hydroxyl radicals. Metals are not selective in their interaction with other molecules helping in a variety of important cellular events, such as chemical reaction catalysis, or electrons transport during energy production. On the other side, however, metal high chemical reactivity can easily become harmful, so sophisticated strategies for a careful tuning of their concentration have been evolutionarily developed in living organisms.

1.1.Metals and brain

Even in the brain metals like copper (Cu), zinc (Zn) and iron (Fe) are normally present at fairly high concentration and there are evidences that a breakdown in metal trafficking regulation (dyshomeostasis) has a significant impact in the development of age-related neurodegenerative diseases [2-4]. During neurotransmission processes high concentrations of Zn (at the level of ~300 μM) and Cu (at the level of ~30 μM) are normally released. Remarkably, release of Cu and Zn has been considered as one of the cause of the precipitation process (which starts in the synapse) leading to amyloid aggregation [5]. The concentration level of these metals was found to be, in fact, especially high in amyloid plaque deposits, reaching 0.4 mM in the case of Cu and 1 mM in the case of Zn [6].

Besides copper and zinc, many other metals (like calcium, magnesium, manganese, iron, cobalt, and molybdenum) are involved in the metabolism of the Central Nervous System (CNS), as catalysts, second messengers, gene expression regulators, *etc.*, and thus play an essential rôle in the correct functioning of the organ. Clearly metals must be supplied to the CNS in an optimally tuned way in order to prevent aberrant behaviours. The transport across the Blood Brain Barrier

(BBB) is the first step in the regulation of their level in the brain [7]. In this context it is interesting to note that high aluminium (Al) content was found in temporal cortex and hippocampus and that Al has been demonstrated to significantly alter the BBB permeability [8-10] with the consequence of accelerating amyloid aggregation [11]. Furthermore its *in vitro* co-incubation with either Zn^{2+} or Cu^{2+} ions was shown to promote precipitation, though possibly not amyloid fibrils formation [12].

In a recent structural study of metal binding to Prion Protein (PrP) [13], the misfolding and aggregation of which is the hallmark of Prion diseases, the existence of a possibly general mechanism for a Cu *vs.* Zn peptide binding competition has been demonstrated. This finding may be taken as an indirect confirmation of a (more general) correlation among failure of metal homeostasis, protein misfolding, and neurodegenerative disease development [14].

1.2. Amyloidosis and Neurodegenerative Diseases

The term *amyloidosis* indicates a family of pathologies caused by the transition of endogenous proteins and peptides from the physiological globular configuration to a (misfolded) harmful fibrillar state. It describes a heterogeneous group of diseases (more than 20) characterized by the extracellular deposition of fibrillar proteic material [15]. Regardless of the nature of the amyloid protein by which they are formed, fibrils have a common ultra-structure. They grow, unbranched, to a variable length that may reach several microns, with a diameter of 7-10 nanometers (1 nm $=10^{-9}$ meters). They are organized in a characteristic helicoidal β-structure and are able to bind to Congo Red and Thyoflavin dyes that are commonly used to detect their presence.

In many, if not in all, of the so-called neurodegenerative disorders, the phenomenon of abnormal protein aggregation is present. Among the many disorders with this aetiology in the present work we will focus our attention on the Alzheimer disease (AD). Our aim is to review some of the most recent structural studies on β-amyloid peptides (Aβ-peptides), whose aggregation is the hallmark of the AD development. The importance of any progress in understanding the biochemical basis of this devastating disease affecting an increasingly large portion of the aged population [16], can hardly be underestimated, given the enormous medical and economical impact that AD has in the society.

1.2.1. Aβ-Peptides and Alzheimer's Disease

The typical AD amyloid plaques are formed by aggregates of Aβ-peptides. These are fragments that originate from the proteolytic cleavage of a membrane protein called Amyloid Precursor Protein (APP). They have a variable length between 39-43 residues owing to the heterogeneity of the cleavage position, localized at the C-terminus. The physiological rôle of cellular APP is still unknown.

The formation of AD plaques is a complex process: the proteolytic cleavage, performed by β- and γ-secretases, generates an intracellular pool of Aβ-peptides that may diffuse in the extracellular space. Soluble Aβ fragments assemble into small nascent β-amyloid fibrils with neurotoxic effects. Aβ fibrils deposit in cerebral tissues, forming highly ordered structures that constitute the nuclei of the typical plaques associated to the disease. At the basis of fibril formation there is a conformational change of the peptide that leads to the creation of an extended β-sheet like structure, capable of aggregating other peptides to form long antiparallel β-sheets with intra-molecular binding.

As we said, it has been observed that plaques contain large amounts of transition metals like Cu^{+2}, Fe^{+3} and Zn^{+2} (the latter being the most abundant). Their rôle is not yet fully understood but it has been conjectured to be crucial in the development of the AD pathology. The interest of elucidating the rôle of metals strongly increased after noticing that Cu^{+2} and Zn^{+2} chelators can be used to solubilize Aβ aggregates [17]. It is clear enough that the nature of the metal binding process can have significant consequences on the protein folding/unfolding and aggregation processes.

1.3. Content and Outline of the Review

The purpose of this review work is twofold. On the one hand we wish to present a fairly complete account of the important results that X-ray Absorption Spectroscopy (XAS) has provided in the years on the atomic structure of the metal binding site in Aβ-peptides metal complexes. On the other we want to discuss how theoretical considerations, based on "*first principle*" simulations of realistic atomic models of these systems, can be of help in interpreting experimental data, thus leading to important insights into the physico-chemical properties of the metal-protein interaction.

The outline of the review is as follows. We start in sect. 2 with a general introduction on the XAS technique, that has been largely employed to investigate the geometry of the metal binding site in metal-protein complexes, and on the parallel complementary use of *ab initio* simulations developed to determine the detailed atomic structural arrangement characterizing not only the metallic site but also the peptide at large. In sect. 3 we describe in some detail the structural information that have been collected in the years, both through XAS (sect. 3.1) and through *ab initio* simulations (sect. 3.2), about the structure of the binding site of Cu and Zn, when these metals are in complex with Aβ-peptides. Conclusions and an outlook of future lines of investigations can be found in sect. 4. Few useful formulae are collected in two Appendices. The list of the abbreviations used in this review is given at the end of the main text.

2. EXPERIMENTAL AND THEORETICAL METHODS

Many experimental techniques have been employed during the last decade in an effort to try to characterize the structure of the metal binding site in proteins, among which Electron Paramagnetic Resonance (EPR) [18], Nuclear Magnetic Resonance (NMR) [19, 20], Circular Dichroism (CD) [18, 20], and XAS [21, 22] are the most prominent ones.

In particular, the availability of a new generation of synchrotron radiation sources has greatly enlarged the range of applications of XAS in the investigation of structural properties of biological systems. Reliable data for a wide range of absorbing atoms, even if very diluted (as it is frequently the case in biological samples), are now accessible. Indeed, XAS can be successfully used to study the environment of metal ions complexed with proteins and peptides in their physiological environment, owing to its chemical selectivity and sensitivity to the local atomic environment around the absorber. An accurate analysis of the extended X-ray absorption fine structure (EXAFS) region of the spectrum in terms of single plus multiple scattering (MS) events allows a clear-cut identification of the amino acid (a.a.) residues primarily bound to the metal. A well-known example of application of this technique is to metal-enzymes, where the metal either acts as a catalytic center or plays a structural rôle in maintaining the protein active conformation [23-27].

As for the theoretical interpretation of the large body of available experimental data, routine techniques used to model atomic interactions (like Monte Carlo and Molecular Dynamics simulations, Quantum chemistry calculations), though yet limited by the insufficient accuracy of present computational methods, are increasing their capability of investigating the supra-molecular level. Indeed, advances in algorithm development, software implementation and computer hardware are rapidly improving the situation in a promising way.

Understanding the peculiar electronic properties of metal complexes is a necessary step to clarify the role played by metal ions in biochemical reactions. This means that the electronic structure of the compound need to be described at the quantum level, *i.e.* in the framework of the density functional theory (DFT) [28-30] with the special adaptations necessary to cope with applications to bio-molecules. In particular, when dealing with delocalized systems like organo-metallic molecules *ab initio* molecular dynamics simulations of the Car-Parrinello (CP) type [31, 32] are especially well suited.

2.1. X-ray Absorption Spectroscopy

From the experimental point of view, this review will be focused on the XAS technique, as the latter displays a number of very interesting features when it is employed in investigating biological systems, and especially in the study of metal-proteins [27, 33-37]. Perhaps the most important of them is that XAS can be used for samples in any state of aggregation. A further advantage with respect to other spectroscopic techniques is that there are no selection rules that would extinct the signal in unlucky circumstances, with the result that a XAS signal is always non-vanishing. Finally XAS is very sensitive to the nature of the metal absorber. It allows extracting structural information about the absorber atomic environment through the study of the oscillations of the absorption coefficient originating from the interference between the outgoing electron wave, kicked-off from the metal, and the back-scattered waves emerging from the surrounding atoms (see Appendix A). This interference spectrum contains detailed information about scatterer-absorber relative positions, from which the geometrical and structural arrangement of the a.a.'s that are coordinated to the metal can be inferred with fairly good accuracy. Data analysis requires a rather sophisticated theory, where single and multiple scattering contributions [38, 39] have to be taken into account. For a pictorial description of the behaviour of the electron wave function and the corresponding measured XAS signal see Fig. **1** in [40] in the case of an isolated atomic absorber (left panel), and in the case of an absorber surrounded by other atoms acting as scattering centers (right panel).

2.1.1. Generalities

XAS uses Synchrotron Radiation as source of photons. We recall that for an absorption process the following very general law holds

$$I(E) = I_0 e^{-\mu(E)d} \;, \qquad \textbf{(1)}$$

where $E = h\nu$ is the energy of the incident photon, $I(E)$ is the intensity of the transmitted radiation, I_0 is the intensity of the incident radiation, $\mu(E)$ is the absorption coefficient characteristic of the system in consideration and d is the thickness of the sample traversed by the photons (see Appendix A for other definitions and more details).

The behaviour of the absorption coefficient, $\mu(E)$, with the photon energy is monotonically decreasing except where the photon energy corresponds to the photo-ionization energy, E_0, of an inner electron of the absorbing atom. Around this energy the absorption coefficient rapidly increases and, if the absorbing atom is isolated (for example when a mono-atomic gas is considered), it starts decreasing soon after the edge energy (see the left panel of Fig. **1** in [40]).

The ionization energy of an inner electron is usually referred to as the "edge energy", or simply the "edge". The K-edge corresponds to the ionization of one of the innermost electrons, while the L-edges correspond to the ionization of the electrons belonging to the next shell, and so on.

At a sufficiently high atomic number the edge energies of the various atoms are well separated, so that the absorbing spectrum of a complex system shows characteristic and well separated peaks. Just to give an idea, the K-edges of Fe, Cu and Zn are located at 7112, 8979 and 9659 eV, respectively. This is the reason that makes XAS such a highly selective technique and allows getting detailed local structural information around a selected atomic absorber.

In a multi-atomic system the value of the absorption coefficient does not decrease monotonically after the edge, as it does for an isolated atom, but it has an oscillating behaviour. As we recalled above (see right panel of Fig. **1** in [40]), the physical explanation for the oscillating behaviour of $\mu(E)$ has its roots in the quantum interference phenomenon. To a very good approximation the wave function of the ionized electron (*photo-electron* in the following) can be described as an outgoing spherical wave centered on the absorber. The atoms surrounding it act as diffusion centers (scatterers) for the impinging wave. In turn the back-scattered waves from the atoms around the absorber interfere with the outgoing spherical wave of the photo-electron, giving rise to the interference phenomenon observed at the absorber location, where the photo-electron wave function is mostly concentrated. The interference will result in a modulation of the modulus square of the total amplitude of the wave function of the photo-electron. As a result the probability of the photon to be absorbed shows maxima or minima, according to whether the outgoing and scattered waves are *in phase* or *out of phase*. Amplitudes and phases of undulations depend on the kind and relative position of absorber and scatterers or, in other words, on the chemical and structural (three-dimensional) arrangement of the absorber atomic environment. This is the same as saying that the interference signal contains information about the local geometrical structure around the absorber.

2.1.2. Analyzing the XAS Spectrum

The XAS spectrum is commonly separated into two energy regions

1. XANES (X-ray Absorption Near Edge Structure) region starting a few eV before the edge energy, E_0, and extending some few tenths of eV above it;

2. EXAFS (Extended X-ray Absorption Fine Structure) region following the XANES region and extending some few hundreds eV above the edge.

3. The XANES region is dominated by a variety of very complicated low energy transfer events. Although this part of the spectrum in principle contains many detailed information about the local atomic structure around the absorber, its theoretical analysis is still at a semi-qualitative level [see, however, the works of refs. [38, 41-44] and limited to cases where quite a precise knowledge about the geometrical arrangement around the absorber is available [45-47].

4. The kinetic energy, $E = h\nu - E_0$, of the photo-electron in the EXAFS region is definitely larger than in the XANES region. At these comparably higher energies, single scattering events are dominant, although MS contributions, that are richer in structural information, are still present and must be taken into account for an accurate analysis of experimental data.

Theoretical approaches [38, 48] giving a rigorous quantum mechanical description of the EXAFS signal, including both single and multiple scattering terms, have been implemented in a number of packages among which we may mention gnXAS [49], FEFF [50] and EXCURV [51, 52] (for a comprehensive review see ref. [53]).

The inclusion of MS terms in the analysis of XAS data is especially important in investigating the structure of the active site in a metal-protein. Amino acidic residues are, in fact, almost completely made of "light" atoms (*i.e.* nitrogen, oxygen and carbon) and their contributions to the total XAS signal are indistinguishable from one another, if the analysis is performed in the single scattering approximation.

Including MS contributions removes to a large extent this limitation. The magnitude of the contributions coming from the presence of a.a.'s around the metal absorber, in fact, turns out to depend not only on the kind and mean distance of the atomic scatterers, but also on the specific geometrical arrangement of the a.a. lateral chain. A well-known and biologically very important example of this situation is represented by the case of the Histidine (His). The presence of this residue bound to a metal can be fairly well identified in a XAS spectrum because the contribution it gives rise to the signal through MS events is strongly enhanced, owing to the positive interference of amplitudes (focusing effect) resulting from the quasi-collinearity of the atoms belonging to the His imidazole ring with the absorbing atom[1] [54].

2.2. *Ab initio* Simulations

A rigorous and reliable understanding of spectroscopic data can only come from a Quantum Mechanical (QM) approach. In this respect *ab initio* simulations - in particular of the CP type - can be used to extract structural information and discriminate among different models thanks to the detailed atomic knowledge that numerical methods can provide. In this review we will briefly outline the theoretical foundations of such *ab initio* methods (see also Appendix B) and discuss some applications to the case of Aβ-peptide in interaction with metals.

2.2.1. Generalities

The program of *ab initio* simulations is conceptually rather simple but epistemologically very ambitious. In a nutshell it consists in the idea of deriving and studying the physico-chemical (or more modestly the structural) properties of a system starting solely from the knowledge of the fundamental interactions among its elementary constituents (atoms). The beauty and the strength of this approach is that in principle there will be no free parameters to play with, as everything will be finally expressed in terms of fundamental physical constants. The price to pay is the enormously large number of degrees of freedom that should be taken into account in the simulation to get a realistic description of the system, especially if, as it is the case of interest here, one is dealing with biological systems. The necessarily limited computer resources available at any time puts severe bounds to the size (hence to the nature) of the systems that can be attacked and studied in this way. Despite these undeniable difficulties, the recent

[1] A remarkable example of this situation is represented by the interplay between the structure of the active site in a metal-protein and its functionality as discussed, for instance, in ref. [27].

enormous advances in computer design and algorithm development have made this kind of *first principle* approach a really viable and useful computational tool [55].

Indeed, taking inspiration from the general ideas and concepts of Statistical Mechanics, many powerful techniques ranging from deterministic Molecular Dynamics (MD) simulations to stochastic Monte Carlo (MC) and Hybrid MC methods have been set up and numerically implemented [56]. The success of this computational strategy is so big that today one can hope to push simulations into the realm of some of the most difficult, still open biophysical problems, like immunological recognition, drug design or protein folding.

A crucial issue in this field is to decide whether one can deal with classical Newtonian Mechanics and potential theory or whether instead a QM approach is necessary. The nature of the problem one wants to tackle dictates the answer to this question. Simple considerations show that, given the values of pressure and temperature which are of interest in biology, it is perfectly well appropriate to treat atoms as classical particles, provided the potential in which they move is computed at the QM level, *i.e.* by solving the Schrödinger equation for the (outermost) electrons of the atoms which make up the system under study.

The CP method [31] couples in a very elegant and computationally efficient way the classical equations that describe the motion of the atoms of the system to the Schrödinger equation for the associated electrons, with the electrons in turn determining the force field experienced by atoms. In other words, the atoms move classically in the QM potential self-consistently generated by the electrons (see Appendix B). MD simulations of this kind are inherently based on the adiabatic decoupling between atomic and electronic degrees of freedom (*i.e.* on the so-called Born-Oppenheimer approximation). This separation is justified by the observation that the characteristic frequencies of the atomic motion are much smaller (by a factor $\sim 10^3$) than the typical electronic frequencies.

2.2.2. Car-Parrinello Molecular Dynamics

Car-Parrinello molecular dynamics (CP-MD) simulations for complex systems have been largely and very successfully used in many research areas ranging from solid-state physics to biological systems. Among the numerous papers in these areas see, for instance, those quoted in refs. [57] and [58], respectively. In applications to the study of metal-protein complexes CP-MD was employed and validated in a detailed structural investigation of the Cu binding sites located in the unfolded PrP octarepeat region [59, 60].

The use of QM methods (as opposed to purely classical MD approaches) for computing the force field felt by atoms is dramatically needed in the study of metal-protein complexes for two reasons. One is of a technical nature and has to do with the presence of a (doubly charged) metal ion in the system, which makes much safer the use of *first principle* simulations, for they embody charge polarization and screening, rather than that of classical MD which would require employing one of the rather sophisticated, but still not fully satisfactory, algorithmic tricks that have been developed to deal with the situation where the long range Coulomb interactions are present [61]. The second reason is more fundamental and it is related to the fact that it is the main purpose of all structural studies to identify the nature of metal ligands. This is of course something that is not known *a priori* and should be the main outcome of the investigation rather than an input as would be the case if one decides to employ classical atomic force fields.

An obvious limitation to the use of QM numerical simulations is the foreseeable very short length of the CP-MD trajectories (few picoseconds - 1 ps $=10^{-12}$ secs) for systems of the size one is interested in in biology, that certainly can never be as extended as one would like it to be. A possible way to cope, at least partially, with the difficulties related to the conflict between the need to deal with a realistically large system and the consequent limitation concerning the length of the simulated trajectory could be to exploit the possibilities offered by the recently developed mixed classical/quantum mechanical methods, like Quantum Mechanics/Molecular Mechanics (QM/MM) [62].

In any case there are good reasons (supported by quite a long experience in the field of CP-MD simulations) that make one to believe that already a few ps trajectory can give useful information on structural problems like those we are interested in this review (*i.e.* identification of primary metal ligands). The argument is based on the observation that CP-MD simulations can be thought of as a way of successively computing the electronic density while atoms move around. From this perspective CP-MD may be considered not so terribly different from genuine DFT or quantum chemistry computations [28-30], provided one could live with the two well-known problems of the CP-MD method. Namely, the fact that excited electronic states are essentially inaccessible and that atoms will only be able to explore a region of the phase space not too distant from their initial configuration.

It is interesting to note that the application of CP-MD methods to the study of metal-proteins is not set back by any of these two limitations. In fact, what one wants to identify and compare are the coordination modes of different ions (mostly copper and zinc) when complexed with various kinds of amyloid peptides. Indeed, we are only concerned here in understanding what could be the specific rôle of metals just in the very first steps of a possible aggregation process, where statistical equilibrium is not yet an issue. This more modest approach is still of great relevance because it looks that only the compounds that are formed in the very early stage of the aggregation process are pathological. The subsequent steps of mesoscopic fibril formation may on the contrary have a protective effect against neurodegenerative processes [63-65]. In any case fibril formation is driven by an extremely complicated dynamics that at the moment is beyond any possible atomistic description.

A parallel version of the freely-available Quantum-ESPRESSO package (opEn-Source Package for Research in Electronic Structure, Simulation, and Optimization [32, 66]) was used for most of the *ab initio* CP-MD simulations discussed in this review.

To minimize finite volume effects periodic boundary conditions are routinely imposed to the system. The simulated peptide is inserted in a super-cell (filled with water molecules at 1 gr/cm^3 density) with sufficiently large linear dimensions to ensure replicas to have negligible spurious self-interactions. For neutral systems a separation of 4.5-5 Å is considered to be sufficient. For charged systems a separation of at least 8 Å is required.

CP-MD calculations are often performed ignoring the electron spin degree of freedom, *i.e.* in the so-called spin-restricted conditions. This approximation is adequate for the kind of systems we are interested in here.

Before moving to the presentation of the results that have been obtained, it is convenient to provide a few more general information about the CP-MD simulation strategy.

A key issue in CP-MD is the structure of the atomic configuration that is used to start the simulation. Given the effectively rather short time duration of any CP trajectory, it is, in fact, mandatory to start from a very accurately equilibrated and thermalized configuration to avoid biases and instabilities. Usually good initial configurations are those coming from crystallographic or NMR data. If no such structural data are available, one must very carefully prepare the system performing preliminary adequately long (of the order of a few nanoseconds (1 ns = 10^{-9} secs)) classical MD simulations. For this purpose any of the currently available MD codes (like GROMACS [67], Amber [68], *etc.*) can be equally well employed.

At this point the CP-MD procedure can be started. According to a well-established experience, which was thoroughly tested in the works of refs. [59, 60], one has to begin by minimizing again stresses and strains among atoms while electrons are pushed to vanishing "temperature". In summary the CP-MD simulations must be carried out according to the general protocol outlined below.

1. Minimization of electronic energy with fixed atomic positions.
2. Minimization of total energy as a function of both atomic and electronic degrees of freedom of the system.
3. A few short preliminary sequential CP-MD simulations at increasing (say, in step of 50 K or 100K) atomic temperatures up to 300 K, using a Nosé-Hoover thermostat [69] coupled to the atomic degrees of freedom, and kept at the desired temperature.
4. Final CP-MD simulations of appropriate length at an atomic temperature of 300 K with the use of the same thermostat as in 3.

Thermalization in step 3. is necessary to slowly attain room temperature, thus avoiding that temperature oscillations affect in an uncontrolled way the approach of electrons to their ground state. The velocity Verl*et al*gorithm [70] for integrating the CP equations of motion is most commonly used.

The key question at this point is how long the simulated CP-MD trajectories can be. The answer depends obviously on the size of the system (*i.e.* volume, number of atoms, N_A, and number of electrons, N_e) and the CPU power of the available machines. A careful analysis of the dynamics underlying CP-MD [71, 72] reveals that an acceptable time step for the atomic dynamics and the iterative solution of Kohn and Sham (KS) [29] equations for the electrons (see Appendix B) turns out to be extremely small, namely of the order of 0.10-0.15 femptoseconds (1 fs = 10^{-15} secs). Thus one immediately comes to the conclusion that, at the moment, it is very hard to get trajectories longer than ~ 10 ps for the kind of systems we are discussing in this review, where a few 10^2 atoms and up to 10^3 electrons are involved.

3. Aβ-Peptides

In this section we present and discuss the results of the extensive study[2] carried out on a set of selected fragments of the Aβ-peptide complexed with either Cu^{2+} or Zn^{2+} [74].

3.1. XAS Experiments

The particular fragments that have been considered in [74] are listed in Table **1**. They have been selected for a number of different reasons. $A\beta_{1\text{-}16}$ is the minimal fragment which contains the three His's (His_6, His_{13} and His_{14}) that have been identified as metal ligands [18, 20], while $A\beta_{17\text{-}40}$ is the complementary sequence where none of these His's is present. In the $A\beta_{1\text{-}28}$ fragment a long hydrophobic region, believed to be relevant in the aggregation processes, is also contained. Finally the $A\beta_{5\text{-}23}$ fragment was measured with the main purpose of trying to answer the question on whether or not the N-terminal region of the Aβ-peptide in involved in the metal binding process.

Besides confirming the general results of [22] concerning the existence of important structural differences between Cu^{2+} and Zn^{2+} coordination modes, XAS

---

[2] All the XAS data presented in this section have been collected at the D2 bending magnet beam line of the EMBL Outstation Hamburg at DESY [73]. The X-ray spectra of the samples were recorded in fluorescence mode.

experiments have been able to elucidate the special rôle played by the N-terminal region in binding the metal. In particular, it was found that only two His residues remain coordinated to Cu^{2+} when the first four a.a. residues are cut out (as is the case in the Cu-$A\beta_{5-23}$ sample). The natural explanation for this peculiar feature is that, among the three His residues (His_6, His_{13} and His_{14}) generally relevant in metal coordination, it is His_6 that is no more available for Cu binding, because binding with the latter is now hindered by the proximity of the dissociated N-terminus.

The situation with Zn-Aβ complexes is somewhat different. It is, in fact, observed that cutting out the first four a.a. residues of the peptide does not modify the number of coordinated His's, as was the case of Cu complexes. The spectrum in the EXAFS region remains unaltered and XAS results are in all cases compatible with four coordinated His's, indicating that each metal ion is shared by two Aβ-peptides. The absence of the first four a.a. residues only affects the local geometry around the Zn absorber, as it is demonstrated by the, instead, markedly different structure of the XANES region of the spectrum of the Zn-$A\beta_{5-23}$ sample with respect to that of all the others.

Table 1: The amino acidic sequence of the five Aβ oligopeptides under consideration.

Oligopeptide	a.a. Sequence
$A\beta_{1-16}$	H_3N^+-DAEFRHDSGYEVHHQK-COO^-
$A\beta_{1-28}$	H_3N^+-DAEFRHDSGYEVHHQKLVFFAEDVGSNK-COO^-
$A\beta_{5-23}$	H_3N^+-RHDSGYEVHHQKLVFFAED-$COOH_3N^+$
$A\beta_{17-40}$	H_3N^+-LVFFAEDVGSNKGAIIGLMVGGVV-COO^-
$A\beta_{1-40}$	H_3N^+-DAEFRHDSGYEVHHQKLVFFAEDVGSNKGAIIGLMVGGVV-COO^-

3.1.1. Data Analysis

As we mentioned at the beginning of sect. 2.1.2, XAS spectra are normally analyzed by separating out the XANES region of the spectrum, from the EXAFS region that extends from about a few tens of eV's beyond the edge onward. In fact, the difficulty of getting a reliable theoretical description of the very complicated electronic processes affecting the low-energy part of the spectrum makes its quantitative interpretation very problematic [38, 41-44]. At the same time, however, the structure of this small slice of the spectrum is very sensitive to the electronic structure of the absorber and the symmetry of the local environment around it, and can yield valuable information on similarities and differences when relative local geometries of structurally similar samples are compared [33]. At variance with this situation, valuable quantitative structural information can be more easily extracted from the EXAFS region, even starting with limited a priori knowledge on the atomic structural environment around the absorbing metal. For these reasons in this review we will limit the discussion to the EXAFS region of the measured spectra.

From a general comparison of the EXAFS portions of the spectra of the 10 samples (*i.e.* five Aβ fragments complexed with either Cu or Zn) that have been subjected to XAS measurements reported in ref. [74], an interesting pattern of strong similarities and differences emerge that are summarized below where the equality sign means identity (within errors) of spectral features (see Figs. (**2**) and (**3**) in [40]).

- (Dis-)similarities among EXAFS spectra of Cu complexes

$$\text{Cu-A}\beta_{1\text{-}16} = \text{Cu-A}\beta_{1\text{-}28} = \text{Cu-A}\beta_{1\text{-}40} \neq \text{Cu-A}\beta_{5\text{-}23} \neq \text{Cu-A}\beta_{17\text{-}40}$$

- (Dis-)similarities among EXAFS spectra of Zn complexes

$$\text{Zn-A}\beta_{1\text{-}16} = \text{Zn-A}\beta_{1\text{-}28} = \text{Zn-A}\beta_{1\text{-}40} = \text{Zn-A}\beta_{5\text{-}23} \neq \text{Zn-A}\beta_{17\text{-}40}$$

On the basis of the previous comparison, discussion and fitting of the data have been limited to the following samples

1. Cu-Aβ_{1-16}, as a prototype of Cu-Aβ_{1-16}, Cu-Aβ_{1-28} and Cu-Aβ_{1-40} samples.

2. Cu-Aβ_{5-23}, as its EXAFS spectrum is different from that of Cu samples above.

3. Zn-Aβ_{1-16}, as a prototype of Zn-Aβ_{1-16}, Zn-Aβ_{1-28}, Zn-Aβ_{1-40} and Zn-Aβ_{5-23} samples.

No fitting of the Cu-A$\beta_{17\text{-}40}$ and Zn-A$\beta_{17\text{-}40}$ data was carried out because the EXAFS spectra of these samples are identical to those of Cu and Zn in their respective buffers ($CuSO_4$ and $ZnCl_2$). This spectral equality is simply interpreted as a signal of the fact that the A$\beta_{17\text{-}40}$ fragments are not able to bind the metal[3].

3.1.2. EXAFS Results

EXAFS data have been analyzed and fitted employing the EXCURV98 package [52]. The procedure implemented in the code is essentially fully automated except for the crucial question of how to choose the initial configuration that should be used to start the fitting algorithm. Concerning this point, as recommended in the literature [19, 20, 22, 75, 76], the strategy that was followed in ref. [74] was to try out various initial geometrical models, differing in the number of His's involved in the metal coordination, with structures taken among the many collected in the Metalloprotein Database and Browser (MDB) [77].

Best fit parameters are listed in Table **2**[4]. It should be remarked that the distance, r, reported there, refers to the position of either the coordinated atom or the "leading" atom of the corresponding a.a. residue. By "leading" atom of His (or Tyrosin, Tyr) we mean the N-imidazole (or the O-hydroxyl) atom through which the residue is bound to the absorber. It is important to note here that, even if in general it is not possible to distinguish among light scatterers (like N, O and C) only on the basis of their individual contribution to the EXAFS signal, when acting as leading atoms, they can be generally identified in a unambiguous way because they are tightly anchored to a large and well ordered bunch of other atoms.

Oxygen atoms, that are simply indicated by O in Table **2**, belong to a water molecule or to a.a.'s other than His or Tyr. As for the quality of the fits, we see that in all cases experimental data are rather well reproduced with values of the r, N and σ_{DW} parameters that are fairly accurate and physically very reasonable. This consistency pattern is confirmed by the nice correspondence between the location and the height of the peaks of the FT of experimental and theoretical signals.

---

[3] It should be remarked that the harmless α- and γ-secretases cleavage of APP precisely cuts out the first 16 a.a.'s of Aβ-peptide.

[4] Experimental and theoretical spectra are shown in Figs. (**4**), (**5**) and (**6**) of Ref. [40].There the left panel of show the fitted (black line) and experimental (grey line) spectrum of the Cu-A$\beta_{1\text{-}16}$, Cu-A$\beta_{5\text{-}23}$, and Zn-A$\beta_{1\text{-}16}$ samples. The modulus of the Fourier Transform (FT) of both the experimental and theoretical spectrum is reported in the right panel.

Table 2: Best fit parameters characterizing the atomic arrangement around the absorber in the Cu-$A\beta_{1\text{-}16}$, Cu-$A\beta_{5\text{-}23}$ and Zn-$A\beta_{1\text{-}16}$ samples. First and second columns show type and number, *N*, of coordinated chemical groups (atom or residue). Third and fourth column show distance, *r*, from the absorber of the coordinated atom or the leading atom of the coordinated residue and corresponding value of Debye-Waller (DW) factors, σ^2. Errors are only statistical. In the last row we report for each sample the Fermi energy shift, ΔE_F, and the fit quality factor, *R*.

Coord. Residue/Atom	N	$r \pm \Delta r$ Å	$\sigma^2 \pm \Delta\sigma^2$ Å^2
Cu-$A\beta_{1\text{-}16}$			
His	3	1.95 ± 0.01	0.002 ± 0.001
Tyr	1	2.06 ± 0.01	0.002 ± 0.001
O	1	1.95 ± 0.01	0.002 ± 0.001
ΔE_F = -10.2 ± 0.7 eV R = 28%			
Cu-$A\beta_{5\text{-}23}$			
His	2	1.99 ± 0.01	0.003 ± 0.001
Tyr	1	1.99 ± 0.01	0.003 ± 0.001
N (terminus)	1	1.99 ± 0.01	0.003 ± 0.001
O	1	2.27 ± 0.01	0.003 ± 0.001
ΔE_F = -13.8 ± 0.4 eV R = 40%			
Zn-$A\beta_{1\text{-}16}$			
His	2	1.96 ± 0.01	0.003 ± 0.001
His	2	2.00 ± 0.01	0.003 ± 0.001
O	1	2.00 ± 0.01	0.003 ± 0.001
ΔE_F = -6.5 ± 0.2 eV R = 23%			

Cu complexes - The best fit for the Cu-$A\beta_{1\text{-}16}$ sample corresponds to a site configuration in which three His's and one Tyr are included in the Cu coordination sphere, plus an oxygen possibly belonging to a water molecule or to an a.a. other than His or Tyr. This structure is the one already proposed in [22] for the Cu-$A\beta_{1\text{-}40}$ peptide. However, it should be pointed out that in the case of the Cu-$A\beta_{1\text{-}16}$ complex the model, in which the Tyr oxygen is replaced by the nitrogen of the N-terminus, gives rise to a fit only marginally worse than the one whose structural parameters are reported in Table **2**. Consequently one cannot completely rule out the possibility of a Cu coordination with the N-terminal nitrogen replacing the Tyr residue.

The situation one encounters here is an important example of a case where *ab initio* simulations can be of help in answering the question whether it is the Tyr oxygen or the N-terminal nitrogen which is coordinated to Cu. We will take back this point in sect. 3.2.

Moving now to the Cu-$A\beta_{5\text{-}23}$ sample, one realizes that a satisfactory fit cannot be obtained if the coordinated residues are the same as for Cu-$A\beta_{1\text{-}16}$ and only their geometrical parameters are left free to move. A good fit is instead found starting from a configuration, inspired by the work of ref. [78], in which His_6 is replaced by the N-terminal amino group. In this model Cu^{2+} is coordinated to two His's, one Tyr, the nitrogen belonging to the N-terminal amino group, and one oxygen. The fact that, by cutting out the first four a.a.'s, the number of coordinated His's is reduced from three to two, is a strong indication that His_6 is the third residue normally bound to the metal. The loss of the His_6-metal bond is to be ascribed to the strains induced by steric hindrance effects when a.a.'s from 1 to 4 are missing.

Zn complexes - Just like in the case of Cu complexes, the Zn-$A\beta_{17\text{-}40}$ spectrum is almost identical to that of Zn in buffer. This identity confirms that the absence of the first 16 a.a.'s prevents metal binding. However, at variance with Cu complexes, here it turns out that also the EXAFS spectrum of Zn-$A\beta_{5\text{-}23}$ is very similar to the spectrum of the three other Zn-samples (*i.e.* Zn-$A\beta_{1\text{-}16}$, Zn-$A\beta_{1\text{-}28}$ and Zn-$A\beta_{1\text{-}40}$) comprising the first four a.a.'s of the Aβ-peptide sequence. Then, as a prototype of the above four (almost) identical Zn complex spectra, only Zn-$A\beta_{1\text{-}16}$ EXAFS data were considered and subjected to a quantitative analysis. The best fit to the data is obtained by including in the Zn coordination sphere four His's and one oxygen. This structure is of particular relevance and it is perhaps one of the most interesting results obtained in these experiments. Recalling, in fact, that each Aβ-peptide at most contains three His's, this finding means that in order for the metal to be coordinated to four His's, at least two different peptides must be involved in the Zn binding mode.

This conclusion should be considered an extremely important result which points in the direction of a propensity of Zn (at variance with Cu) to form a sort of a network of Aβ-peptides with the metal stabilizing the whole structure by binding His's belonging to adjacent peptides (see also [79]). In the next section we will see that these conclusions are nicely confirmed by *ab initio* simulation results.

3.2. CP-MD

In this part of the review we want to discuss how *ab initio* simulations (in particular CP-MD simulations) can be used to interpret experimental results and possibly discriminate among different models owing to the detailed atomic information that numerical methods can provide[5].

In the following sections we want to show how to set up an effective strategy to investigate, in the important instance of Aβ-peptides, the rôle played by metallic ions (specifically Cu and Zn) in giving the protein its functionality or, on the contrary, in transforming it into a pathogenic conformer. For this study the knowledge of the structure of the metal-Aβ binding site is a key prerequisite.

3.2.1. Cu-Aβ-Peptides

We start to discuss the case of Cu. The experimental situation is not completely satisfactory here as there are in the literature somewhat conflicting results about the Cu coordination mode in Aβ-peptides. On the one hand, in fact, NMR data on Cu complexed with $A\beta_{1-28}$ [18] and $A\beta_{1-40}$ [76] peptides suggest that three His's (His_6, His_{13} and His_{14}) are coordinated to the metal with the fourth ligand being a nitrogen from the N-terminus. On the other, XAS experiments on various portions of the $A\beta_{1-40}$ peptide [22, 74] and NMR/EPR experiments on the $A\beta_{1-28}$ peptide [82], as well as NMR data on the $A\beta_{1-16}$ [20] fragment, all point to the conclusion that, besides the above three His's, the fourth Cu ligand is the Tyr_{10} oxygen.

In these circumstances a natural application of the CP-MD theoretical approach is thus to compare the two structural situations where, besides His_6, His_{13} and His_{14}, either the N-terminus or the Tyr_{10} oxygen is coordinated to Cu, with the aim of determining which one of the two atomic arrangements is the physically realized one. This is done by studying the stability properties of the two configurations along the simulated CP-MD trajectories.

We stress that clarifying this point is not without interest, as it is expected that the more or less open structure of the peptide can strongly influence its aggregation

---

[5]Although a QM approach is the method of choice for this kind of problems, we wish to mention that there have been interesting classical MD simulations of stacks of β-amyloid peptides (in the absence of metals) confirming experimental indications [80] about the peculiar way in which in their early stage of aggregation peptides may be packed and structured [81].

propensity. One may suspect that a coordination mode where the N-terminus is not bound to Cu will typically give rise to a more open geometry, which would probably be more prone to aggregation.

3.2.1.1. Models Construction

In order to tackle the structural problem described above three specific Cu-Aβ complex model systems (denoted by S_1-Cu, S_2-Cu and S_3-Cu in the following and described below) have been set up for CP-MD simulations [83]. For reasons we have already explained, their detailed atomic structure is constrained by a compromise between the need of having a sufficiently realistic description of the actual physical system and the impossibility of dealing with too many atoms and electrons. According to this criterion the simulated model systems have been built up as follows. First of all, attention was limited to the $A\beta_{1-14}$ segment (see Table **1**) where the Cu binding site is known to be located. Secondly, since the His_6, His_{13} and His_{14} residues have been positively identified as Cu ligands, they are all explicitly included with the full atomic structure of their lateral chains. As for the other a.a.'s, somewhat different choices for the S_1-Cu, S_2-Cu and S_3-Cu systems (see below) are considered. In all cases the C-terminus is capped in the usual way (*i.e.* by an $NHCH_3$ group), while the N-terminus of the fragment is left open (with an ending NH_2 group) to allow for possible Cu binding accompanied by the loss of the amine hydrogen. Periodic boundary conditions are used and the size of the box was chosen in such a way that the distance between any atom and its nearest image is at least 5 Å. The whole system is neutral as the double positive charge of Cu^{+2} is balanced by the sum of the negative charges of Asp_1 and Glu_3. The detailed structures of the three model systems are described here below and sketched in Fig. **1**.

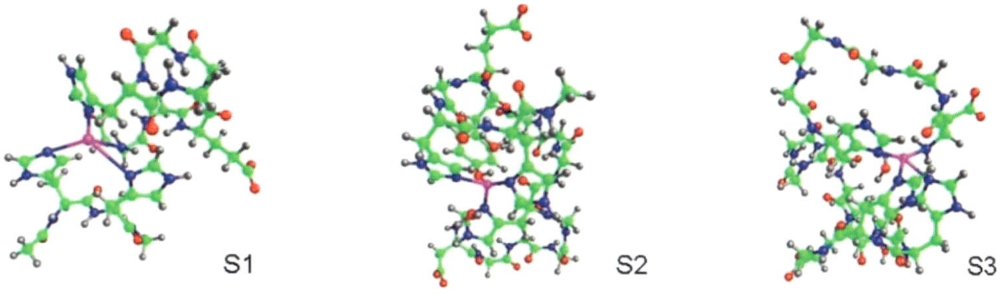

Figure 1: The atomic structure of the S_1-Cu, S_2-Cu and S_3-Cu model systems (denoted S_1, S_2 and S_3 in the figure). Colors are as follows: gray is H, red is O, green is C, blue is N, and magenta is Cu.

• S_1-Cu System

Of the first six a.a.'s (from 1 to 6), besides the backbone, only the lateral chains of Asp_1, Glu_3, and His_6 are retained. Among the remaining a.a.'s (from 7 to 14) only His_{13} and His_{14} with their lateral chains are explicitly included. The His_{13}-His_{14} dipeptide is capped with a CH_3CO group at its N-terminus and by an $NHCH_3$ group at its C-terminus. The system, solvated with 125 water molecules, is contained in a box of volume V=14×19×19 Å^3. In this way density is equal to 1 g/cm_3. All in all, the system (including Cu and water molecules) is made by 494 atoms. The number of KS (see Appendix B) electrons (*i.e.* the electrons that are considered relevant in determining the inter-atomic potential) is 1369. The initial peptide configuration for the CP-MD simulations was taken from the PBD file of [75] with Cu replacing Zn.

• S_2-Cu System

The backbone of the whole 1-14 peptide is retained together with the full lateral chains of Asp_1, His_6, Tyr_{10}, Glu_{11}, His_{13}, and His_{14}. The system, solvated with 225 water molecules, is contained in a box of volume V=22×23×20 Å^3. In this way density is equal to 1 g/cm^3. All in all, the total number of atoms of the system (including Cu and water molecules) is 838 and the number of KS electrons is 2311. The initial configuration for the CP-MD simulations has been taken from a 8 ns long classical MD simulation of the whole Cu-$A\beta_{1\text{-}16}$ peptide in water with His_6, His_{13}, His_{14} and Tyr_{10} bound to Cu. For this step the GROMACS package [67] was used.

• S_3-Cu System

The backbone of the whole 1-14 peptide is retained together with the lateral chains of Asp_1, His_6, Tyr_{10}, Glu_{11}, His_{13}, and His_{14}. The system, solvated with 223 water molecules, is contained in a box of volume V=20×24×20 Å^3. In this way density is equal to 1 g/cm^3. All in all, the total number of atoms of the system (including Cu and water molecules) is 832, and the number of KS electrons is 2295. The initial configuration for the CP-MD simulations has been taken from a 6 ns long classical MD simulation of the whole Cu-$A\beta_{1\text{-}16}$ peptide in water with His_6, His_{13}, His_{14} and the N-terminus bound to Cu. For this step the GROMACS package [67] was used.

Comparing the various model systems, we observe that the S_1-Cu model is a rather crude approximation of the Cu-A$\beta_{1\text{-}14}$ peptide. The S_2-Cu and S_3-Cu models are more realistic and differ only for the fact that besides His_6, His_{13}, His_{14}, in the case of S_2-Cu the fourth Cu ligand is Tyr_{10}, while in the case of S_3-Cu the fourth ligand is the N-terminus. In all cases a water molecule is present in the Cu coordination sphere as a fifth ligand.

3.2.1.2. Results

• S_1-Cu System

Starting from the atomic configuration suggested by the NMR experiments of ref. [75], a thermalization step consisting of two simulations of 0.6 ps at 100 and 200 K was first carried out. After that, a CP-MD trajectory of 1.4 ps at room temperature (300 K) was generated. The main outcome of the simulation is that, starting from a configuration where, besides the imidazole rings of His_6, His_{13} and His_{14}, the nitrogen of the N-terminus was lying inside the Cu coordination sphere, the system ended up in a state where only the three His's remained coordinated to Cu, while the N-terminal nitrogen had moved far out from it[6].

• S_2-Cu and S_3-Cu Systems

The S_1-Cu simulations indicate that the tentative conclusion drawn from the NMR measurements of refs. [18] and [76] according to which the N-terminal nitrogen is one of the Cu ligand, is not tenable. In order to try to reliably identify the structure of the Cu site, simulations of the more realistic systems S_2-Cu and S_3-Cu were carried out with the purpose of comparing the two situations where the oxygen of Tyr_{10} (S_2-Cu) or the N-terminus (S_3-Cu) is coordinated to Cu at the initial step of their respective CP-MD trajectory. The possibility that the Tyr_{10} oxygen is a Cu ligand was suggested in [20] and confirmed in [22, 74], but criticized in [84, 85].

To prepare the systems for the successive *ab initio* calculations, the S_2-Cu and S_3-Cu systems have been first submitted to classical MD simulations in order to obtain well-equilibrated atomic configurations. From these configurations the

[6] This feature is clearly visible when comparing Figs. (**10**) and (**11**) in [40], where as functions of time (for completeness also the history of the initial thermalization steps is reported) the distances from Cu of the nitrogen atoms of the N-terminus and of $N_\delta(His_6)$, $N_{\square}(His_{13})$ and $N_\delta(His_{14})$ are displayed. From the same figures it is clear that the N-terminal nitrogen moves quickly away from Cu reaching a distance of about 7 Å at the end of the simulation.

long procedure for CP-MD simulations described at the beginning of this Section is started. Already at the end of the two minimization steps (steps 1 and 2 above) some interesting differences between the two systems are visible. Namely, in spite of the fact that at the beginning of the classical MD step the $N_\delta(His_6)$, $N_\varepsilon(His_{13})$, and $N_\delta(His_{14})$ atoms were located at the same positions around Cu in the two systems, at the end of classical MD and after the atomic energy minimization step, quite different geometrical arrangements are reached. In fact, the system S_3-Cu ends up with a characteristic planar geometry around Cu, similar to the one we saw in the case of the S_1-Cu system. This is not so in the case of the S_2-Cu system, where the dihedral angle $N_\delta(His_6)$-Cu-$N_\varepsilon(His_{13})$-$N_\delta(His_{14})$ is always pretty far from 180°.

It is interesting to note that in ref. [86] the structure of the Cu^{2+}-imidazole complex in water was studied by a combined theoretical analysis of EXAFS and XANES data, coming to the conclusion that a square-pyramidal geometry around Cu is preferred (over the planar or octahedral one) and persists through other Cu complexes like $[Cu^{2+}(H_2O)_5]$ and $[Cu^{2+}(NH_3)_4(H_2O)]$ (see refs. [87] and [88]). Remarkably, the *ab initio* simulations of the S_2-Cu model system, besides confirming this conclusion, are able to give us the extra information that the Cu ligands in the Cu-$A\beta_{1-14}$ complex are the His_6, His_{13}, His_{14} and Tyr_{10} residues, through the N_δ, N_ε, N_δ and O atoms, respectively.

3.2.2. Zn-Aβ-Peptides

The importance of studying Zn-Aβ complexes stems from the observation that Zn is seen to induce Aβ aggregation more effectively than Cu [89, 90]. From a structural point of view, while to date most of the experimental results [19, 91] and numerical simulations [92, 93] converge to the conclusion of a stable intra-molecular Cu coordination, the situation appears to be much more complicated for Zn^{2+}-Aβ-peptide complexes where several Zn^{2+} coordination modes have been proposed [74, 76, 79, 94].

Thus it appears to be of the utmost importance to understand and clarify whether and how Cu^{2+} and Zn^{2+} differ in their way of interacting with amyloidogenic peptides in general, and Aβ-peptides in particular. For Zn, NMR investigations have suggested a variety of inter- and intra-molecular [19, 75, 76] metal binding modes involving, besides other ligands, different numbers of His's. The existence of a variety of inter-molecular binding modes was put in evidence by XAS studies [21, 22, 74], among which a rather peculiar and somewhat unusual four-His Zn binding mode. It should be stressed, in fact, that over 5854 PDB entries containing at least one Zn only one case is found [95] where Zn is coordinated to four His side-chains belonging to the same protein monomer (PDB code 1PB026). In a second case the four His side-chains coordinated to Zn belong to different monomers (PDB codes 1HWT and 1QP927).

There is another worth mentioning feature of Zn binding to Aβ-peptides that should be stressed. Experimental data suggest that the four involved His's are made by the two pairs of consecutive, His_{13} and His_{14}, residues coming from two adjacent Aβ-peptides. This structure gives rise to a very special arrangement, as structural databases report one single instance where a metal (actually Cu) is bound to two His's that are one next to the other along the protein sequence [96]. There are instead many cases where Cu is coordinated to four His's side-chains belonging to the same monomer, but all of them concern proteins belonging to the wide class of Cu,Zn-superoxide dismutase (Cu,Zn-SOD) proteins. Actually a fully Zn-substituted SOD enzyme (encoded by the human SOD1 gene) has been shown to be at least as stable as the wild-type heterodinuclear protein [97].

The coordination of Zn by four neutral imidazolyl groups is infrequent even within non-protein coordination complexes. A search for this coordination in the Cambridge structural data- base (CSD) [98] yields, with the exception of tetraimidazole Zn^{2+} perchlorate, only structures in which the imidazolyl group is either deprotonated (imidazolate) or N-methyl protected.

One might be tempted to conclude that the peculiar Zn binding mode found in recent experimental data is a hallmark of peptide aggregation. Although XAS data certainly give a significant indication in this direction, their consideration alone is not enough to reach such a conclusion. In fact, it is certainly true that the strength of XAS resides in its sensitivity to short-range order as it allows us to reliably identify at atomic resolution the average structure around the metal absorber for systems in any state of aggregation. But this same feature seems to result in a significant limitation in this case, where in order to fully understand the complicated peptide aggregation mechanism assisted by metals, one must be able to reconstruct the structure of the system at distances larger than 6 Å from the absorber. It appears, in fact, that *in vivo* rather large oligomeric or polymeric structures get formed.

3.2.2.1. Models Construction

For the purpose of investigating fibril aggregation, it is not enough to "simply" reproduce the Zn-K-edge XAS spectra (for which, as we just said, the knowledge of the atomic geometry in a small sphere of radius, say, 5-6 Å is enough). Rather it is necessary to be able to identify what are the stable Zn-Aβ-peptide organized structures (for which the knowledge of the geometry of the sample at large is required). For this reason one is led to the use a combined two-step strategy (XAS data fitting plus *ab initio* simulations) to pass from local structural geometry to large scale modeling [99].

In order to build a model of the Zn-Aβ-peptide complex compatible with the experimental XAS data, a number of systems were constructed and submitted to simulations. In particular, based on general structural information and more or less sophisticated numerical methods (ranging from empirical modeling of single and multiple peptide compounds to small truncated *first principle* simulations - the latter being dealt with at the level of the density functional theory), four models (S_i-Zn, i=1,2,3,4) are constructed and then optimized (*i.e.* fitted) against the available XAS data. The four models are assembled by putting together two identical $A\beta_{1\text{-}16}$ chains (A e B in the following), with the two nitrogen atoms, $N_\delta(His_{14}{}^{(A)})$ and $N_\delta(His_{14}{}^{(B)})$, bound to a single Zn. After a first energy minimization, this initial configuration is further relaxed by a Monte Carlo random walk [100] (MCRW) method. The method consists in randomly changing all the dihedral angles of the two peptide chains, with the exception of those belonging to the two His_{14} side chains that were held fixed to keep the $N_\delta(His_{14}{}^{(A)})$-Zn-$N_\delta(His_{14}{}^{(B)})$ motif blocked in space. Among the many configurations produced in this way a few of them are retained, those that appear to fulfill the required geometrical and structural constraints. The virtue of the random walk sampling method is that no configurations of the Zn-bridging dimer with ''bad'' contacts between pairs of atoms are ever accepted.

• S_1-Zn Model

This model corresponds to one particular configuration of MCRW trajectory in which Zn is closer than 3 Å from $N_\varepsilon(His_{13})$ in both monomers. The reason for this choice is that, among the other possible four-fold metal coordinations, the configuration in which Zn is coordinated to $N_\varepsilon(His_{13}^{(A)})$, $N_\delta(His_{14}^{(A)})$, $N_\varepsilon(His_{13}^{(B)})$ and $N_\delta(His_{14}^{(B)})$ is, according to NMR data [75] and Car-Parrinello (CP-MD) simulations, [94] the most stable one.

• S_2-Zn Model

Along the MCRW trajectory a configuration is selected where Zn is coordinated to three His imidazole rings in a 3N1O configuration (with the oxygen coming from the main chain of one of the bound His's). This model was built with the purpose of testing whether a three-imidazole Zn geometry can be compatible with the XAS results of ref. [74]. The reason for binding the oxygen of His_{14} is that the resulting geometry mimics a sort of "half-His" structure, in the sense that from the XAS point of view only half of the pathways available to the photo-electron, compared to the situation in which the metal is bound to an imidazole ring, are now allowed.

The Zn-bridged $A\beta_{1\text{-}16}$ dimers of S_1-Zn and S_2-Zn models were truncated down to systems affordable by semi-empirical and *first principle* methods. In particular the segments 1-10 of both peptide chains were removed and the Glu_{11} N-terminal was capped with the usual acetyl group. Since, as also suggested by the analysis of XAS data, Zn is preferably penta-coordinated, the oxygen of a water molecule is brought at a binding distance from the metal as a fifth Zn ligand. Each truncated dimer was merged into an orthorhombic cell whose dimensions were determined in order for the periodic replicas to be separated by 0.5 nm. The cell is filled with 376 TIP3P [101] water molecules.

In order to check for the stability of the Zn coordination, the resulting configurations of the S_1-Zn and S_2-Zn models were finally subjected to a full quantum-mechanical step using CP-MD [31]. It is a well recognized fact that classically unnoticed instabilities are easily amplified to a visible magnitude by even very short (of the order of a few picoseconds) quantum-mechanical simulations of the CP-MD type [102].

• S_3-Zn Model

A third model was designed, slightly modifying the S_1-Zn model, by substituting the H_ε atom of $His_{14}^{(A)}$ with a second Zn ion. In the following we will refer to the two Zn atoms as Zn_a and Zn_b. The extra Zn_b, coordinated to one nitrogen from the His bridging the two Zn ions and two oxygens from the Glu_{11} side-chain, is added to check whether its presence is able to stabilize the four-His coordination of Zn_a.

• S_4-Zn Model

A final model, intended to represent a hypothetic, perhaps more realistic situation, is obtained by adding a third peptide fragment (chain C, truncated down to a 11-16 fragment, as it was done for chains A and B), with $N_\varepsilon(His_{13}^{(C)})$ and $N_\delta(His_{14}^{(C)})$ in the same positions as the two water molecules that were bound to the second Zn site (Zn_b site) in model S_3-Zn at the end of the CP-MD simulation (see Table **3** below).

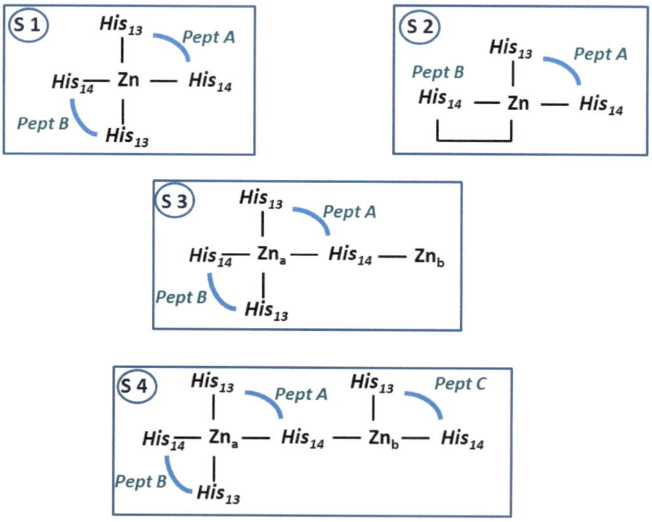

Figure 2: Schematic view of the Zn site in the four models we have constructed. His's connected by blue bands belong to the same peptide. The staple comprising His_{14} and Zn in the S_2-Zn model (in the figure the four S_i-Zn models (i=1,2,3,4) are simply denoted S_i) is there to recall that, besides three imidazoles, the oxygen of the His_{14} main chain is also bound to the metal.

In Fig. **2** for the reader's convenience we sketch the structure of the metal binding site in the four different models we have described. In particular we show which of the the His's are bound to which Zn ion.

3.2.2.2. Results

The relevant features of the evolution of the configurations of the S_i-Zn, i=1,2,3,4 models during the thermalization process are summarized in Table **3**. In the second column of Table **3** (starting configuration) the Zn coordination modes of the four systems before CP-MD (for models S_1-Zn, S_2-Zn and S_3-Zn) or Born-Oppenheimer molecular dynamics (for model S_4-Zn) simulations are listed. Heating the systems from 0 to 250 K (third column), one notices that in both the S_1-Zn and S_2-Zn models Zn loses one ligand and ends up in a tetrahedral 3N1O coordination. For what concerns model S_3-Zn, it is very remarkable that the unlikely initial three-fold coordination of the extra Zn_b readily becomes a more realistic tetra-coordination owing to the oxygen of a water molecule that is attracted within its coordination shell (2.5 Å). Interestingly enough the Zn coordination of both metal sites in model S_4-Zn remains stable along the whole simulation. In the last column, we report the final modifications (when they occur) that take place when the systems are brought to room temperature. We see that the only thing that happens is that in model S_3-Zn one of the two Zn_b-coordinated $O(Glu_{11})$ atoms is replaced by the oxygen of a second water molecule attracted within the coordination shell.

Table 3: For each system in the first column, we report in the second column the atoms that lie within 2.5 Å from Zn (*i.e.* inside the Zn-coordination shell) before the CP-MD or BO-MD simulations. The subscripts (His, Glu, W) denote the residue/molecule to which the atom belongs (W stands for water). In S_3-Zn and S_4 -Zn models the two Zn atoms are denoted Zn_a and Zn_b. In the third and fourth columns the structural variations observed at the end of the simulations at temperatures up to 250 K and at 300 K, respectively, are reported. A''minus'' indicates that a ligand leaves the Zn coordination sphere, while ''plus'' that it enters it.

		Zn-binding modification	
Name	Starting configuration	0–250 K	300 K
S1	Zn: $4N_{His} + 1O_W$	$-1N_{His}$	None
S2	Zn: $3N_{His} + 1O_{His} + 1O_W$	$-1O_{His}$	None
S3	Zn_a: $4N_{His} + 1O_W$ Zn_b: $1N_{His} + 2O_{Glu}$	Zn_b: $+1O_W$	Zn_b: $-1O_{Glu} + 1O_W$
S4	Zn_a: $4N_{His} + 1O_W$ Zn_b: $3N_{His} + 1O_{Glu}$	None	None

The detailed analysis of the four S_i-Zn models carried out in [99] shows that the S_4-Zn model is not only able to nicely fit the experimental findings of ref. [74], but it remains with the Zn ions in a stable coordination mode all along the numerical simulation steps. The stable geometry of the model is displayed in Fig. **3**. We see that Aβ-peptides are pairwise cross-linked by Zn ions, with one Zn bonded by two pairs of adjacent His's (His_{13} and His_{14}) from two peptides, and a second Zn, replacing the proton in the NH group of one of the involved imidazolyl side-chains, necessary to stabilize the whole system. This pattern can possibly repeat itself thus including a large number of monomers. Indeed, the extensive *first principle* (CP-MD) and semi-empirical (tight-binding methods and Born-Oppenheimer molecular dynamics) combined simulations that have been performed support the picture of a Zn-assisted deprotonation of (at least) one of the His side-chains of the peptide leading to the formation of aggregated complexes.

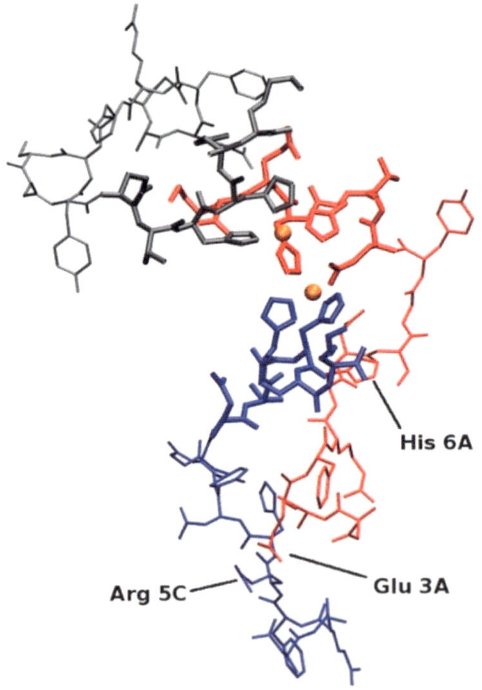

Figure 3: Final MD (t = 500 ps, T = 300 K) configuration of the S_4-Cu model (in which the full $A\beta_{1-16}$ peptide is shown). Zn atoms are displayed in orange, atoms are displayed with sticks, hydrogen atoms are not shown. Chain A is in red, B is in gray and C is in blue. Bonds in the 11-16 residue regions are thicker than those in the 1-10 regions.

4. CONCLUSIONS AND OUTLOOK

Although we are still far from a clear understanding of the rôle of metals in protein misfolding and/or aggregation, experimental and theoretical studies have enormously increased our knowledge in this exploding research area.

In the case of Aβ-peptides experimental information [22, 74] point to a markedly different behaviour depending on whether Cu or Zn is involved in the game. While Cu is bound to Aβ-peptides in rather packed and stable configurations, Zn binding is more flexible and seems to be able to give rise to networks of cross-linked peptides [19].

Detailed *ab initio* studies of the mechanical stability of different models of Zn-Aβ-peptide complexes have been carried out that have led to the identification of a very peculiar arrangement of Zn ions and Aβ-peptides whose stability largely depends on the formation of a Zn-His-Zn bridge assisted by an unusual deprotonated imidazole ring (imidazolate). This sort of imidazolate configuration is very similar to the one it is found in Cu,Zn-SOD (see Fig. **4**) even at mild acidic conditions.

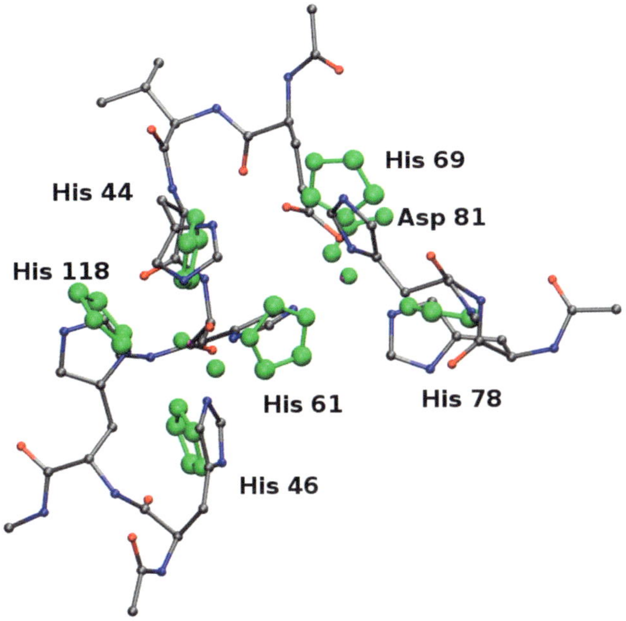

Figure 4: Comparison between S4 truncated energy-minimized model with the structure of reduced bovine SOD enzyme (PDB 1SXA) in green.

Extensive XAS studies have also been carried out on various portions of the PrP tetra-octarepeat peptide in complexes with Cu^{2+} ions, both in the presence and in the absence of Zn^{2+}. A careful analysis of these data shows that Zn acts by directly interacting with the peptide, in this way competing with Cu for binding with His. This finding suggests that metal binding competition can be important in the more general context of metal homeostasis.

Naturally the ultimate goal of the kind of complementary experimental and theoretical investigations we have illustrated in this review is to provide an understanding of the fundamental biochemical processes which are at the basis of metal metabolism, with the hope of finding new treatments for the devastating neurodegenerative diseases associated to protein aggregation and fibril formation.

ACKNOWLEDGEMENTS

We would like to thank all the many collaborators that have directly or indirectly contributed to the many of the work reported in this review. Among them special thanks are due to G. La Penna, V. Minicozzi, G.C. Rossi and F. Stellato. Fruitful discussions with F. Guerrieri and S. Furlan are also acknowledged. This work was partially supported by INFN TO61 project and PRIN project 20083Y34Y7.

CONFLICT OF INTEREST

The authors confirm that this chapter content has no conflict of interest.

DISCLOSURE

This chapter is an update of our previous publication in CAR "The Role of Metals in β-Amyloid Peptide Aggregation: X-Ray Spectroscopy and Numerical Simulations" published in 'CAR', Volume 5, Number 6, December, pp. 508 to 524.

ABBREVIATIONS

AD = Alzheimer's disease

Al = Aluminium

a.a	=	Amino acid
APP	=	Amyloid Precursor Protein
BBB	=	Blood Brain Barrier
CD	=	Circular Dichroism
CNS	=	Central Nervous System
CP	=	Car-Parrinello
CP-MD	=	Car-Parrinello Molecular Dynamics
Cu	=	Copper
DFT	=	Density Functional Theory
EPR	=	Electron Paramagnetic Resonance
EXAFS	=	Extended X-ray Absorption Fine Structure
Fe	=	Iron
fs	=	Femptosecond
FT	=	Fourier Transform
Gly	=	Glycine
His	=	Histidine
KS	=	Kohn and Sham
MC	=	Monte Carlo
MCRW	=	Monte Carlo Random Walk
MD	=	Molecular Dynamics

MDB	=	Metal-protein Database and Browser
MS	=	Multiple Scattering
NMR	=	Nuclear Magnetic Resonance
ns	=	Nanosecond
PrP	=	Prion Protein
ps	=	Picosecond
QM	=	Quantum-Mechanical
QM/MM	=	Quantum Mechanics Molecular Mechanics
SOD	=	Superoxide Dismutase
TSE	=	Transmissible Spongiform Encephalophaty
Tyr	=	Tyrosine
XANES	=	X-ray Absorption Near Edge Structure
XAS	=	X-ray Absorption Spectroscopy
Zn	=	Zinc

Appendix A

In this Appendix we recollect a few standard XAS formulae useful to recall the meaning of the physical quantities and symbols used in the text.

1) The so-called EXAFS signal, $\chi(k)$, is defined through the measured total absorption coefficient, $\mu(E)$, and the absorption coefficient of the isolated absorber, $\mu_0(E)$, *via* the relation

$$\chi(k) = \frac{\mu(E) - \mu_0(E)}{\mu_0(E)}, \quad \textbf{(1)}$$

$$\hbar k = \sqrt{2m(E - E_0)}, \quad \textbf{(2)}$$

where m is the electron mass, $\hbar$ the (reduced) Planck constant and k the wave vector of the extracted electron. The wave vector is related to the incident photon energy, E, and the ionization energy, E_0 as shown in eq. (2).

2) For completeness and to fix the notation we recall how the parameters introduced in Table **2** enter the theoretical formula representing the EXAFS signal. For simplicity we report equations valid in the single scattering approximation. In this case the theoretical EXAFS signal has the rather simple expression

$$\chi(k) = S_0^2 \sum_{\ell} \frac{N_\ell}{kr_\ell^2} |f_\ell(k,\pi)| \sin(2kr_\ell + \phi_\ell(k)) e^{-\sigma_\ell^2 k^2} e^{-2r_\ell/\lambda(k)}, \quad \textbf{(3)}$$

where the sum over ℓ runs over the different coordination shells around the absorber. N_ℓ is the number of scatterers in the ℓ-th shell, located at a distance r_ℓ from the absorber and σ_ℓ^2 is the associated Debye-Waller factor. $|f_\ell(k,\pi)|$ is the modulus of the back-scattering amplitude and $\phi_\ell(k)$ the total scattering phase. Finally S_0^2 is an empirical (positive) quantity that accounts for all the many-body losses in photo-absorption processes and $\lambda(k)$ is the photo-electron mean free path. For MS processes a formally similar expression can be derived, in which r_ℓ represents the length of the full MS path. Modulus and phase functions have now more complicated expressions that depend on all the scattering events occurring along the MS path [38, 41-44].

3) The quality factor of a fit, R, is computed according to the formula

$$R = \sum_{i=1}^{P} \frac{1}{w_i} \left| \chi^{\exp}(k_i) - \chi^{th}(k_i) \right| \,, \tag{4}$$

where $\chi^{\exp}(k_i)$ and $\chi^{th}(k_i)$ are the experimental and theoretical data points, respectively, and the sum is over the number, P, of the k-values at which data were collected. The "weighting" parameter w_i is given by

$$w_i = \frac{1}{k_i^n} \sum_{j=1}^{P} k_j^n \left| \chi^{\exp}(k_j) \right| \tag{5}$$

where the integer n is selected in such a way that the amplitude of the EXAFS oscillations in the combination $k^n \left| \chi^{\exp}(k) \right|$ does not die away at large values of k. In the analysis presented in this work the rather standard value $n = 3$ was taken. As for the size of R, it is a consolidated experience that for complex biological molecules a fit can be considered adequately good when R takes a value that it isn't larger than 20% ÷ 40% [52].

Appendix B

In this Appendix we want to give the fundamental formulae that underlay CP-MD simulations. The CP-MD method [31, 71, 72] is based on the DFT theory the foundations of which have been laid out in the seminal papers of refs. [28, 29] (see ref. [30] for recent reviews and applications to quantum chemistry).

The N_A atoms of the system, identified by the Cartesian coordinates $\{\vec{R}\} = \{\vec{R}_I, I = 1, \ldots, N_A\}$, move (in the standard Born-Oppenheimer approximation) according to the classical equations of motion

$$M_I \frac{d^2 \vec{R}_I}{dt^2} = -\frac{\partial V_T\left(\{\vec{R}\}\right)}{\partial \vec{R}_I}, \quad I = 1, \ldots, N_A \,, \tag{6}$$

where M_I is the mass of the I -th atom and $V_T\left(\left\{\vec{R}\right\}\right)$ is the total atomic potential energy

$$V_T\left(\left\{\vec{R}\right\}\right)=\frac{1}{2}\sum_{I\neq J=1}^{N_A}\frac{Z_I Z_J e^2}{\left|\vec{R}_I-\vec{R}_J\right|}+E_{QM}\left(\left\{\vec{R}\right\}\right). \quad \textbf{(7)}$$

The first term of eq. (7) is the Coulomb potential between pairs of atoms endowed with electric charge $Z_I e$ and $Z_J e$. The second term, $E_{QM}\left(\left\{\vec{R}\right\}\right)$, is the piece of the atomic potential energy generated by the electrons according to the general principles of Quantum Mechanics. For simplicity we will assume here that the system is electrically neutral. This means that the total number of electrons, N_e, participating in the dynamics and generating the potential $E_{QM}\left(\left\{\vec{R}\right\}\right)$ is

$$N_e=\sum_{I=1}^{N_A}Z_I \quad \textbf{(8)}$$

The most difficult part of the method is the determination of $E_{QM}\left(\left\{\vec{R}\right\}\right)$. In principle this can be done by first solving the Kohn and Sham (KS) [29] equations

$$H\psi_i(\vec{r})=\varepsilon_i\psi_i(\vec{r}),\ i=1,\ldots,N_e\ , \quad \textbf{(9)}$$

$$H=-\frac{\hbar^2}{2m}\vec{\nabla}^2-\sum_{I=1}^{N_A}\frac{Z_I e^2}{\left|\vec{r}-\vec{R}_I\right|}+\int d\vec{r}^{\,'}\frac{n(\vec{r}^{\,'})}{\left|\vec{r}^{\,'}-\vec{r}\right|}+\frac{\delta E_{xc}\left[n\right]}{\delta n(\vec{r}^{\,'})}\ , \quad \textbf{(10)}$$

where $\vec{\nabla}^2=\partial^2/\partial x^2+\partial^2/\partial y^2+\partial^2/\partial z^2$ is the three-dimensional Laplace differential operator, $E_{xc}\left[n\right]$ is the exchange and correlation functional and $n(\vec{r})$ is the electronic density which in turn can be expressed in terms of the KS wave-functions through the formula

$$n(\vec{r})=\sum_{i=1}^{N_e}\left|\psi_i(\vec{r})\right|^2. \quad \textbf{(11)}$$

The KS equations have a precise physical meaning. They represent, in fact, the minimization condition for the following functional of the electronic density

$$E(n;\{\vec{R}\}) = -\frac{\hbar^2}{2m}\sum_{i=1}^{N_e}\int d\vec{r}\psi_i^*(\vec{r})\vec{\nabla}^2\psi_i(\vec{r}) - \int d\vec{r} n(\vec{r})\sum_{I=1}^{N_A}\frac{Z_I e^2}{|\vec{r}-\vec{R}_I|} +$$
$$+\frac{1}{2}\int d\vec{r}\int d\vec{r}'\frac{n(\vec{r})n(\vec{r}')}{|\vec{r}'-\vec{r}|} + E_{xc}[n] \tag{12}$$

Once the N_e orthonormal KS wave-functions, ψ_i, and eigenvalues, ε_i, have been determined by solving eq. (9), they can be substituted back in eq. (12) leading to the formula

$$E_{QM}(\{\vec{R}\}) = \sum_{i=1}^{N_e}\varepsilon_i - \frac{1}{2}\int d\vec{r}\int d\vec{r}'\frac{n(\vec{r})n(\vec{r}')}{|\vec{r}'-\vec{r}|} + E_{xc}[n] - \int d\vec{r}\frac{\delta E_{xc}[n]}{\delta n(\vec{r})}n(\vec{r}) \ . \tag{13}$$

Eq. (13) yields the desired expression of the QM atomic potential generated by the electrons appearing in eq. (7).

There are two problems with the approach we have described. The first is of a conceptual nature and has to do with the lack of a precise knowledge of the $E_{xc}[n]$ functional, which is only approximate. The second is more practical and has to do with the observation that in the way things are formulated one would have to solve the KS equations every time the atomic coordinates change as a consequence of the time evolution (6). This makes the whole procedure of simulating the dynamics of the system impossibly long and slow.

The first problem has been pragmatically solved in the literature where many, more or less sophisticated, examples of exchange and correlations functionals have been constructed in correspondence with the various specific problems that have been considered (some instances are recalled in refs. [71, 72]). The common starting point for all these formulae is the one derived from the local density approximation (LDA) equation

$$E_{xc}^{LDA}[n] = -\frac{3}{4\pi}\int d\vec{r}[3\pi^2 n(\vec{r})]^{1/3}n(\vec{r}) \ , \tag{14}$$

that is valid in the regime of slowly varying electron density [28, 29, 94]. It may be useful to recall that the kinetic energy of a gas of free electrons is given by the following functional of the electron density

$$T^{free}[n] = \frac{3}{10}\int d\vec{r}[3\pi^2 n(\vec{r})]^{2/3} n(\vec{r}) \ . \tag{15}$$

The second problem has been brilliantly solved by Car and Parrinello in their seminal '85 paper [31]. The idea is to adiabatically move the atoms in the force field generated by the current value of the functional (12), while the latter is minimized. The minimization procedure is carried out by letting the wave functions, ψ_i, to depend on a fictitious time, *t*, and solving for the electrons the Newton-like equations of motion

$$\mu_i \frac{\partial^2 \psi_i(\vec{r},t)}{\partial t^2} = H\psi_i(\vec{r},t) - \varepsilon_i \psi_i(\vec{r},t) \ , \ i = 1,\ldots,N_e \ , \tag{16}$$

while at the same time the "electron kinetic energy", $2E_{kin} = \sum_i \mu_i \,|\, d\psi_i \,/\, dt\,|^2$ is slowly driven to zero. In eq. (14) μ_i is a parameter with the dimensions of a mass that is tuned so as to make the typical frequencies associated with the fictitious motion of the electrons of the same order of magnitude as the typical frequencies associated with the classical motion of the atoms described by eq. (6). In this way both equations can be solved employing the same time step, which for the systems of interest here turns out to be rather small, *viz.* of the order of 0.1 fs.

We conclude by observing that the set of atomic and electronic equations (eqs. (6) and (16)) can be elegantly derived from the effective Lagrangian

$$L(\{\psi\},\{\vec{R}\}) = \frac{1}{2}\sum_{I=1}^{N_A} M_I \left(\frac{d\vec{R}_I}{dt}\right)^2 + \frac{1}{2}\sum_{i=1}^{N_e} \mu_i \left|\frac{d\psi_i}{dt}\right|^2 - \frac{1}{2}\sum_{I\neq J=1}^{N_A} \frac{Z_I Z_J e^2}{\left|\vec{R}_I - \vec{R}_J\right|} + \\ - E[n;\{\vec{R}\}] + \sum_{ij=1}^{N_e} \lambda_{ij}\left(\int d\vec{r}\psi_j^*(\vec{r},t)\psi_i(\vec{r},t) - \delta_{ij}\right) \tag{17}$$

where the last term is necessary to ensure the orthonormality of the KS wave-functions (with the ε_i in eq. (14) the eigenvalues of the symmetric matrix λ_{ij}) and the functional $E[n;\{\vec{R}\}]$ is defined in eq. (12).

REFERENCES

[1] Schläfer HL and Gliemann G. 'Basic Principles of Ligand Field Theory'. Wiley Interscience. New York (1969); Miessler GL and Tarr DA. 'Inorganic Chemistry', 3rd Ed., Pearson/Prentice Hall publisher.

[2] Bush AI. The metallobiology of Alzheimer's disease. Trends Neurosci 26: 207-214 (2003).

[3] Barnham KJ, Masters CL and Bush AI. Neurodegenerative diseases and oxidative stress. Nat Rev Drug Disc 3: 205-214 (2004).

[4] Wang H, Wang M, Li M, Chen H, Yu X, Zhao Y, Feng W, Chai Z. The distribution profile and oxidation states of biometals in APP transgenic mouse brain: dyshomeostasis with age and as a function of the development of Alzheimer's disease. Metallomics 4(3):289-296 (2012).

[5] Therry RD. The pathogenesis of Alzheimer disease: an alternative to the amyloid hypothesis. J Neuropathol Exp Neurol 55: 1023-1025 (1996).

[6] Lovell MA, Robertson JD, Teesdale WJ, Campbell JL and Markesbery WR. Copper, iron and zinc in Alzheimer's disease senile plaques. J Neurol Sci 158: 47-52 (1998).

[7] Zheng W, Aschner M and Ghersi-Egea JF. Brain barrier systems: a new frontier in metal neurotoxicological research. Toxicol Appl Pharmacol 192: 1-11 (2003).

[8] Banks WA, Kastin AJ and Zatta P. The blood-brain barrier in aluminum toxicity and Alzheimer's disease. In 'Non-neuronal cells in Alzheimer disease' (Eds: Zatta P and Nicolini M) World Scientific, Singapore, p. 1-12 (1995).

[9] Yokel RA. Brain uptake, retention, and efflux of aluminum and manganese. Environ Health Perspect (Suppl.) 5: 699-704 (2002).

[10] Bala Gupta V, Anitha S, Hedge ML, Zecca L, Garruto RM, Ravid R, Shankar SK, Stein R, Shanmugavelu P and Jagannatha Rao KS. Aluminum in Alzheimer's disease: are we still at a crossroad? Cell Mol Life Sci 62: 143-158 (2005).

[11] Drago D, Folin M, Baiguera S, Tognon G, Ricchelli F and Zatta P. Comparative effects of Aβ(1-42)-Al complex from rat and human amyloid on rat endothelial cell cultures. J Alzheimer's Dis 11: 33-44 (2007).

[12] Khan A, Ashcroft AE, Korchazhkina OV and Exley C. Metal-mediated formation of fibrillar Aβ-amyloid. J Inorg Biochem 98: 2006-2010 (2004).

[13] Morante S, González-Iglesias R, Potrich C, Meneghini C, Meyer-Klaucke W, Menestrina G, Gasset M. Inter- and intra- octarepeat Cu(II) site geometries in the prion protein. Implication in Cu(II) binding cooperativity and Cu(II)-mediated assemblies. J Biol Chem 279:11753-11759 (2004).

[14] Leal SS, Botelho HM, Gomes CM. Metal ions as modulators of protein conformation and misfolding in neurodegeneration. Coordination Chemistry available online (2012).

[15] Pepys MB. Pathogenesis, diagnosis and treatment of systemic amyloidosis. Philos Trans R Soc Lond B Biol Sci 356: 203-210 (2001).

[16] Selkoe DJ. Alzheimer's disease: genes, proteins, and therapy. Physiol Rev 81: 741-766 (2001).

[17] Cherny RA, Atwood CS, Xilinas ME, Gray DN, Jones WD, McLean CA, Barnham KJ, Volitakis I, Fraser FW, Kim YS, Huang X, Goldstein LE, Moir RD, Lim JT, Beyreuther K, Zheng H, Tanzi RE, Masters CL and Bush AI. Treatment with a copper-zinc chelator

markedly and rapidly inhibits beta-amyloid accumulation in Alzheimer's disease transgenic mice. Neurol 30: 665-676 (2001).

[18] Syme CD, Nadal RC, Rigby SEJ and Viles JH. Copper binding to the amyloid-beta (Abeta) peptide associated with Alzheimer's disease: folding, coordination geometry, pH dependence, stoichiometry, and affinity of Abeta-(1-28): insights from a range of complementary spectroscopic techniques. J Biol Chem 279: 18169-18177 (2004).

[19] Syme CD and Viles JH. Solution 1H NMR investigation of Zn2+ and Cd2+ binding to amyloid-beta peptide (Abeta) of Alzheimer's disease. Biochim Biophys Acta 1764: 246-256 (2006).

[20] Ma QF, Hu J, Wu WH, Liu HD, Du JD, Fu Y, Wu YW, Lei P, Zhao YF and Li YM. Characterization of copper binding to the peptide amyloid-beta(1-16) associated with Alzheimer's disease. Biopolymers 83: 20-31 (2006).

[21] Dong J, Shokes JE, Scott RA and Lynn DG. Modulating amyloid self-assembly and fibril morphology with Zn(II). J Am Chem Soc 128: 3540-3542 (2006).

[22] Stellato F, Menestrina G, Dalla Serra M, Potrich C, Tomazzolli R, Meyer-Klaucke W and Morante S. Metal binding in amyloid beta-peptides shows intra- and inter-peptide coordination modes. Eur Biophys J 35: 340-351 (2006).

[23] Strange RW, Blackburn NJ, Knowles PF and Hasnain SS. X-ray Absorption Spectroscopy of Metal-Histidine Coordination in Metalloproteins. Exact Simulation of the EXAFS of Tetrakis(imidazole)copper(II) Nitrate and Other Copper-Imidazole Complexes by the Use of a Multiple-Scattering Treatment. J Am Chem Soc 109: 7157-7162 (1987).

[24] Bianconi A, Di Cicco A, Pavel NV, Benfatto M, Marcelli A, Natoli CR, Pianetta P and Woicik J. Multiple-scattering effects in the K-edge x-ray-absorption near-edge structure of crystalline and amorphous silicon. Phys Rev B 36: 6426-6433 (1987).

[25] Filipponi A, Evangelisti F, Benfatto M, Mobilio S and Natoli CR. Structural investigation of a-Si and a-Si:H using x-ray-absorption spectroscopy at the Si K edge. Phys Rev B 40: 9636-9643 (1989).

[26] Zhang HH, Filipponi A, Di Cicco A, Scott MJ, Holm RH, Hedman B and Hodgson KO. Multiple-Edge XAS Studies of Cyanide-Bridged Iron-Copper Molecular Assemblies Relevant to Cyanide-Inhibited Heme-Copper Oxidases Using Four-Body Multiple-Scattering Analysis. J Am Chem Soc 119: 2470-2478 (1997) and references therein.

[27] Meneghini C and Morante S. The active site structure of tetanus neurotoxin resolved by multiple scattering analysis in X-Ray absorption spectroscopy. Biophys J 75: 1953-1963 (1998).

[28] Hohenenberg P and Kohn W. Inhomogeneous Electron Gas. Phys Rev 136: 864-871 (1964).

[29] Kohn W and Sham LJ. Quantum Density Oscillations in an Inhomogeneous Electron Gas. Phys Rev 137: 1697-1705 (1965); Kohn W and Sham LJ. Self-Consistent Equations Including Exchange and Correlation Effects. Phys Rev 140: 1133-1138 (1965).

[30] Parr RG and Yang W. 'Density Functional Theory of Atoms and Molecules'. Oxford University Press. Oxford, (1989); Dreizler RM and Gross EKU. 'Density functional theory'. Springer-Verlag, Berlin (1990); 'Primer in Density Functional Theory'. (Eds: Fiolhais C, Nogueira F and Marques MAL). Lecture Notes in Physics, Springer-Verlag, Berlin (2003).

[31] Car R and Parrinello M. Unified approach for molecular dynamics and density functional theory. Phys Rev Lett 55: 2471-2474 (1985).

[32] Giannozzi P, de Angelis F and Car R. First-principle molecular dynamics with ultrasoft pseudopotentials: parallel implementation and application to extended bio-inorganic system. J Chem Phys 120: 5903-5914 (2004).

[33] Bianconi A., Congiu-Castellano A, Dell'Ariccia M, Giovannelli A, Morante S, Burattini E and Durham PJ. 'Local Fe site structure in the tense-to-relaxed transition in carp deoxyhemoglobin: a XANES (x-ray absorption near edge structure) study'. Proc Natl Acad Sci USA 83: 7736-7740 (1986).

[34] Morante S, Gonzalez-Iglesias R, Potrich C, Meneghini C, Meyer-Klaucke W, Menestrina G and Gasset M. Inter- and intra-octarepeat Cu(II) site geometries in the prion protein: implications in Cu(II) binding cooperativity and Cu(II)-mediated assemblies. J Biol Chem 279: 11753-11759 (2004).

[35] Redecke L, Meyer-Klaucke W, Koker M, Clos J, Georgieva D, Genov N, Echner H, Kalbacher H, Perbandt M, Bredehorst R, Völter W and Betzel C. Comparative analysis of the human and chicken prion protein copper binding regions at pH 6.5. J Biol Chem 280: 13987-13992 (2005).

[36] Mentler M, Weiss A, Grantner K, Del Pino P, Deluca D, Fiori S, Renner C, Meyer-Klaucke W, Moroder L, Bertsch U, Kretzschmar HA, Tavan P and Parak FG. A New Method to determine the Structure of the Metal Environment in Metalloproteins: Investigation of the Prion Protein Octapeptide Repeat Cu(2+) Complex. Eur Biophys J 34(2): 97-112 (2005).

[37] Del Pino P, Weiss A, Bertsch U, Renner C, Mentler M, Grantner K, Fiorino F, Meyer-Klaucke W, Moroder L, Kretzschmar HA and Parak FG. The Configuration of the Cu(2+) Binding Region in Full-Length Human Prion Protein. Eur Biophys J 36: 239-252 (2007).

[38] Benfatto M, Natoli CR, Bianconi A, Garcia J, Marcelli A, Fanfoni M and Davoli I. Multiple-scattering regime and higher-order correlations in x-ray-absorption spectra of liquid solutions. Phys Rev B34: 5774-5781 (1986).

[39] Lee PA, Citrin PH, Eisenberg P and Kinkaid BM. Extended x-ray absorption fine structure: its strengths and limitations as a structural tool. Rev Mod Phys 53: 769-806 (1981).

[40] Morante S. The rôle of metals in β-amyloid peptide aggregation: X-ray spectroscopy and numerical simulations. Current Alzheimer Research 5/6: 508-524 (2008).

[41] Lee PA and Pendry JB. Theory of the extended X-ray absorption fine structure. Phys Rev 11: 2795-2811 (1975).

[42] Gurman SJ, Binsted N and Ross I. A rapid, exact, curved-wave theory for EXAFS calculations. II. The multiple-scattering contributions. J Phys C19: 1845-1861 (1986).

[43] 'X-ray Absorption. Principles, applications, techniques of EXAFS, SEXAFS and XANES'. (Eds: Koningsberger DC and Prins R) John Wiley & Sons (1988) and references quoted therein.

[44] Rehr JJ and Albers RC. Scattering-matrix formulation of curved-wave multiple-scattering theory: Application to x-ray-absorption fine structure. Phys Rev B41: 8139-8149 (1990).

[45] Benfatto M and Della Longa S. Geometrical fitting of experimental XANES spectra by a full multiple-scattering procedure. J Synchrotron Rad 8: 1087-1094 (2001).

[46] Della Longa S, Arcovito A, Girasole M, Hazemann JL and Benfatto M. Quantitative analysis of x-ray absorption near edge structure data by a full multiple scattering procedure: the Fe-CO geometry in photolysed carbonmonoxy-myoglobin single crystal. Phys Rev Lett 87: 155501-155504 (2001).

[47] Benfatto M, Della Longa S, Qin Y, Li Q, Pan G, Wu Z and Morante S. The rôle of Zn in the interplay among Langmuir-Blodgett multilayer and myelin basic protein: a quantitative analysis of XANES spectra. Biophys Chem 110: 191-201 (2004).

[48] Filipponi A, Di Cicco A and Natoli CR. X-ray-absorption spectroscopy and n-body distribution functions in condensed matter. I. Theory. Phys Rev B52: 15122-15134 (1995).

[49] Filipponi A and Di Cicco A. X-ray-absorption spectroscopy and n-body distribution functions in condensed matter. II. Data analysis and applications. Phys Rev B52: 15135-15149 (1995).

[50] Ankudinov AL, Ravel B, Rehr JJ and Conradson SD. Real Space Multiple Scattering Calculation of XANES. Phys Rev B58: 7565-7576 (1998).

[51] Binsted N, Strange RW and Hasnain SS. Constrained and restrained refinement in EXAFS data analysis with curved wave theory. Biochemistry 31: 12117-12125 (1992).

[52] Binsted N. EXCURV98: CCLRC Daresbury Laboratory computer program (1998).

[53] Rehr JJ and Albers RC. Theoretical approaches to x-ray absorption fine structure. Rev Mod Phys 72: 621-654 (2000).

[54] Bunker G, Stern EA, Blankeship RE and Parson WW. An x-ray absorption study of the iron site in bacterial photosynthetic reaction center. Biophys J 37: 539-551 (1982); Blackburn NJ, Hasnain SS, Diakun GP, Knowles PF, Binsted N and Garner CD. An extended x-ray absorption fine structure study of the copper and zinc sites of freeze-dried bovine superoxide dismutase. Biochem J 213: 765-768 (1983).

[55] Rossi GC. Theories, models, simulations: A computational challenge. e-print: arXiv: 0607211 [hep-th].

[56] Allen MP and Tildesley DJ. 'Computer Simulation of Liquids'. Clarendon Press, Oxford, UK (1990); Frenkel D and Smit B. 'Understanding Molecular Simulations'. Academic Press, San Diego, USA (1996).

[57] Martonak R, Laio A and Parrinello M. Predicting crystal structures: the Parrinello-Rahman method revisited. e-print: arXiv: 0211551 [cond-mat]; Kuo I-FW, Mundy CJ, McGrath MJ, Siepmann JI, VandeVondele J, Sprik M, Hutter J, Chen B, Klein ML, Mohamed FR, Krack M and Parrinello M. Liquid Water from First Principles: Investigation of Different Sampling Approaches. J Phys Chem B108: 12990-12998 (2004); Aktah D, Passerone D and Parrinello M. Insights into the Electronic Dynamics in Chemical Reactions. J Phys Chem A108: 848-854 (2004); Kühne TD, Krack M, Mohamed FR and Parrinello M. An Efficient and Accurate Car-Parrinello-like Approach to Born-Oppenheimer Molecular Dynamics. Phys Rev Lett 98: 066401-4 (2007).

[58] Carloni P, Blochl P and Parrinello M. Electronic structure of the Cu, Zn superoxide dismutase active site and its interactions with the substrate. J Phys Chem 99: 1338-1348 (1995); Hutter J, Carloni P and Parrinello M. Nonempirical Calculations of a Hydrated RNA Duplex. J Am Chem Soc 118: 8710-8712 (1996); Carloni P. Density Functional Theory-Based Molecular Dynamics of Biological Systems. Quant Struct Act Relat 21: 166-172 (2002); Piana S, Bucher D, Carloni P and Rothlisberger U. Reaction Mechanism of HIV-1 Protease by Hybrid Car-Parrinello/Classical MD Simulations. J Phys Chem B108: 11139-11149 (2004); Sharma M, Resta R and Car R. Intermolecular Dynamical Charge Fluctuations in Water: A Signature of the H-Bond Network. Phys Rev Lett 95: 187401-4 (2005).

[59] Furlan S, La Penna G, Guerrieri F, Morante S and Rossi GC. *Ab initio* simulations of Cu binding sites on the N-terminal region of prion protein. J Biol Inorg Chem 12: 571-583 (2007).

[60] Furlan S, La Penna G, Guerrieri F, Morante S and Rossi GC. Studying the Cu binding sites in the PrP N-terminal region: a test case for *ab initio* simulations. Eur Biophys J 36: 841-845 (2007).

[61] Ewald PP. Die Berechnung optischer und elektrostatischer Gitterpotentiale. Ann Phys 64: 253-287 (1921); Allen MP and Tildesley DJ. 'Computer simulation of liquids'. Clarendon Press, New York (1988); Darden T, York D and Pedersen L. Particle mesh Ewald: An N-log(N) method for Ewald sums in large systems. J Chem Phys 98: 10089-10092 (1993); Essmann U, Perera L, Berkowitz ML, Darden T, Lee H and Pedersen LG. A smooth particle mesh Ewald potential. J Chem Phys 103: 8577-8592 (1995).

[62] Gao J. Review on QM/MM. Reviews in Comp Chem 7: 119-185 (1996); Assfeld X and Rivail JL. Quantum chemical computations on parts of large molecules: The ab initio Local Self-Consistent Field method. Chem Phys Lett 263: 100-106 (1996); Bash PA, Ho LL, MacKerell ADJ, Levine D and Hallstrom P. Progress toward chemical accuracy in the computer simulation of condensed phase reactions. Proc Natl Acad Sci 93 3698-3703 (1996); Field MJ, Bash PA and Karplus M. A Combined Quantum Mechanical and Molecular Mechanical Potential for Molecular Dynamics Simulations. J Comp Chem 11: 700-733 (1990); Freindorf M and Gao J. Optimization of the Lennard-Jones Parameter for Combined Ab Initio Quantum Mechanical and Molecular Mechanical Potential Using the 3-21G Basis Set. J Comp Chem 17: 386-395 (1996); Gao J. Hybrid Quantum and Molecular Mechanical Simulations: An Alternative Avenue to Solvent Effects in Organic Chemistry. Acc Chem Res 29: 298-305 (1996); Eichinger M, Tavan P, Hutter J and Parrinello M. A hybrid method for solutes in complex solvents: density functional theory combined with empirical force fields. J Chem Phys 110: 10452-10467; Reuter N, Dejaegere A, Maigret B. and Karplus M. Frontier Bonds in QM/MM Methods: A Comparison of Different Methods. J Phys Chem A104 1720-1735 (2000).

[63] Lambert MP, Barlow AK, Chromy BA, Edwards C, Freed R, Liosatos M, Morgan TE, Rozovsky I, Trommer B, Viola KL, Wals P, Zhang C, Finch CE, Krafft GA and Klein WL. Diffusible, nonfibrillar ligands derived from Abeta-42 are potent central nervous system neurotoxins. Proc Natl Acad Sci USA 95: 6448-6453 (1998).

[64] Chromy BA, Nowak RJ, Lambert MP, Viola KL, Chang L, Velasco PT, Jones BW, Fernandez SJ, Lacor PN, Horowitz P, Finch CE, Krafft GA and Klein WL. Self-assembly of Abeta (1-42) into globular neurotoxins. Biochemistry 42: 12749-12760 (2003).

[65] Klein WL. Cytotoxic intermediates in the fibrillation pathway: Aβ-oligomers in Alzheimer's disease as a case study. In 'Protein Misfolding, Aggregation and Conformational diseases. Part A' (Eds: Uversky VN and Fink AL) p. 61-81 Springer-Verlag, Berlin (2006).

[66] Baroni S, Dal Corso A, de Gironcoli S, Giannozzi P, Cavazzoni C, Ballabio G, Scandolo S, Chiarotti G, Focher P, Pasquarello A, Laasonen K, Trave A, Car R, Marzari N and Kokalj A. http://www.pwscf.org/.

[67] Van der Spoel D, van Buuren AR, Apol E, Meulenhoff PJ, Tieleman DP, Sijbers ALTM, Hess B, Feenstra KA, Lindhal E, van Drunen R and Berensden HJC. 'Gromacs User Manual' version 3.1.1; Nijenborgh 4, 9747 AG Groningen: The Netherlands, 2002; http://www.gromacs.org.

[68] http://amber.scripps.edu/

[69] Nosé S. A molecular dynamics method for simulations in the canonical ensemble. Molec Phys 52: 255-268 (1984); Hoover WG. Canonical dynamics: equilibrium phase-space distributions. Phys Rev A 31: 1695-1697 (1985).

[70] Frenkel D and Smit B. 'Understanding molecular simulation' Academic Press, San Diego (1996).

[71] Payne MC, Teter MP, Allan DC, Arias TA and Joannopoulos JD. Iterative minimization techniques for ab initio total-energy calculations: molecular dynamics and conjugate gradients. Rev Mod Phys 64: 1045-1097 (1992).

[72] Mark D and Hutter J. in 'Modern Methods and Algorithms of Quantum Chemistry' (Ed. Grotendorst J.), John von Neumann Institute for Computing, Jülich, http://www.fz-juelich.de/nic-series.

[73] http://www.embl.org/

[74] Minicozzi V, Stellato F, Comai M, Dalla Serra M, Potrich C, Meyer-Klaucke W and Morante S. Identifying the minimal Cu and Zn binding site sequence in Amyloid beta peptides. J Biol Chem 283: 10784-10792 (2008).

[75] Zirah S, Kozin SA, Mazur AK, Blond A, Cheminant M, Ségalas-Milazzo I, Debey P and Rebuffat S. Structural Changes of Region 1-16 of the Alzheimer Disease Amyloid-Peptide upon Zinc Binding and *in Vitro* Aging. J Biol Chem 281: 2151-2161 (2006).

[76] Danielsson J, Pierattelli R, Banci L and Graslund A. High-resolution NMR studies of the zinc-binding site of the Alzheimer's amyloid beta-peptide. FEBS J 274: 46-59 (2007).

[77] Castagnetto JM, Hennessy SW, Roberts VA, Getzoff ED, Tainer JA and Pique ME. MDB: the Metalloprotein Database and Browser at The Scripps Research Institute. Nucleic Acids Res 30: 379-382 (2002).

[78] Kowalik-Jankowska T, Ruta M, Wisniewska K and Lankiewicz L. Coordination abilities of the 1-16 and 1-28 fragments of β-amyloid peptide towards copper(II) ions: a combined potentiometric and spectroscopic study. J Inorg Biochem 95: 270-282 (2003).

[79] Miura T, Suzuki K, Kohata N and Takeuchi H. Metal Binding Modes of Alzheimer's Amyloid β-Peptide in Insoluble Aggregates and Soluble Complexes. Biochemistry 39: 7024-7031 (2000).

[80] Kirschner DA, Abraham C and Selkoe DJ. X-ray diffraction from intraneuronal paired helical filaments and extraneuronal amyloid fibers in Alzheimer disease indicates cross-β conformation. Proc Natl Acad Sci USA 83: 503-507 (1986); Kirschner DA, Inouye H, Duffy LK, Sinclair A, Lind M and Selkoe DJ. Synthetic peptide homologous to β protein from Alzheimer disease forms amyloid-like fibrils *in vitro*. Proc Natl Acad Sci USA 84: 6953-6957 (1987); Sunde M, Serpell LC, Bartlam M, Fraser PE, Bepys MB and Blake CCF. Common core structure of amyloid fibrils by synchrotron x-ray diffraction. J Mol Biol 273: 729-739 (1997); Balbach JJ, Ishii Y, Antzutkin ON, Leapman RD, Rizzo NW, Dyda F, Reed J and Tycko R. Amyloid fibril formation by $A\beta_{16\text{-}22}$, a seven-residue fragment of the Alzheimer's β-amyloid peptide, and structural characterization by solid state NMR. Biochemistry 39: 13748-13759 (2000).

[81] Ma B and Nussinov R. Stabilities and conformations of Alzheimers β -amyloid peptide oligomers ($A\beta_{16\text{-}22}$, $A\beta_{16\text{-}35}$ and $A\beta_{10\text{-}35}$: sequence effects. Proc Natl Acad Sci USA 99: 14126-14131 (2002); Rohrig UF, Laio A, Tantalo N, Parrinello M and Petronzio R. Stability and structure of oligomers of the Alzheimer peptide $A\beta_{16\text{-}22}$: From the dimer to the 32-mer. Biophys J 91: 3217-3229 (2006).

[82] Tickler AK, Smith DG, Ciccotosto GD, Tew DJ, Curtain CC, Carrington D, Masters CL, Bush AI, Cherny RA, Cappa R, Wade JD, Barnham KJ. Methylation of the imidazole side chains of the Alzheimer disease amyloid-beta peptide results in abolition of superoxide dismutase-like structures and inhibition of neurotoxicity. J Biol Chem 280: 13355-13363 (2005).

[83] Minicozzi V, Morante S, Rossi GC, Stellato F, Christian N, Jansen K. The rôle of metals in aggregation. Experiments and *ab initio* simulations. Int J Q Chem 108: 1992-2015 (2008).

[84] Karr JW, Akintoye H, Kaupp LJ, Szalai VA. N-terminal deletions modify the Cu^{2+} binding site in amyloid-beta. Biochemistry 44: 5478-5487 (2005).

[85] Karr JW, Szalai VA. Role of aspartate-1 in Cu(II) binding to the amyloid-beta peptide of Alzheimer's disease. J Am Chem Soc 129: 3796-3797 (2007).

[86] Frank P, Benfatto M, Hedman B, Hodgson KO. The X-ray Absorption Spectroscopic model of the Copper (II) imidazole complex ion in liquid aqueous solution: a strongly solvated square pyramid. Inorganic Chemistry 51: 2086-2096 (2012).

[87] Frank P, Benfatto M, Szilagyi RK, D'Angelo P, Della Longa S, Hodgson KO. The Solution Structure of $[Cu(aq)]^{2+}$ and Its Implications for Rack-Induced Bonding in Blue Copper Protein Active Sites. Inorg Chem 44: 1922-1933 (2005).

[88] Frank P, Benfatto M, Hedman B, Hodgson KO. Solution $[Cu(amm)]^{2+}$ is a strongly solvated square pyramid: a full account of the copper K-edge XAS spectrum within single-electron theory. Inorg Chem 47: 4126-4139 (2008).

[89] Atwood CS, Moir RD, Huang X, Scarpa RC, Bacarra NM, Romano DM, Hartshorn MA, Tanzi RE, Bush AI. Dramatic aggregation of Alzheimer abeta by Cu(II) is induced by conditions representing physiological acidosis. J Biol Chem 273: 12817-12826 (1998).

[90] Atwood CS, Scarpa RC, Huang X, Moir RD, Jones WD, Fairlie DP, Tanzi RE, Bush AI. Characterization of copper interactions with alzheimer amyloid beta peptides: identification of an attomolar-affinity copper binding site on amyloid beta1-42. J Neurochem 75: 1219-1233 (2000).

[91] Faller P, Hureau C. Bioinorganic chemistry of copper and zinc ions coordinated to amyloid-beta peptide. Dalton Trans 21:1080-1094 (2009).

[92] Mantri Y, Fioroni M, Baik MH. Computational study of the binding of CuII to Alzheimer's amyloid-beta peptide: do Abeta42 and Abeta40 bind copper in identical fashion? J Biol Inorg Chem 13:1197-1204 (2009).

[93] Raffa DF, Gomez-Balderas R, Brunelle P, Rickard GA, Rauk A. Ab initio model studies of copper binding to peptides containing a His-His sequence: relevance to the beta-amyloid peptide of Alzheimer's disease. J Biol Inorg Chem 10: 887-902 (2005).

[94] Furlan S, La Penna G. Modeling of the Zn2+ binding in the 1-16 region of the amyloid beta peptide involved in Alzheimer's disease. Phys Chem Chem Phys 11: 6468-6481 (2009).

[95] Peters MB, Yang Y, Wang B, Füsti-Molnár L, Weaver MN, Merz KMJ. Structural Survey of Zinc Containing Proteins and the Development of the Zinc AMBER Force Field (ZAFF). J Chem Theory Comput 6: 2935-2947 (2010).

[96] Siebert X, Eipper BA, Mains RE, Prigge S, Blackburn NJ, Amzel LM. The catalytic copper of peptidylglycine alpha-hydroxylating monooxygenase also plays a critical structural role. Biophys J 89: 3312-3319 (2005).

[97] Strange RW, Antonyuk SV, Hough MA, Doucette PA, Valentine JS, Hasnain SS. Variable metallation of human superoxide dismutase: atomic resolution crystal structures of Cu-Zn, Zn-Zn and as-isolated wild-type enzymes. J Mol Biol 356:1152-1162 (2006).

[98] Allen FH. The Cambridge Structural Database: a quarter of a million crystal structures and rising. Acta Crystallogr Sect. B: Struct Sci. 58: 380-388 (2002).

[99] Giannozzi P, Jansen K, La Penna G, Minicozzi V, Morante S, Rossi GC, Stellato F. Proving metal involvement in beta-amyloid aggregation by ab-initio simulations and XAS measurements. Metallomics 4(2):156-165 (2012).

[100] La Penna G, Morante S, Perico A, Rossi GC. Designing generalized statistical ensembles for numerical simulations of biopolymers. J Chem Phys 121:10725-10741 (2004).
[101] Jorgensen WL, Chandrasekhar J, Madura JD, Impey RW, Klein MJ. Comparison of simple potential functions for simulating liquid water. J Chem Phys 79: 926-935 (1983).
[102] Minicozzi V, Morante S. Is Cu involved in prion oligopeptide stability? Experiments and numerical simulations. Int J Quantum Chem 110: 656-680(2010).

CHAPTER 5

Increased CRMP-2 Phosphorylation is Observed in Alzheimer's Disease: Does This Tell Anything about Disease Development?

Marc P.M. Soutar, Paul Thornhill, Adam R. Cole and Calum Sutherland*

Medical Research Institute, University of Dundee, Ninewells Hospital, Dundee DD1 9SY, Scotland, United Kingdom

Abstract: Collapsin response mediator protein-2 (CRMP-2) is a physiological substrate for GSK3 and Cdk5, two protein kinases suggested to exhibit greater activity in Alzheimer's disease (AD). Indeed, phosphorylation of CRMP-2, at the residues targeted by GSK3 and Cdk5, is relatively high in cortex isolated from human AD brain, as well as in the brains of animal models of AD, while phospho-CRMP-2 is found in neurofibrillary tangles. In mouse models of AD, increased phosphorylation occurs prior to pathology, and abnormal phosphorylation is not seen in other forms of human dementia. Although CRMP-2 has no known enzymatic activity, a great deal of information is appearing on its importance in neuronal development and polarity, as well as in axon growth and guidance. In this mini-review, we examine what is known about CRMP-2 function, how that is controlled by phosphorylation, what alterations in molecular mechanisms could lead to the abnormally high CRMP-2 phosphorylation in AD, and whether this is likely to be specific to AD or occur in other forms of neurodegeneration. This will include discussion of the evidence for increased GSK3 or Cdk5 activity, for decreased phosphatase activity, or the upregulation of other CRMP-2 protein kinases in AD. Importantly, we will compare the processes that may contribute to increased CRMP-2 phosphorylation with those known to increase tau hyperphosphorylation in AD, and whether these are likely to be part of disease development or a useful early marker for AD.

Keywords: Biomarker, collapsin response mediator protein, microtubule transport, neuronal polarity, phosphorylation.

INTRODUCTION

Alzheimer's disease (AD) is characterised by the formation of amyloid plaques (aggregated β amyloid protein cleaved from the amyloid precursor protein) and

***Corresponding author Calum Sutherland:** Medical Research Institute, University of Dundee, Ninewells Hospital, Dundee DD1 9SY, Scotland, United Kingdom; Tel: 01382 383098; E-mail: c.d.sutherland@dundee.ac.uk

D.K. Lahiri (Ed)

neurofibrillary tangles (aggregated Tau in a hyperphosphorylated state) in the brain. For several years, many groups have attempted to establish the molecular mechanisms involved in the development of AD pathology, in order to understand the processes that result in the associated memory and cognitive defects. Many studies have implicated the abnormal regulation of an abundant brain-enriched protein called Collapsin Response Mediator Protein 2 (CRMP-2) in AD pathogenesis and the development of neurofibrillary tangles [1-5]. In this mini-review we summarise what is known about the biology and regulation by phosphorylation of this novel AD associated protein.

COLLAPSIN RESPONSE MEDIATOR PROTEIN

Discovery

CRMP-2 (gene name, DPYSL2) was identified in 1995 as an intracellular component of Semaphorin 3A (Sema3A) growth cone collapse signalling in the chick dorsal root ganglion (DRG) [6]. It is also known as dihydropyrimidinase-related protein (DRP)-2, due to its primary structure having homology to the enzyme that catalyses the second step of pyrimidine degradation. However CRMP-2 has no known catalytic activity [7]. CRMP-2 is a mammalian homologue of the *C.elegans* gene *unc-33* [8]. Loss or mutation of *unc-33* results in axonal growth and guidance defects, as well as protein sorting [9], which severely attenuate the movement of the worm. Three other CRMP family members have been identified in mammals (CRMP-1, CRMP-3, and CRMP-4) although CRMP-2 remains the most extensively characterised family member to date. More recently, a CRMP3-associated protein (CRAM) was designated as a fifth member of the family (now termed CRMP5) [10]. The CRMP isoforms 1 through 4 share >68% cDNA sequence identity, whereas CRMP-5 is more phylogenetically divergent (Table **1**), and CRMP-2 has 51.9% DNA sequence identity to dihydropyrimidinase (58% identity at the protein level). Meanwhile, CRMP-2 is highly conserved from rodents to man (Table **1**), with 33% sequence identity between human CRMP2 and *unc-33* cDNA.

Table 1: **A**- Percentage sequence identities (cDNA) between CRMP family members and dihydropyrimidinase (DPYS). **B**- CRMP2 percentage sequence identities (cDNA/protein) between human, mouse, rat and *C.elegans*.

A

	CRMP1	CRMP2	CRMP3	CRMP4	CRMP5	DPYS
CRMP1	-	73.9	68.5	71.0	55.4	52.2
CRMP2	73.9	-	71.6	72.7	56.0	51.9
CRMP3	68.5	71.6	-	67.9	57.3	53.3
CRMP4	71.0	72.7	67.9	-	55.4	52.4
CRMP5	55.4	56.0	57.3	55.4	-	56.9
DPYS	52.2	51.9	53.3	52.4	56.9	-

B

	hCRMP2 cDNA/prot	mCRMP2 cDNA/prot	rCRMP2 cDNA/prot	Unc-33 cDNA/prot
hCRMP2	-	91/99	91/98	33/37
mCRMP2	91/99	-	96/100	34/35
rCRMP2	91/98	96/100	-	35/36
Unc-33	33/37	34/34	35/36	-

Structure and Expression

CRMP isoforms are found exclusively as homo- and hetero-tetramers [7, 11-14], and each CRMP can exist as at least two variants due to differential use of first exons, with the A-isoform having an N-terminal extension resulting in a larger protein product (approximately 73kDa) than the B-isoform (the predominant isoform), which has an apparent Mol Wt of approximately 62kDa [15]. CRMP's are expressed in post-mitotic neurons [16, 17], however each isoform displays variations in spatial and temporal expression throughout the adult brain and during development [18]. For example, CRMP-2 is highly expressed in the cerebellum, hippocampus and hypothalamus in late stage embryos, declining somewhat after birth, while CRMP3 mRNA expression is enriched in cerebellum, with high levels persisting through to adulthood [16-18]. Interestingly, in adult brain, CRMP2 and CRMP4 account for approximately 1% and 0.4% of total triton X100 soluble brain protein, respectively (MS unpublished data). In the worm,

Unc-33 is expressed in axonal processes from early embryogenesis through larval and adult stages [18]. Similarly, mammalian CRMPs are predominantly expressed within the brain, although expression has been reported in peripheral tissues such as the testis (CRMP-1, 4 and 5), monocytes during maturation (CRMP-2), lung tissue (CRMP-2, mRNA only) and T lymphocytes [19] (reviewed in [20]).

Immunocytochemical studies in hippocampal and dorsal root ganglion (DRG) neurones indicate CRMP-2 is distributed throughout the cell body and axonal processes with higher levels of staining in growth cones and the distal axon [21-24]. CRMP-2 is enriched at the centre of the growth cone, in close proximity to microtubules and actin, whereas CRMP-2 phosphorylated at the C-terminal region, has a more punctate staining throughout the growth cone and filopodia [24]. Gauchy and colleagues found distinct intracellular distributions of CRMP-1, -2A, -2B and -5, dependent on cell type and developmental stage [25]. In cortical neurons CRMP-1 is distributed throughout the cell body and within neuronal shafts and actin-rich protrusions on dendritic processes [26], while in chick DRG neurons it is localised mainly in the proximal axonal shafts of growth cones [27]. In chick DRG neurons, CRMP-4 (TUC-4) is expressed at high levels both along neurites and throughout growth cones however the long isoform of CRMP-4A (TUC-4b) has a more restricted expression, concentrated in the growth cones. Within the growth cone itself, CRMP-4A is associated with vesicles in the central region, whereas CRMP-4B (shorter isoform) is expressed throughout the growth cone and filopodia [28].

Function

Since CRMP proteins have no known catalytic activity their potential functions are inferred from knockout/overexpression studies, or through their interaction with proteins of known function. Neurons injected with antibodies to CRMP-2 no longer exhibit a response to Sema 3A (originally known as collapsin) [6]. Meanwhile, overexpression of CRMP-2 in mammalian primary neurons or neuroblastoma cells, induces axon or neurite outgrowth, respectively, and can induce the formation of more than one axon [2, 21, 22]. More recently a critical role for CRMP-2 was demonstrated in CNP/cGMP regulation of axonal development [29]. This suggests an important general function in neurite growth and guidance as well as neuronal polarity. In accordance, mutation of *unc-33*, the *C. elegans* homologue of CRMP2, impairs axonal outgrowth in chemosensory neurons [8], while CRMP-2 binds to α/β tubulin heterodimers in preference to preformed microtubules (10 times higher affinity) and promotes the oligomerization of tubulin heterodimers to form microtubules *in vitro* [30-32]. However, it is not yet known if CRMP-2 can bind pre-formed microtubules and stabilize their structural integrity *in vivo*, in a similar fashion to other microtubule-associated proteins, such as Tau and MAP-2 [31]. CRMP-2 can also associate with the kinesin network to facilitate anterograde protein cargo transport along microtubules [32, 33].

Another function ascribed to CRMP is the regulation of surface expression of cell adhesion molecules. CRMP-2 binds to Numb, a carrier protein for the cell adhesion molecule, L1 [34]. L1 co-localizes with the NP-1 receptor, which regulates the internalization of L1 during growth cone modulation [34]. Endocytosis of L1 promotes its accumulation in the cytoplasm. Subsequent association with Numb, and transportation along the microtubule network *via* a kinesin/CRMP-2 complex, allows it to be recycled back into the neuronal growth cone [35]. The sra-1/WAVE complex, which is required for regulation of the actin cytoskeleton during lamellipodia formation, is also transported along the microtubule network in a CRMP-2 and kinesin-dependent manner [31, 33]. CRMP-2 is bidirectionally regulated by N-type voltage-gated Ca(2+) channels (CaV2.2) [36, 37], while presynaptically CRMP-2 interacts with hippocampal cholinergic neurostimulating peptide (HCNP), a protein involved in the synthesis of acetyl choline [38]. Finally CRMP-2 was recently found to be critical for formation of primary cilia in fibroblasts [39]. Therefore CRMP-2 appears crucial to the integrity of many polarized cell structures.

Regulation

CRMP-2 is a phosphoprotein but has also been found to contain O-linked N-acetyl glucosamine [3, 40] and to be oxidised [41]. The posttranslational modification of the other CRMP isoforms is less well characterised, however many of the known phosphorylated motifs found in CRMP-2 are conserved, particularly in CRMP1 and CRMP-4, Fig. (**1**).

	509 514 518 522
CRMP1	$_{504}$**YEVPATPKYATPAPSAKS*S*PSKHQ**$_{527}$
CRMP2	$_{504}$**CEVSVTPKTVTPASSAKT*S*PAKQQ**$_{527}$
CRMP3	$_{504}$**HEVMVPAKPGSGAPARASCPGKIS**$_{527}$
CRMP4	$_{504}$**FDLTTTPKGGTPAGSTRG*S*PTRPN**$_{527}$
CRMP5	$_{504}$**KKEMGTPLADTPTRPVTRHGGMRD**$_{527}$

Figure 1: Human CRMP isoform sequence alignments (residues 504–527). Residues confirmed as GSK3 phosphorylation sites within this region are underlined, while the priming site is in *italic*.

The protein tyrosine kinase Fes/Fps can complex with CRMP family members [42]. CRMP-2 and the distant relative, CRMP-5, can be phosphorylated by Fes *in vitro* and when co-expressed in cells [42], while Sema 3A can alter the phospho-tyrosine status of CRMP-2 and CRMP-5 in neurons, as well as regulate Fes/Fps activity. This suggests a pathway from Sema 3A to CRMP through Fes, however the exact residues targeted by the tyrosine kinase remain to be determined, along with the stoichiometry of phosphorylation or the effect of mutation of the targeted tyrosine. In addition, the Fes related kinase Fer, can phosphorylate CRMP-2 *in vitro* and is regulated by Sema 3A [43], but again the exact details of the phosphorylation are not known. Interestingly, Fes/Fps/Fer may actually lie downstream of CRMP-2, since their activity can be reduced by expression of CRMP-2 [43]. The phosphorylation of CRMP-5 may mediate its interaction with the neuronal glycine transporter GlyT2, since phosphatase inhibitors increase the complex formation in cells [44].

Kaibuchi and colleagues established that CRMP-2 is phosphorylated by Rho kinase at Thr555 *in vitro* and in co-expression studies, while this modification occurs in response to LPA treatment of neurons [45]. Importantly, inhibitors of Rho kinase or dominant negative Rho kinase mutants that block Thr555 phosphorylation, also reduce LPA induced growth cone collapse, while mutation of Thr555 to alanine reduces LPA regulation of growth cone collapse. In contrast, Sema3A treatment of cells does not regulate Thr555 phosphorylation and inhibition of Rho kinase has no effect on growth cone collapse induced by this agent [45]. This suggests a role for Rho kinase and Thr555 phosphorylation in LPA but not Sema3A induced growth cone collapse.

The phosphorylation of a C-terminal domain of CRMP-2 was first identified in protein isolated from neurofibrillary tangles [3, 5]. Glycogen Synthase Kinase 3 (GSK3) was then identified as the kinase responsible for phosphorylation of CRMP1, 2 and 4 at Ser518, Thr514 and Thr509 *in vitro* and *in vivo* [2, 27, 46]. GSK3 will phosphorylate CRMP-1, 2 and 4 *in vitro*, while phosphorylation of these residues in cells exposed to any one of several different selective inhibitors of GSK3 is greatly reduced ([46] and CS unpublished data). Finally, IGF-1 induced dephosphorylation of these sites is lost in neurons that express a form of GSK3 that is insensitive to IGF-1 [47]. GSK3 is relatively active in cells, however most GSK3 substrates require prior phosphorylation by another protein kinase in order to be phosphorylated efficiently by GSK3; a process known as priming. Neurons lacking Cyclin Dependant Kinase 5 (Cdk5) express CRMP1 and CRMP-2 that are poorly phosphorylated at the GSK3 target sites [46]. However CRMP-4 phosphorylation is normal in the absence of Cdk5. Cdk5 will phosphorylate CRMP1, 2 and 4 at Ser522 *in vitro*, priming for subsequent phosphorylation by GSK3, Fig. (**2**). In addition, CRMP-2 interacts with Cdk5 and alpha2-chimaerin, and this complex is required for Sema 3A induced growth cone collapse [23]. The α2-chimaerin regulates bipolar transition and neuronal migration through modulating the activity of CRMP-2 [48].

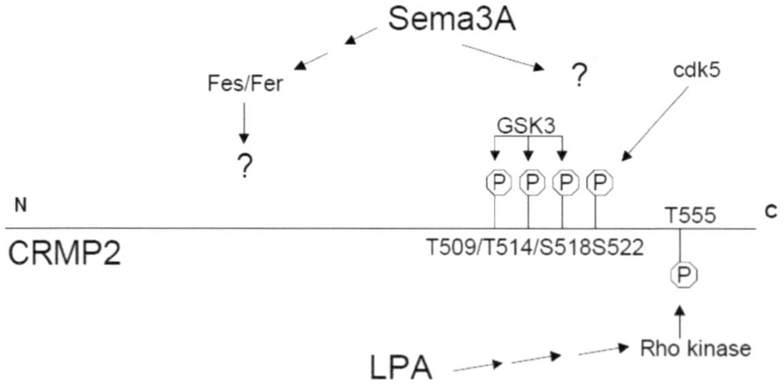

Figure 2: Independent mechanisms of growth cone collapse, mediated through phosphorylation of CRMP-2. Lysophosphatidic acid (LPA) can induce axon growth cone collapse *via* activation of Rho kinase and its subsequent phosphorylation of CRMP-2 at Thr555. This phosphorylation of CRMP-2 does not occur during Sema3A induced growth cone collapse. Sema3A signalling in neurons is not fully understood, however it is postulated to involve the activation of several kinases and the phosphorylation of CRMP-2 at Ser522 (Cdk5), Ser518, Thr514, and Thr509 (GSK3), as well as undefined tyrosine residues (Fer/Fes).

All of the above data argues that Cdk5 primes CRMP1 and 2 at Ser522 *in vivo* but that it is not required for the priming of CRMP-4. Interestingly, Dual Specificity Tyrosine phosphorylation Regulated Kinase (DYRK) can prime CRMP-4 *in vitro* (but not CRMP-2) allowing subsequent phosphorylation of Ser518, Thr514 and Thr509 by GSK3 [46], however it has yet to be confirmed whether DYRK is required for priming *in vivo*.

Neurons are polarized cells possessing a single axon and many dendrites. Over expression of CRMP-2 in primary neurons and neuroblastoma cells altered axon elongation [2, 22] and induced the development of multiple axons from previously established dendrites [21]. Overexpression of truncated CRMP-2 (DC381 or DC350), lacking the C-terminus (including the GSK3 and Cdk5 phosphorylation sites), suppressed axon growth, suggesting that this region is key to the stimulatory effects of CRMP-2 on axonal growth [21, 31]. The overexpression of a non-phosphorylatable point mutant of CRMP-2 in neurons had distinct effects on axon growth compared to wild-type protein, and regulation of axon growth by GSK3 is altered when CRMP-2 is removed [49], establishing the importance of phosphorylation of CRMP-2 by Cdk5 and GSK3 in this function of the protein [2, 50]. The exact molecular mechanisms underlying this effect are not yet clear, although it is reasonable to predict that phosphorylation of CRMP-2 will regulate its ability to bind to a protein vital for microtubule reorganisation or transport. For example, a CRMP-2 Ser514Asp mutant (that mimics phosphorylation at this site [51]) has lower CRMP-2/tubulin binding stoichiometry compared to wild type CRMP-2 (0.05 and 0.3 mol/mol respectively) [50]. Alternatively, phosphorylation of CRMP-2 by Cdk5/GSK3 might regulate the release of cargo from the CRMP-2/kinesin transport complex at the appropriate location (*e.g.* tubulin, L1). Indeed, phosphorylated forms of CRMP-2 are enriched at the distal tips of elongating axons [50], and are increased by stimulation of cells with extracellular cell growth guidance molecules, such as Sema3A [23, 27, 46]. Similarly, the CNP/cGMP regulation of axonal development also requires the phosphorylation of CRMP-2 by GSK3 [29], and the interaction of CRMP-2 with HCNP is regulated in a reciprocal fashion by phosphorylation at Ser522 and Thr514 [38] while the CRMP-2/CaV2.2 interaction is regulated by Ser522 phosphorylation [37]. Finally, the regulation of primary cilia formation in fibroblasts by CRMP-2 is also controlled by GSK3 [39].

Of course, the full compliment of CRMP-2 (and other CRMP isoforms) binding proteins is not yet known and this would be of great benefit in elucidating the precise mechanisms that CRMP-2 uses to control cell structure. We recently reported a method for enriching and identifying CRMP-2 and CRMP-4 binding proteins that were specifically regulated by the phosphorylation of CRMP by GSK3 [52]. In this preliminary analysis, b-tubulin was confirmed as a dephospho-CRMP-2 and CRMP-4 binding protein, while novel proteins were also identified.

CRMP and Alzheimer's Disease

Neurofibrillary tangles (NFT) are a pathological feature of a number of neurodegenerative disorders, including Alzheimer's diseases (AD), Pick's disease (PiD), progressive supranuclear palsy and familial frontotemporal dementia and parkinsonism linked to chromosome 17 (FTDP-17) (for review see [53]). NFT's consist primarily of hyperphosphorylated tau. Interestingly, the antibody 3F4, raised against purified preparations of NFT's from cortices of AD patients, reacts strongly with CRMP-2 [5]. The 3F4 epitope was later found to encompass the phosphorylated C-terminal residues Thr509, Ser518 and Ser522 of CRMP-2 [3]. More recently, CRMP-2 was shown to be hyperphosphorylated at residues Thr509, Thr514, Ser518 and Ser522 in protein lysates (Triton X100-soluble fraction) generated from both human AD cortex (Table **2**) and animal models of AD (Table **3**), while the expression and phosphorylation of CRMP-4 was not altered [54]. This demonstrated that not only was phospho-CRMP-2 present in tangles, but the relative level of phosphorylation of CRMP-2 actually increases in brain areas associated with AD pathology.

CRMP2 phosphorylation is also increased in cortices and hippocampi from double transgenic (PS1 (M146V) KI; Thy1.2-APP (swe) - develop plaques) and triple transgenic mice (PS1 (M146V) KI; Thy1.2- APP (swe); Thy1.2tau (P301L) - develop plaques and tangles), but not in Tg2576 APP(swe)/ABAD (develop plaques) and P301L or P301S tau mutant mice (develop tangles) (Table **3**). These data suggest it is the increase in APP expression and proteolytic processing by PS-1 that leads to CRMP-2 hyperphosphorylation. Consistent with this, mice that over-express the amyloid intracellular C terminal domain (AICD) with Fe65 also

Table 2: CRMP phosphorylation in animal models of Alzheimer's disease. An increase in CRMP2 phosphorylation is observed in models possessing increased Cdk5 activity or increased APP processing (details in Cole *et al.* 2007).

Protein	Phosphorylation Sites Analysed (Probable Kinases)	Analysis in AD Tissue	Other Neuro-Degenerative Conditions
CRMP2	T509/514 (GSK3) S522 (Cdk5)	Increased 1.4 fold in AD frontal cortex Increased 2.0 fold in AD frontal cortex	Not changed in frontotemporal lobar degeneration associated with mutations in MAPT or with Pick bodies
CRMP4	T509 (GSK3) S522 (DYRK)	No change in AD frontal cortex No change in AD frontal cortex	Not Determined
tau	Up to 45 different phosphorylation sites have been identified including clusters described below: 202-217 (multiple including PKA, CaMKII/Cdk5/GSK3/CK-I) 231-238 (multiple including PKA, CaMKII/Cdk5/GSK3) S262/S356 (BRSK/ CaMKII/Cdk5/GSK3/CK-I) S396/T403/S404 (multiple including PKA, CaMKII/Cdk5/GSK3)	All phosphosites are present in PHF/AD tissue. Overall tau phosphorylation increases from around 3 to 9 mol/mol in AD tissue compared to control. 231 increases in CSF from AD	Increased overall phosphorylation can been seen in all tauopathies. 202 and 217 increased in Progressive Supranuclear Palsy (PSP) 231 and 235 increased in PSP little change in Pick Bodies 396 increased in PSP

exhibit CRMP-2 hyperphosphorylation [4]. The increase in CRMP-2 phosphorylation (at the GSK3-sites) in the double and triple transgenic mice was 1.5 - 2 fold higher than control brains, similar to that observed in human AD. In healthy brain, 30 - 50% of neuronal CRMP-2 is phosphorylated at Ser518 and Thr514/509 (MS, unpublished data), suggesting phosphorylation in AD may be reaching its maximum. Importantly, hyperphosphorylation in the double and triple transgenic mice was detected at 2 months of age, well before plaque or tangle formation, therefore, like tau hyperphosphorylation, it may be an early event in AD pathogenesis [54]. It is reasonable to speculate that the same upstream signalling events initiated during early AD development, lead to the abnormal phosphorylation of both tau and CRMP-2. As such, both of these protein modifications represent potential points for early diagnosis of molecular development of AD, prior to any pathology and hence neurodegeneration.

Table 3: CRMP phosphorylation in animal models of Alzheimer's disease.

	Genotype	Phenotype	CRMP2 Phosphorylation	Brain Region
Tg2576 Single Transgenic	Express a mutated form of human APP (APP695, K670M, N671L - Swedish mutation)	Long-term potentiation deficits, with synaptic, cognitive, and memory dysfunction (5 months). Plaques (12–18 months)	No change in phosphorylation at Thr509/514	Cortex Hippocampus
TASTPM	Tg2576 plus mutated form of Presenilin-1 (M146V); (Component of γ secretase complex)	Similar spectrum as above but more severe.	Phosphorylation at Thr509/514 and Ser522 is significantly increased.	Cortex Hippocampus
Triple Transgenic	TASTPM plus expression of mutant tau (Thy1.2-tauP301L).	Exhibits both plaque (6-9 m) and NFT pathology (10-18 m). Displays multiple neurological deficits.	Phosphorylation at Thr509/514 and Ser522 is significantly increased.	Cortex Hippocampus
APP/ABAD	Mice over-express mutated forms of human APP (APP695, 751/APP770, K670M/N671L) and ABAD	Learning and memory dysfunction at 5 months of age. Increased levels of Aβ in cortex at 3 months	No change in phosphorylation at Thr509/514	Cortex
Human Tau Mutants	P301L and P301S	Display mild to severe NFT pathology	No change in phosphorylation at Thr509/514	Cortex Hippocampus
GSK3β Over-expression	Insertion of tet-off GSK3β gene in brain. Removal of tetracycline results in over-expression of GSK3β.	Increased levels of phosphorylated tau and AD like pre-tangles. No neurodegeneration or motor deficits.	No change in phosphorylation at Thr509/514	Hippocampus
GSK3α/β Ser21/9 Ala Knock-in	Ser21 (GSK3alpha) and Ser9 (GSK3beta) mutated to Ala. GSK3 expressed normally but cannot be regulated by growth factors/insulin.	No neurodegeneration or motor deficits. Normal neuronal development.	No change in phosphorylation at Thr509/514	Whole Brain
p25-Tg Over-expression	33% over-expression of the p25 Cdk5 subunit, increases endogenous Cdk5 activity.	Increase in tau phosphorylation in old but not young mice. No neurodegeneration or motor deficits.	Phosphorylation at Thr509/514 and Ser522 is significantly increased	Hippocampus

SIMILARITIES BETWEEN TAU AND CRMP

Tau is a brain-enriched, microtubule associated protein that is expressed in adult brain as 6 alternatively spliced isoforms from a single gene. In normal brain, tau contains 2-3 moles of phosphate per mole of tau. In AD brain, where over 30 phosphorylation sites have been identified [55, 56], there is an increase of phosphate to around 9-10 mol/ mol of tau [57], similar to the level found in fetal tau [58]. This abnormal phosphorylation of tau in adult brain is proposed to alter its conformation resulting in dissociation from the microtubules, although it remains possible that release of tau from microtubules by a distinct mechanism, may result in subsequent abnormal phosphorylation of the protein in the cytoplasm. That said, the binding of tau clearly stabilises microtubules *in vitro* and in cells, while phosphorylation of tau by kinases including Cdk5, GSK3 and DYRK, promotes its release from microtubules to allow dynamic rearrangement of neurite structure/morphology [59]. Loss of the stabilizing interaction between tau and microtubules is thought to weaken the structural integrity of microtubules and the neurites they support, impairing the efficiency of communication between neurons. In addition, excessive/abnormal phosphorylation converts the normally soluble tau into an insoluble form that promotes aggregation into paired helical filaments within the cell cytoplasm, the primary constituent of NFT's [60, 61]. Alzheimer-related changes in activity of several tau kinases have been reported, including GSK3, Cdk5, DYRK, cAMP-dependent protein kinase (PKA) and p38 MAP kinase (for review see [62]), and most of these can be linked to the development of NFT like structures [61]. Thus, the finer details of the causes of tau hyperphosphorylation in AD, its influence on microtubule stability and NFT formation remain incomplete.

Therefore, tau and CRMP-2 have striking functional and pathological similarities in that both regulate polymerization/stability of microtubules [31, 63], both respond to the growth cone guidance molecule Sema3A [46, 64], and they are both phosphorylated by Cdk5 and GSK3, negatively regulating their ability to bind to tubulin [2, 12, 27, 52, 53, 65]. In addition, abnormal phosphorylation of these two structural proteins is associated with the development of AD (Tables **2** and **3**).

DEFECTIVE SIGNALLING UPSTREAM OF TAU AND CRMP-2 IN AD

GSK- 3 and Cdk5

Several studies have implicated alterations in the activity and/or expression levels of Cdk5 [66] and GSK3 [67, 68] in AD that might account for the high phosphorylation of CRMP2 in this disease. However, in GSK3β over expressing mice and GSK3α/β knock-in (Ser21/9Ala) mice, we found no evidence of hyperphosphorylation of CRMP-2 at the GSK3 phosphorylation sites, Thr509, 514, and Ser518 [46]. This suggests that an increase in GSK3 activity or loss of negative regulation of GSK3 is insufficient to increase CRMP-2 phosphorylation (Table **3**). Similarly, phosphorylation of tau does not increase in concert with GSK3 activity [69, 70]. Therefore, priming of CRMP-2 by Cdk5 at Ser522 (and potentially tau at an unidentified site), prior to GSK3 phosphorylation, is a limiting factor. Consistent with this, CRMP2 is also hyperphosphorylated at the Cdk5 priming site (Ser522) in human AD cortex and in the double and triple Tg mouse models. Together, these observations suggest that increased GSK3 activity is unlikely to be the single cause of CRMP-2 or tau hyperphosphorylation in AD. Cdk5 activity could be increased following abnormal processing of APP, accumulation of Aβ oligomers, a subsequent increase in the calcium concentration within neurons, calpain induction, and the cleavage of the Cdk5 regulatory subunit p35 (required for Cdk5 activity) to p25 [71]. p25 retains the ability to bind to Cdk5, however this cleavage disrupts its membrane anchorage *via* removal of the myristoylation sequence thereby increasing and prolonging Cdk5 activation (p25 has a half life 5-fold higher than p35) [66]. CRMP-2 phosphorylation increases at both the Cdk5 site (Ser522), as well as the GSK3 sites Ser518, Thr514, and Thr509, in transgenic mice overexpressing p25 [54]. Therefore, induced or dysregulated activity of Cdk5 is sufficient to increase phosphorylation of CRMP-2. That said, we could find no evidence for significant changes in Cdk5 activity or Cdk5/p25/p35 expression levels in the mouse models of AD that displayed hyperphosphorylation of CRMP-2 [54].

CRMP-2 Phosphatases

Protein phosphorylation is a reversible event, regulated by the balance of the activity of protein kinases *and* protein phosphatases. Therefore, lower activity or expression of the phosphoserine/threonine phosphatase (PPase) responsible for removing phosphate from these residues on CRMP-2 and/or tau would lead to the increased phosphorylation of these proteins in AD. There are 4 major classes of mammalian serine/threonine phosphatases (PP1, PP2A, PP2B and PP2C) and several minor classes (*e.g.* PP5), ubiquitously expressed within the brain (reviewed in [72]). PP1, PP2B and PP5 have the ability to dephosphorylate many tau epitopes *in vitro*, however PP2A appears to be the major phosphatase responsible for the dephosphorylation of key AD-related tau phosphorylation sites *in vivo* [73], while down regulation of PP2A activity has been proposed as a major factor in the development of AD [74].

In contrast, the PP1 family is the major PPase class involved in the dephosphorylation of Ser518, Thr514, and Thr509 of CRMP-2 *in vitro* and *in vivo* [47]. Interestingly, the Cdk5 site (Ser522) is relatively resistant to dephosphorylation *in vitro* by any of these major PPase classes [47]. This is likely to be due to the presence of basic lysine residues located at positions -2 (Ser520) and +3 (Ser525) of the priming site, promoting an ionic interaction with the phosphorylated Ser522, and stabilising the phosphorylation. Interestingly, pThr231 and pSer404 on tau lie in a similar sequence, with a +3 basic residue, and both of these phosphorylated residues are resistant to dephosphorylation *in vitro*, even with PP2A [47]. It is possible to reduce Ser522 phosphorylation in cells by incubation with a Cdk5 inhibitor [47], therefore a phospho-Ser522 PPase activity is present in cells. This may be a highly specific and/or rare PPase, or alternatively the activity may require the presence of a PPase cofactor. For example, the peptidyl prolyl isomerase Pin1 binds to phosphorylated tau at phosphoThr231Pro232, altering its conformation resulting in an increase in dephosphorylation [75, 76]. However, loss of Pin1, or overexpression of active Pin1, has no effect on Ser522 phosphorylation *in vivo* or in cells [47]. The identification of the Ser522 PPase (which may also target Thr231 and Ser404 in Tau) would provide a novel target for reversing the abnormal phosphorylation of CRMP-2 observed in AD, and help establish the importance of the modification in the disease process.

Novel AD Associated CRMP-2 and Tau Kinases

It is quite possible that Ser522 kinase(s) other than Cdk5 become up regulated in AD and are responsible for shifting the balance of Ser522 phosphorylation.

Microglial cells have many supportive functions within the brain, one of which is the release of pro-inflammatory cytokines involved in an immune response. Aβ accumulation within the brain causes persistent activation of these cells and the generation of Reactive Oxygen Species (ROS), both of which have been implicated in the pathogenesis of AD (reviewed in [77]). There are several lines of evidence for the activation of stress-activated protein kinase(s) (*e.g.* p38 MAPK or JNK) and mitogenic pathways (*e.g.* ERK), subsequent to the production of Aβ (reviewed in [78]). p38 MAPK, JNK and ERK are all proline directed Ser/ Thr protein kinases of the mitogen activated protein kinase family, and are therefore Ser522 kinase candidates. It will be of interest to establish whether inhibitors of these pathways block the increase in Ser522 phosphorylation associated with the development of AD, or whether Ser522 phosphorylation is a general marker of neuronal inflammation.

CRMP PHOSPHORYLATION IN OTHER NEURODEGENERATIVE DISORDERS

Hyperphosphorylation of tau has been reported in a number of neurodegenerative disorders in addition to AD (Table **3**), in particular in tauopathies such as Progressive Supranuclear Palsy (PSP) [79] and FTDP-17 (see [80] for recent review). The measurement of tau (phosphorylation and amount) in CSF samples may be beneficial for the differential diagnosis of vascular dementia and fronto-temperal dementia, and could contribute to a diagnosis of mild cognitive impairment (MCI) [81]. Although PHF-tau phosphorylation analysis in CSF [81] or post-mortem tissue [82] is not, on its own, able to predict MCI, high phosphorylation of Thr231 of tau correlates with cross over from MCI to AD [83, 84].

Increased phosphorylation of CRMP2 is a relatively early characteristic of certain animal models of AD [54], therefore it will be of great interest to examine human post-mortem and CSF samples to establish whether this modification will be of use in the diagnosis of MCI. However, as yet we have not observed any increase in CRMP2 phosphorylation in other forms of neurodegeneration including other tauopathies [85]. This suggests that CRMP2 hyperphosphorylation could be a more specific marker of AD than tau hyperphosphorylation, and may provide a means for differential diagnosis of the tauopathies. In that case it is unlikely to be a marker of MCI, other than in patients likely to go on to AD.

CRMP expression/stability is also linked to specific forms of neurodegeneration. Abnormal CRMP2, CRMP3 and CRMP4 expression has been reported in embryonic Downs Syndrome brain [86], while CRMP2 expression is dramatically altered in a mouse expressing the neuroprotective slow Wallerian degeneration (Wld(s)) gene [87]. However overexpression of a CRMP2 mutant that cannot undergo phosphorylation provides greater neuroprotection in the Wlds model than wild type CRMP-2 [88] suggesting phosphorylation also contributes to this function of CRMP-2. Abnormal CRMP2 processing resulting in increases in a truncated form of CRMP (58kDa) have been found in ischemic brain [89] and traumatic brain injury [90], while this truncation may be reduced in Mesial Temporal Epilepsy [91]. Glutamate induces calpain mediated cleavage of the C-terminus of CRMP-2 [92] and CRMP-4 [93], which reduces kinesin transport of the NR2B subunit of the NMDA receptor along the microtubule network, affecting its appearance at the cell surface [92, 93]. It is hypothesised that this is a protective mechanism against glutamate toxicity [92]. The exact location of the proteolytic cleavage has not yet been reported however the size of the truncated protein would predict that it will lie very close to the Thr509-Ser522 phosphorylation domain. It remains to be seen whether phosphorylation affects the truncation of CRMPs.

FUTURE PERSPECTIVES

Alzheimer's disease is a progressive neuronal disorder of old-age, making it extremely difficult to study in humans. Indeed, it remains rather difficult to even diagnose accurately in its early stages and one of the major goals of AD research is to develop accurate and specific markers of early disease. Whether the multiple protein modifications and accumulations observed in pathological structures of AD contribute to disease progression or constitute responses to the molecular changes ongoing remains unclear. Clearly the answer to this question dictates whether such modifications are markers of disease or potential therapeutic targets.

The abnormal phosphorylation of specific members of the CRMP family (CRMP-1 and CRMP-2) in human AD, as well as in specific models of AD, may represent a symptom of the disease. As such, its early appearance, prior to cognitive decline, suggests that it, or the processes that lead to its abnormal modification (*e.g.* increased kinase or decreased PPase) are candidate markers for early diagnosis. Indeed, a complete understanding of the signalling processes that lead to the abnormal modification of CRMP-2 (and similar phosphorylation motifs such as on tau) will provide clues as to the initial molecular pathology of this disorder. Alternatively, due to the important role that CRMP-2 plays in neuronal polarity and axon guidance, one could envision a contribution of abnormal CRMP-2 regulation to the severity of neurodegeneration associated with AD. In that case, CRMP-2 function itself would be a worthwhile target for intervention.

In summary, CRMP-2 is a phosphoprotein, recently identified as abnormally regulated in human brain during AD but not other tauopathies, as well as in the brain of animals expressing human proteins associated with the development of AD pathology. As such it represents a novel and potentially specific marker of AD, and a complete understanding of its regulation should provide key information on the signalling processes that are responsible for disease progression.

ACKNOWLEDGEMENT

MS is the recipient of a Medical Research Council Capacity Building Studentship, while research in the lab of CS is primarily supported by the Alzheimer's Research UK and Diabetes UK.

CONFLICT OF INTEREST

Declared None.

DISCLOSURE

This chapter is an update of our previous publication in CAR "Increased CRMP2 Phosphorylation is Observed in Alzheimer's Disease; Does this Tell us Anything About Disease Development?" published in 'CAR', Volume 6, Number 3, June, pp. 269 to 278.

REFERENCES

[1] Cole AR, Astell A, Green C, and Sutherland C, Molecular connexions between dementia and diabetes. Neurosci Biobehav Rev 31(7): p. 1046-63 2007.

[2] Cole AR, Knebel A, Morrice NA, Robertson LA, Irving AJ, Connolly CN, *et al.*, GSK-3 phosphorylation of the Alzheimer epitope within collapsin response mediator proteins regulates axon elongation in primary neurons. J Biol Chem 279(48): p. 50176-80 2004.

[3] Gu Y, Hamajima N, and Ihara Y, Neurofibrillary tangle-associated collapsin response mediator protein-2 (CRMP-2) is highly phosphorylated on Thr-509, Ser-518, and Ser-522. Biochemistry 39(15): p. 4267-75 2000.

[4] Ryan KA and Pimplikar SW, Activation of GSK-3 and phosphorylation of CRMP2 in transgenic mice expressing APP intracellular domain. J Cell Biol 171(2): p. 327-35 2005.

[5] Yoshida H, Watanabe A, and Ihara Y, Collapsin response mediator protein-2 is associated with neurofibrillary tangles in Alzheimer's disease. J Biol Chem 273(16): p. 9761-8 1998.

[6] Goshima Y, Nakamura F, Strittmatter P, and Strittmatter SM, Collapsin-induced growth cone collapse mediated by an intracellular protein related to UNC-33. Nature 376(6540): p. 509-14 1995.

[7] Wang LH and Strittmatter SM, Brain CRMP forms heterotetramers similar to liver dihydropyrimidinase. J Neurochem 69(6): p. 2261-9 1997.

[8] Hedgecock EM, Culotti JG, Thomson JN, and Perkins LA, Axonal guidance mutants of Caenorhabditis elegans identified by filling sensory neurons with fluorescein dyes. Dev Biol 111(1): p. 158-70 1985.

[9] Maniar TA, Kaplan M, Wang GJ, Shen K, Wei L, Shaw JE, *et al.*, UNC-33 (CRMP) and ankyrin organize microtubules and localize kinesin to polarize axon-dendrite sorting. Nat Neurosci 15(1): p. 48-56 2012.

[10] Inatome R, Tsujimura T, Hitomi T, Mitsui N, Hermann P, Kuroda S, *et al.*, Identification of CRAM, a novel unc-33 gene family protein that associates with CRMP3 and protein-tyrosine kinase(s) in the developing rat brain. J Biol Chem 275(35): p. 27291-302 2000.

[11] Deo RC, Schmidt EF, Elhabazi A, Togashi H, Burley SK, and Strittmatter SM, Structural bases for CRMP function in plexin-dependent semaphorin3A signaling. Embo J 23(1): p. 9-22 2004.

[12] Li T, Hawkes C, Qureshi HY, Kar S, and Paudel HK, Cyclin-dependent protein kinase 5 primes microtubule-associated protein tau site-specifically for glycogen synthase kinase 3beta. Biochemistry 45(10): p. 3134-45 2006.

[13] Majava V, Loytynoja N, Chen WQ, Lubec G, and Kursula P, Crystal and solution structure, stability and post-translational modifications of collapsin response mediator protein 2. Febs J 2008.

[14] Ponnusamy R and Lohkamp B, Insights into the oligomerization of CRMPs: crystal structure of human collapsin response mediator protein 5. J Neurochem 2013.

[15] Yuasa-Kawada J, Suzuki R, Kano F, Ohkawara T, Murata M, and Noda M, Axonal morphogenesis controlled by antagonistic roles of two CRMP subtypes in microtubule organization. Eur J Neurosci 17(11): p. 2329-43 2003.

[16] Minturn JE, Fryer HJ, Geschwind DH, and Hockfield S, TOAD-64, a gene expressed early in neuronal differentiation in the rat, is related to unc-33, a C. elegans gene involved in axon outgrowth. J Neurosci 15(10): p. 6757-66 1995.

[17] Minturn JE, Geschwind DH, Fryer HJ, and Hockfield S, Early postmitotic neurons transiently express TOAD-64, a neural specific protein. J Comp Neurol 355(3): p. 369-79 1995.
[18] Wang LH and Strittmatter SM, A family of rat CRMP genes is differentially expressed in the nervous system. J Neurosci 16(19): p. 6197-207 1996.
[19] Vincent P, Collette Y, Marignier R, Vuaillat C, Rogemond V, Davoust N, *et al.*, A role for the neuronal protein collapsin response mediator protein 2 in T lymphocyte polarization and migration. J Immunol 175(11): p. 7650-60 2005.
[20] Charrier E, Reibel S, Rogemond V, Aguera M, Thomasset N, and Honnorat J, Collapsin response mediator proteins (CRMPs): involvement in nervous system development and adult neurodegenerative disorders. Mol Neurobiol 28(1): p. 51-64 2003.
[21] Inagaki N, Chihara K, Arimura N, Menager C, Kawano Y, Matsuo N, *et al.*, CRMP-2 induces axons in cultured hippocampal neurons. Nat Neurosci 4(8): p. 781-2 2001.
[22] Fukata Y, Kimura T, and Kaibuchi K, Axon specification in hippocampal neurons. Neurosci Res 43(4): p. 305-15 2002.
[23] Brown M, Jacobs T, Eickholt B, Ferrari G, Teo M, Monfries C, *et al.*, Alpha2-chimaerin, cyclin-dependent Kinase 5/p35, and its target collapsin response mediator protein-2 are essential components in semaphorin 3A-induced growth-cone collapse. J Neurosci 24(41): p. 8994-9004 2004.
[24] Arimura N, Ménager C, Kawano Y, Yoshimura T, Kawabata S, Hattori A, *et al.*, Phosphorylation by Rho kinase regulates CRMP-2 activity in growth cones. Mol. Cell Biol. 25(22): p. 9973-9984 2005.
[25] Bretin S, Reibel S, Charrier E, Maus-Moatti M, Auvergnon N, Thevenoux A, *et al.*, Differential expression of CRMP1, CRMP2A, CRMP2B, and CRMP5 in axons or dendrites of distinct neurons in the mouse brain. J.Comp.Neurol. 486(1): p. 1-17 2005.
[26] Yamashita N, Morita A, Uchida Y, Nakamura F, Usui H, Ohshima T, *et al.*, Regulation of spine development by semaphorin3A through cyclin-dependent kinase 5 phosphorylation of collapsin response mediator protein 1. J. Neurosci. 27(46): p. 12546-12554 2007.
[27] Uchida Y, Ohshima T, Sasaki Y, Suzuki H, Yanai S, Yamashita N, *et al.*, Semaphorin3A signalling is mediated *via* sequential Cdk5 and GSK3beta phosphorylation of CRMP2: implication of common phosphorylating mechanism underlying axon guidance and Alzheimer's disease. Genes Cells 10(2): p. 165-79 2005.
[28] Quinn CC, Chen E, Kinjo TG, Kelly G, Bell AW, Elliott RC, *et al.*, TUC-4b, a novel TUC family variant, regulates neurite outgrowth and associates with vesicles in the growth cone. J. Neurosci. 23(7): p. 2815-2823 2003.
[29] Xia C, Nguyen M, Garrison AK, Zhao Z, Wang Z, Sutherland C, *et al.*, CNP/cGMP signaling regulates axon branching and growth by modulating microtubule polymerization. Dev Neurobiol 2013.
[30] Gu Y and Ihara Y, Evidence that collapsin response mediator protein-2 is involved in the dynamics of microtubules. J Biol Chem 275(24): p. 17917-20 2000.
[31] Fukata Y, Itoh TJ, Kimura T, Menager C, Nishimura T, Shiromizu T, *et al.*, CRMP-2 binds to tubulin heterodimers to promote microtubule assembly. Nat Cell Biol 4(8): p. 583-91 2002.
[32] Kimura T, Watanabe H, Iwamatsu A, and Kaibuchi K, Tubulin and CRMP-2 complex is transported *via* Kinesin-1. J Neurochem 93(6): p. 1371-82 2005.

[33] Kawano Y, Yoshimura T, Tsuboi D, Kawabata S, Kaneko-Kawano T, Shirataki H, *et al.*, CRMP-2 is involved in kinesin-1-dependent transport of the Sra-1/WAVE1 complex and axon formation. Mol Cell Biol 25(22): p. 9920-35 2005.

[34] Castellani V, Falk J, and Rougon G, Semaphorin3A-induced receptor endocytosis during axon guidance responses is mediated by L1 CAM. Mol Cell Neurosci 26(1): p. 89-100 2004.

[35] Nishimura T, Fukata Y, Kato K, Yamaguchi T, Matsuura Y, Kamiguchi H, *et al.*, CRMP-2 regulates polarized Numb-mediated endocytosis for axon growth. Nat Cell Biol 5(9): p. 819-26 2003.

[36] Chi XX, Schmutzler BS, Brittain JM, Wang Y, Hingtgen CM, Nicol GD, *et al.*, Regulation of N-type voltage-gated calcium channels (Cav2.2) and transmitter release by collapsin response mediator protein-2 (CRMP-2) in sensory neurons. J Cell Sci 122(Pt 23): p. 4351-62 2009.

[37] Brittain JM, Wang Y, Eruvwetere O, and Khanna R, Cdk5-mediated phosphorylation of CRMP-2 enhances its interaction with CaV2.2. FEBS Lett 586(21): p. 3813-8 2012.

[38] Mizuno M, Kato D, Kanamori T, Toyoda T, Suzuki T, Ojika K, *et al.*, Phosphorylation of collapsin response mediator protein-2 regulates its localization and association with hippocampal cholinergic neurostimulating peptide precursor in the hippocampus. Neurosci Lett 535: p. 122-7 2013.

[39] Ou Y, Zhang Y, Cheng M, Rattner JB, Dobrinski I, and van der Hoorn FA, Targeting of CRMP-2 to the primary cilium is modulated by GSK-3beta. PLoS One 7(11): p. e48773 2012.

[40] Akimoto Y, Comer FI, Cole RN, Kudo A, Kawakami H, Hirano H, *et al.*, Localization of the O-GlcNAc transferase and O-GlcNAc-modified proteins in rat cerebellar cortex. Brain Res 966(2): p. 194-205 2003.

[41] Morinaka A, Yamada M, Itofusa R, Funato Y, Yoshimura Y, Nakamura F, *et al.*, Thioredoxin mediates oxidation-dependent phosphorylation of CRMP2 and growth cone collapse. Sci Signal 4(170): p. ra26 2011.

[42] Mitsui N, Inatome R, Takahashi S, Goshima Y, Yamamura H, and Yanagi S, Involvement of Fes/Fps tyrosine kinase in semaphorin3A signaling. Embo J 21(13): p. 3274-85 2002.

[43] Shapovalova Z, Tabunshchyk K, and Greer PA, The Fer tyrosine kinase regulates an axon retraction response to Semaphorin 3A in dorsal root ganglion neurons. BMC Dev Biol 7: p. 133 2007.

[44] Horiuchi M, Loebrich S, Brandstaetter JH, Kneussel M, and Betz H, Cellular localization and subcellular distribution of Unc-33-like protein 6, a brain-specific protein of the collapsin response mediator protein family that interacts with the neuronal glycine transporter 2. J Neurochem 94(2): p. 307-15 2005.

[45] Arimura N, Inagaki N, Chihara K, Menager C, Nakamura N, Amano M, *et al.*, Phosphorylation of collapsin response mediator protein-2 by Rho-kinase. Evidence for two separate signaling pathways for growth cone collapse. J Biol Chem 275(31): p. 23973-80 2000.

[46] Cole AR, Causeret F, Yadirgi G, Hastie CJ, McLauchlan H, McManus EJ, *et al.*, Distinct priming kinases contribute to differential regulation of collapsin response mediator proteins by glycogen synthase kinase-3 *in vivo*. J Biol Chem 281(24): p. 16591-8 2006.

[47] Cole AR, Soutar MP, Rembutsu M, van Aalten L, Hastie CJ, McLauchlan H, *et al.*, Relative Resistance of Cdk5-phosphorylated CRMP2 to Dephosphorylation. J Biol Chem 283(26): p. 18227-18237 2008.

[48] Ip JP, Shi L, Chen Y, Itoh Y, Fu WY, Betz A, *et al.*, alpha2-chimaerin controls neuronal migration and functioning of the cerebral cortex through CRMP-2. Nat Neurosci 15(1): p. 39-47 2012.

[49] Tan M, Ma S, Huang Q, Hu K, Song B, and Li M, GSK-3alpha/beta-mediated phosphorylation of CRMP-2 regulates activity-dependent dendritic growth. J Neurochem 2013.

[50] Yoshimura T, Kawano Y, Arimura N, Kawabata S, Kikuchi A, and Kaibuchi K, GSK-3beta regulates phosphorylation of CRMP-2 and neuronal polarity. Cell 120(1): p. 137-49 2005.

[51] Sweeney HL, Yang Z, Zhi G, Stull JT, and Trybus KM, Charge replacement near the phosphorylatable serine of the myosin regulatory light chain mimics aspects of phosphorylation. Proc Natl Acad Sci U S A 91(4): p. 1490-4 1994.

[52] Rembutsu M, Soutar MP, Van Aalten L, Gourlay R, Hastie CJ, McLauchlan H, *et al.*, Novel procedure to investigate the effect of phosphorylation on protein complex formation *in vitro* and in cells. Biochemistry 47(7): p. 2153-61 2008.

[53] Lee VM, Goedert M, and Trojanowski JQ, Neurodegenerative tauopathies. Annu Rev Neurosci 24: p. 1121-59 2001.

[54] Cole AR, Noble W, van Aalten L, Plattner F, Meimaridou R, Hogan D, *et al.*, Collapsin response mediator protein-2 hyperphosphorylation is an early event in Alzheimer's disease progression. J Neurochem 103(3): p. 1132-44 2007.

[55] Gong CX, Liu F, Grundke-Iqbal I, and Iqbal K, Post-translational modifications of tau protein in Alzheimer's disease. J Neural Transm 112(6): p. 813-38 2005.

[56] Hanger DP, Byers HL, Wray S, Leung KY, Saxton MJ, Seereeram A, *et al.*, Novel phosphorylation sites in tau from Alzheimer brain support a role for casein kinase 1 in disease pathogenesis. J Biol Chem 282(32): p. 23645-54 2007.

[57] Ksiezak-Reding H, Liu WK, and Yen SH, Phosphate analysis and dephosphorylation of modified tau associated with paired helical filaments. Brain Res 597(2): p. 209-19 1992.

[58] Goedert M, Jakes R, Crowther RA, Six J, Lubke U, Vandermeeren M, *et al.*, The abnormal phosphorylation of tau protein at Ser-202 in Alzheimer disease recapitulates phosphorylation during development. Proc Natl Acad Sci U S A 90(11): p. 5066-70 1993.

[59] Liu F, Li B, Tung EJ, Grundke-Iqbal I, Iqbal K, and Gong CX, Site-specific effects of tau phosphorylation on its microtubule assembly activity and self-aggregation. Eur J Neurosci 26(12): p. 3429-36 2007.

[60] Grundke-Iqbal I, Iqbal K, Tung YC, Quinlan M, Wisniewski HM, and Binder LI, Abnormal phosphorylation of the microtubule-associated protein tau (tau) in Alzheimer cytoskeletal pathology. Proc Natl Acad Sci U S A 83(13): p. 4913-7 1986.

[61] Wang JZ, Grundke-Iqbal I, and Iqbal K, Kinases and phosphatases and tau sites involved in Alzheimer neurofibrillary degeneration. Eur.J.Neurosci. 25(1): p. 59-68 2007.

[62] Goedert M, Klug A, and Crowther RA, Tau protein, the paired helical filament and Alzheimer's disease. J Alzheimers Dis 9(3 Suppl): p. 195-207 2006.

[63] Weingarten MD, Lockwood AH, Hwo SY, and Kirschner MW, A protein factor essential for microtubule assembly. Proc Natl Acad Sci U S A 72(5): p. 1858-62 1975.

[64] Sasaki Y, Cheng C, Uchida Y, Nakajima O, Ohshima T, Yagi T, *et al.*, Fyn and Cdk5 mediate semaphorin-3A signaling, which is involved in regulation of dendrite orientation in cerebral cortex. Neuron 35(5): p. 907-20 2002.

[65] Noble W, Olm V, Takata K, Casey E, Mary O, Meyerson J, *et al.*, Cdk5 is a key factor in tau aggregation and tangle formation *in vivo*. Neuron 38(4): p. 555-65 2003.

[66] Patrick GN, Zukerberg L, Nikolic M, de la Monte S, Dikkes P, and Tsai LH, Conversion of p35 to p25 deregulates Cdk5 activity and promotes neurodegeneration. Nature 402(6762): p. 615-22 1999.
[67] Arioka M, Tsukamoto M, Ishiguro K, Kato R, Sato K, Imahori K, *et al.*, Tau protein kinase II is involved in the regulation of the normal phosphorylation state of tau protein. J Neurochem 60(2): p. 461-8 1993.
[68] Ishiguro K, Shiratsuchi A, Sato S, Omori A, Arioka M, Kobayashi S, *et al.*, Glycogen synthase kinase 3 beta is identical to tau protein kinase I generating several epitopes of paired helical filaments. FEBS Lett 325(3): p. 167-72 1993.
[69] Kerr F, Rickle A, Nayeem N, Brandner S, Cowburn RF, and Lovestone S, PTEN, a negative regulator of PI3 kinase signalling, alters tau phosphorylation in cells by mechanisms independent of GSK-3. FEBS Lett 580(13): p. 3121-8 2006.
[70] Nayeem N, Kerr F, Naumann H, Linehan J, Lovestone S, and Brandner S, Hyperphosphorylation of tau and neurofilaments and activation of CDK5 and ERK1/2 in PTEN-deficient cerebella. Mol Cell Neurosci 34(3): p. 400-8 2007.
[71] Tseng HC, Zhou Y, Shen Y, and Tsai LH, A survey of Cdk5 activator p35 and p25 levels in Alzheimer's disease brains. FEBS Lett 523(1-3): p. 58-62 2002.
[72] Cohen PT, Novel protein serine/threonine phosphatases: variety is the spice of life. Trends Biochem Sci 22(7): p. 245-51 1997.
[73] Liu F, Grundke-Iqbal I, Iqbal K, and Gong CX, Contributions of protein phosphatases PP1, PP2A, PP2B and PP5 to the regulation of tau phosphorylation. Eur J Neurosci 22(8): p. 1942-50 2005.
[74] Goedert M, Cohen ES, Jakes R, and Cohen P, p42 MAP kinase phosphorylation sites in microtubule-associated protein tau are dephosphorylated by protein phosphatase 2A1. Implications for Alzheimer's disease [corrected]. FEBS Lett 312(1): p. 95-9 1992.
[75] Lim J and Lu KP, Pinning down phosphorylated tau and tauopathies. Biochim Biophys Acta 1739(2-3): p. 311-22 2005.
[76] Lu PJ, Wulf G, Zhou XZ, Davies P, and Lu KP, The prolyl isomerase Pin1 restores the function of Alzheimer-associated phosphorylated tau protein. Nature 399(6738): p. 784-8 1999.
[77] Bamberger ME and Landreth GE, Microglial interaction with beta-amyloid: implications for the pathogenesis of Alzheimer's disease. Microsc Res Tech 54(2): p. 59-70 2001.
[78] Zhu X, Lee HG, Raina AK, Perry G, and Smith MA, The role of mitogen-activated protein kinase pathways in Alzheimer's disease. Neurosignals 11(5): p. 270-81 2002.
[79] Wray S, Saxton M, Anderton BH, and Hanger DP, Direct analysis of tau from PSP brain identifies new phosphorylation sites and a major fragment of N-terminally cleaved tau containing four microtubule-binding repeats. J Neurochem 2008.
[80] Alonso AC, Li B, Grundke-Iqbal I, and Iqbal K, Mechanism of tau-induced neurodegeneration in Alzheimer disease and related tauopathies. Curr.Alzheimer Res. 5(4): p. 375-384 2008.
[81] Frankfort SV, Tulner LR, van Campen JP, Verbeek MM, Jansen RW, and Beijnen JH, Amyloid beta protein and tau in cerebrospinal fluid and plasma as biomarkers for dementia: a review of recent literature. Curr Clin Pharmacol 3(2): p. 123-31 2008.
[82] Tremblay C, Pilote M, Phivilay A, Emond V, Bennett DA, and Calon F, Biochemical characterization of Abeta and tau pathologies in mild cognitive impairment and Alzheimer's disease. J.Alz. Dis. 12(4): p. 377-390 2007.

[83] Ewers M, Buerger K, Teipel SJ, Scheltens P, Schroder J, Zinkowski RP, *et al.*, Multicenter assessment of CSF-phosphorylated tau for the prediction of conversion of MCI. Neurology 69(24): p. 2205-12 2007.

[84] Brys M, Pirraglia E, Rich K, Rolstad S, Mosconi L, Switalski R, *et al.*, Prediction and longitudinal study of CSF biomarkers in mild cognitive impairment. Neurobiol Aging 2007.

[85] Williamson R, van Aalten L, Mann DMA, Platt B, Plattner F, Bedford L, *et al.*, CRMP2 hyperphosphorylation is characteristic of Alzheimer's disease and not a feature common to other neurodegenerative diseases. J. Alzheimers Dis. 27(3): p. 615-625 2011.

[86] Lubec G, Nonaka M, Krapfenbauer K, Gratzer M, Cairns N, and Fountoulakis M, Expression of the dihydropyrimidinase related protein 2 (DRP-2) in Down syndrome and Alzheimer's disease brain is downregulated at the mRNA and dysregulated at the protein level. J Neural Transm Suppl 57: p. 161-77 1999.

[87] Wishart TM, Paterson JM, Short DM, Meredith S, Robertson KA, Sutherland C, *et al.*, Differential proteomics analysis of synaptic proteins identifies potential cellular targets and protein mediators of synaptic neuroprotection conferred by the slow Wallerian degeneration (Wlds) gene. Mol Cell Proteomics 6(8): p. 1318-30 2007.

[88] Wakatsuki S, Saitoh F, and Araki T, ZNRF1 promotes Wallerian degeneration by degrading AKT to induce GSK3B-dependent CRMP2 phosphorylation. Nat Cell Biol 13(12): p. 1415-23 2011.

[89] Jiang SX, Kappler J, Zurakowski B, Desbois A, Aylsworth A, and Hou ST, Calpain cleavage of collapsin response mediator proteins in ischemic mouse brain. Eur J Neurosci 26(4): p. 801-9 2007.

[90] Zhang Z, Ottens AK, Sadasivan S, Kobeissy FH, Fang T, Hayes RL, *et al.*, Calpain-mediated collapsin response mediator protein-1, -2, and -4 proteolysis after neurotoxic and traumatic brain injury. J Neurotrauma 24(3): p. 460-72 2007.

[91] Czech T, Yang JW, Csaszar E, Kappler J, Baumgartner C, and Lubec G, Reduction of hippocampal collapsin response mediated protein-2 in patients with mesial temporal lobe epilepsy. Neurochem Res 29(12): p. 2189-96 2004.

[92] Bretin S, Rogemond V, Marin P, Maus M, Torrens Y, Honnorat J, *et al.*, Calpain product of WT-CRMP2 reduces the amount of surface NR2B NMDA receptor subunit. J Neurochem 98(4): p. 1252-65 2006.

[93] Kowara R, Chen Q, Milliken M, and Chakravarthy B, Calpain-mediated truncation of dihydropyrimidinase-like 3 protein (DPYSL3) in response to NMDA and H2O2 toxicity. J Neurochem 95(2): p. 466-74 2005.

CHAPTER 6

N200 Latency and CSF Cytochrome C Levels as Biomarkers for Early Detection of Progression to Alzheimer's Disease in Mild Cognitive Impairment Patients

Vasileios T. Papaliagkas[1,*], Georgios A. Anogianakis[2], Magda N. Tsolaki[1] and Vasileios K. Kimiskidis[3]

[1]Third Department of Neurology, "G. Papanikolaou" Hospital, Aristotle University of Thessaloniki, Exohi Thessaloniki, Greece; [2]Department of Experimental Physiology, Faculty of Medicine, Aristotle University of Thessaloniki, Greece and [3]Clinical Neurophysiology Department, AHEPA University Hospital, Thessaloniki, Greece

Abstract: The role of CSF cytochrome c levels and auditory event-related potentials (AERPs) in the progress of mild cognitive impairment (MCI) to Alzheimer's disease (AD) is investigated. A study sample that consisted of fifty one MCI patients and fourteen healthy individuals that underwent lumbar puncture at baseline was used and their CSF cytochrome c levels were determined. CSF cytochrome c levels were re-examined in 20 patients after a time period of 11 months. During this period five patients progressed to AD. All patients underwent AERP examinations both at baseline and follow-up. MCI patients were found to have significantly higher cytochrome c levels compared to healthy controls (Mann-Whitney test, Z=-2.110, p=0.018). AD-converters, had a higher increase over time in cytochrome c levels (Mann-Whitney test, p=0.002; effect size r=0.63) and significantly prolonged N200 latency (Mann-Whitney test, p<0.001; effect size r=0.50) compared to MCI stable patients. Amongst the ERP wave characteristics that were studied, only N200 amplitude was significantly correlated with CSF cytochrome c levels (r_s=0.310, p=0.03). Both parameters could discriminate AD converters from MCI stable patients, with sensitivity and specificity >75%. When both N200 latency and cytochrome c increase were applied, the prediction of the MCI patients who converted to AD was 100%.

Our results suggest that MCI to AD conversion is associated with a marked elevated N200 latency at baseline and a high increase in cytochrome c levels during a relatively short period of time, and that both parameters could be possibly considered as candidate markers for the discrimination between AD converters and MCI stable patients.

Keywords: Alzheimer's Disease, auditory event-related potentials, cytochrome c, mild cognitive impairment, N200 latency

***Corresponding author Vasileios T. Papaliagkas:** Third Department of Neurology, "G. Papanikolaou" Hospital, Aristotle University of Thessaloniki, Exohi, 57010 Thessaloniki, Greece; Tel: +302310313178; Fax: +302310313178; E-mail: vpapal@auth.gr

D.K. Lahiri (Ed)

INTRODUCTION

Apoptosis is a fundamental biological process essential for the development and tissue homeostasis of multicellular organisms, which is believed according by several studies to be connected to AD pathogenesis [1, 2, 3]. A subfamily of cysteine proteases known as caspases (cysteine containing proteases that cleave proteins at aspartate residues) is involved in the mechanism of apoptosis [4, 5, 6]. One major pathway for caspase activation is a cytochrome c-initiated pathway, where a variety of apoptotic stimuli cause cytochrome c release from mitochondria, which triggers a series of biochemical reactions that result in caspase activation and subsequent cell death [2, 7]. Cytochrome c is a protein loosely attached to the surface of the inner mitochondrial membrane, and is a vital part of the electron transfer chain. Cytochrome c shuttles the electrons in the intermembrane space between adjacent mitochondria. It is coded by ribosomes as apocytochrome c, and then is transported to the mitochondria, with the help of heme attachment synthesizing holocytochrome c [8, 9]. Cytochrome c is a required cofactor for apoptotic protease activating factor 1 (Apaf-1) function. Apaf-1 contains a caspase-recruitment domain (CARD), a nucleotide-binding domain, and 12 WD-40 repeats [10, 11]. An early event in apoptosis is the release of cytochrome c from mitochondria into the cytosol [12] where it binds to Apaf-1, leading to the activation of procaspase 9 and then as a consequence other downstream caspases [13]. Other proteins involved in the apoptotic process also interact with cytochrome c. B-cell leukemia/lymphoma-2 (Bcl-2) and B-cell leukemia/lymphoma –xL (Bcl-xL) bind to the outer mitochondrial membrane and block cytochrome c release both *in vitro* and *in vivo* [14, 15], while pro-apoptotic proteins such as Bcl-2-associated X protein (Bax) and Bcl-2-antagonist/killer (Bak) facilitate the release of cytochrome c from the mitochondrial membrane. It appears that these proteins, through their Bcl-2 Homology 3 (BH3) parts, interact with the mitochondrial membrane and form channels through which cytochrome c is released [16]. High levels of cytochrome c and its release from mitochondria may also result in mitochondrial damage and dysfunction, both of which are related to oxidative stress in normal ageing and AD progression [17]. Mitochondrial dysfunction is one of the early features in AD and reduced number of mitochondria was observed in the hippocampus of AD patients [18-20]. Also,

Abeta inhibits cytochrome c oxidase activity [21] by binding to subunit 1; an event that takes place early in the process of synaptic generation in AD [22]. Cytochrome c has been noted in a subset of plaque-associated dystrophic neurites and possibly a subset of neurons that contain pretangles in AD cases [23]. Beta-amyloid 1-40 and 1-42 induces release of cytochrome c from isolated mouse brain mitochondria, with subsequent activation of the caspase cascade [24, 25]. Furthermore, correlations between decreased cytochrome c oxidase activity and deficits in cognitive abilities have been reported [26-28]. Cytochrome c oxidase was reduced in AD brain compared to normal human brain [29] and in platelets from AD patients [30, 31]. Other studies show that apoptosis is not correlated with AD [17]. No difference in expression of apoptosis-related proteins and apoptotic morphology in control, pathologically aged and Alzheimer's disease cases has been reported [32]. Due to the contradicting results on the relation between apoptosis and AD, it is clear that further investigation of apoptotic-related proteins, such as cytochrome c, in relation to AD progress should be performed.

Cerebrospinal fluid (CSF) is a clear colourless fluid, which is produced in the brain ventricles at a rate of 500ml/24h and bathes the whole central nervous system. CSF is in direct contact with the brain's extracellular space, it is equally distributed therefore it can be assumed that pathological changes observed in the brain are reflected in the distribution of certain biomarkers in the CSF.

Cognitive event-related potentials (ERPs) are recorded in response to specific external stimuli (*e.g.* visual, auditory) to which patients pay attention while they are required to distinguish the target stimulus from other non-target stimuli. The major waves observed in the Auditory AERPs are N200, P300 and Slow Wave. In the current study we focused on N200 wave, which is a negative deflection in the AERPs appearing about 200ms after the stimulus. It is composed of N2a known as mismatch negativity (MMN) and N2b. MMN is present both in attending and non-attending conditions, therefore it is not influenced by attention. It could represent short duration memory functions and preattentive storage taking place in sensory cortex 26 [33]. Auditory temporal cortex, frontal-lobe as well as the thalamus and the hippocampus contribute in the generation of MMN [34].

The aim of the study is to assess the cognitive function of MCI patients with AERPs, and concurrently evaluate the process of apoptosis, with the measurement of CSF cytochrome c levels. Since apoptosis is presumably implicated in the pathogenesis of cognitive impairment in MCI, while abnormal AERPs are the electrophysiological expression of this decline, we hypothesized that cytochrome c levels, a biomarker of apoptosis, may possibly be correlated with AERPs parameters in MCI patients.

MATERIALS AND METHODS

The study sample consists of two groups of MCI patients, selected from the Memory and Dementia Clinic, in "G. Papanikolaou" Hospital, Thessaloniki, Greece. All patients were clinically investigated by health professionals that were specialized in cognitive disorders. The investigation included a medical history, and physical, neurological and neuropsychometric examinations. Baseline cognitive ability was assessed by Mini-Mental State Examination (MMSE) [35, 36]. All patients gave informed consent to participate in the study, which was conducted according to the Declaration of Helsinki and was approved by the ethics committee of the Aristotle University of Thessaloniki, Greece.

Group 1 consisted of 51 MCI patients diagnosed according to the widely used criteria of Petersen *et al.* [37]. CSF samples were collected from all patients, by lumbar puncture, performed at the L3/L4 or L4/L5 interspace. CSF samples were also taken from 14 age-matched healthy subjects, used as the control group.

Group 2 was a sub-group of group 1 which consists of 20 patients, from which a second CSF sample was taken after an average period of 11±5.9 months (range 6-22 months). This group was used in order to gain information on the evolution of certain parameters between baseline and endpoint. All CSF samples were stored at -80 degrees Celsius until analysis, which was performed at a later stage, using the human Cytochrome c ELISA kit from Bender Medsystems GmbH, Vienna, Austria.

During the follow-up period, five of the patients of group 1 (10%), four of them belonging to group 2 as well, developed AD, diagnosed according to the DSM-IV criteria.

AERPs were performed in all patients using a simple discrimination task, the so-called oddball paradigm. Follow up AERPs were also performed in those patients who underwent repeat lumbar puncture and CSF cytochrome c levels measurement. N200, P300 and Slow Wave (SW) latencies and also N200 and P300 amplitudes were determined both at baseline and follow-up. AERPs use two different tones, an interstimulus interval of several seconds, with the target oddball stimulus presented less frequently than the non-target or standard stimulus. In this task, a series of binaural tones at 70-dB sound pressure level (SPL) with a 10 ms rise/fall and a 100ms, plateau time was presented to all subjects. The auditory stimuli were presented in a random sequence with target tones of 2000Hz occurring 20% of the time and standard tones of 1000Hz occurring 80% of the time at a rate of 0.5Hz [38]. The subject was required to distinguish between the two tones by responding to the target (*e.g.* mentally counting,) and not responding to the standard [39]. Patients were instructed to pay attention in distinguishing the tones, count the target tones silently and report the total number at the end of the exam.

ERP activity was recorded (filter bandpass: 0.1-50Hz, analysis time:1sec) from scalp AgCl electrodes at Cz and Pz sites according to the 10/20 system referred to linked earlobe electrodes, with a right forearm ground. Artifacts caused by ocular movement ±50μV were automatically rejected. Each patient was tested twice to ensure that waveform components were reproducible. The peak of the ERP components was determined as follows: if the waveform was smooth, the maximal amplitude point was taken as the peak. Otherwise, the leading and trailing slopes of the waveform were extended, and the intersection point was determined [38]. For the purpose of reduced impedance a special type of paste was used (Elefix Nihon-Kohden, EEG paste Z-401 CE), while the AERPs were analyzed by means of Neuropack 4 (Nihon-Kohden, Tokyo) equipment.

Statistical analysis was performed with SPSS 15.0 for Windows (SPSS Inc). Mann–Whitney *U*-test was used to compare medians of CSF cytochrome c levels and ERP components between stable MCI patients and AD-converters. Wilcoxon matched-pairs signed-rank test was used to compare data between baseline and endpoint. The Spearman's correlation coefficient rho (r_s) was used for correlations. The effect size (Pearson's r) was used for measuring the strength of relationship between two variables. Statistical significance was set at $p<0.05$.

RESULTS

Cytochrome C

The cytochrome c levels measured at baseline for the groups are shown in Tables **1** and **2**. Significant differences in the cytochrome c levels between the control group and groups 1 and 2 were found (group 1: Z=-2.349, p=0.018, group 2: Z=-2.275, p=0.022).

Table 1: Basic Demographics, MMSE scores, cytochrome c levels and ERP components at baseline for Group 1 (medians and interquartile ranges are shown in parentheses)

	Total	**MCI stable**	**AD-converters**
N (female)	51(31)	46(29)	5(2)
Age, Mean ±SD (yrs)	67.7±7.9	67.2±7.6	73.0±9.4
MMSE	28 (26-29)	28(27-29)	26(24-28)
Cytochrome c(ng/ml)	0.131(0.05-0.24)	0.131(0.06-0.22)	0.054(0.03-0.77)
N200 latency (ms)	243(228-276)	240(228-264)	306(296-352)
P300 latency (ms)	400(381-431)	398(376-426)	467(395-490)
SW latency (ms)	524(483-558)	525(484-558)	522(465-578)
N200 amplitude (μV)	7.50(6.25-10.00)	7.50(6.25-10.00)	7.65(6.87-11.87)
P300 amplitude (μV)	14.55(10.32-17.95)	15.30(10.50-18.10)	10.40(7.02-13.75)

In group 1 no significant difference was observed between the cytochrome c levels of MCI stable patients and AD converters (Z=-0.079, p=0.939>0.05). The difference over time measured in patients of group 2 was not significant (Wilcoxon matched-pairs signed-rank test Z=-0.019, p>0.05). Moreover no correlation was found between cytochrome c levels and age (Group 1: r_s=0.08, p>0.05; group 2: r_s=0.05, p>0.05).

In group 2 the cytochrome c levels measured in the AD converters during the study period underwent a 2.5-fold increase (median levels 0.24 ng/ml at baseline and 0.61 ng/ml at follow-up), whereas in the MCI stable patients they decreased from 0.18 to 0.16 ng/ml. However, the difference between baseline and follow-up measurement was not significant. In order to evaluate the change in time course, the difference of the measurement at follow-up minus baseline measurement was calculated for all subjects. The median (IQR) value of the cytochrome c levels of the 16 MCI stable patients was -0.07 (range-0.34 to 0.09), and that of the AD-converters 0.37(range 0.11 to 1.74), (see Fig. **1**). The difference in cytochrome c levels of the AD-converters was found to be significantly higher than that of the MCI stable patients (Mann-Whitney test, Z=-2.646, p=0.005, effect size r=0.59).

Table 2: Basic Demographics, CSF cytochrome c levels and ERP components at baseline and follow up for Group 2 (medians and interquartile ranges are shown in parentheses)

	Total		**MCI stable**		**AD-converters**	
	Baseline	**Follow-up**	**Baseline**	**Follow-up**	**Baseline**	**Follow-up**
N (female)	20(11)		16(9)		4(2)	
Age, Mean±SD, (yrs)	68.1±7.6		67.2 ±7.6		73.0 ±9.4	
Cytochrome c (ng/ml)	0.184 (0.05-0.45)	0.165 (0.10-0.23)	0.184 (0.06-0.43)	0.162 (0.07-0.20)	0.238 (0.03-0.94)	0.607 (0.13-2.68)
N200 latency (ms)	258 (230-288)	251 (234-299)	245 (225-272)	244 (226-276)	304 (293-354)	308 (263-323)
P300 latency (ms)	404 (378-464)	413 (390-464)	400 (372-449)	413 (390-441)	438 (388-477)	431 (390-551)
SW latency (ms)	522 (487-556)	535 (497-605)	496 (526-558)	536 (500-604)	502 (456-542)	524 (450-688)
N200 amplitude (μV)	7.57 (6.25-12.50)	8.75 (5.00-10.00)	7.78 (6.25-12.50)	8.75 (5.00-10.94)	7.57 (6.56-12.22)	7.83 (5.32-9.84)
P300 amplitude (μV)	14.85 (12.07-19.58)	14.50 (10.05-9.90)	16.20 (12.47-1.72)	17.00 (11.58-0.30)	10.44 (6.34-14.37)	9.45 (7.05-11.48)

Despite the small number of subjects of our study, especially of the AD-converting group, receiver operating characteristic (ROC) curve analysis was performed to determine the power of the change in cytochrome c levels to discriminate between AD converters and MCI stable patients. The analysis showed that applying a cutoff value for a cytochrome c level difference of 0.08 ng/ml, we achieved an Area Under Curve (AUC) of 0.938 (95% CI =0.733-0.992) (p=0.008), a sensitivity of 100% (95% CI=40.2-100) and a specificity of 75%

(95% CI=47.6-92.6). The results suggest that MCI conversion to AD is associated with a high increase in cytochrome c levels over a time period of one year.

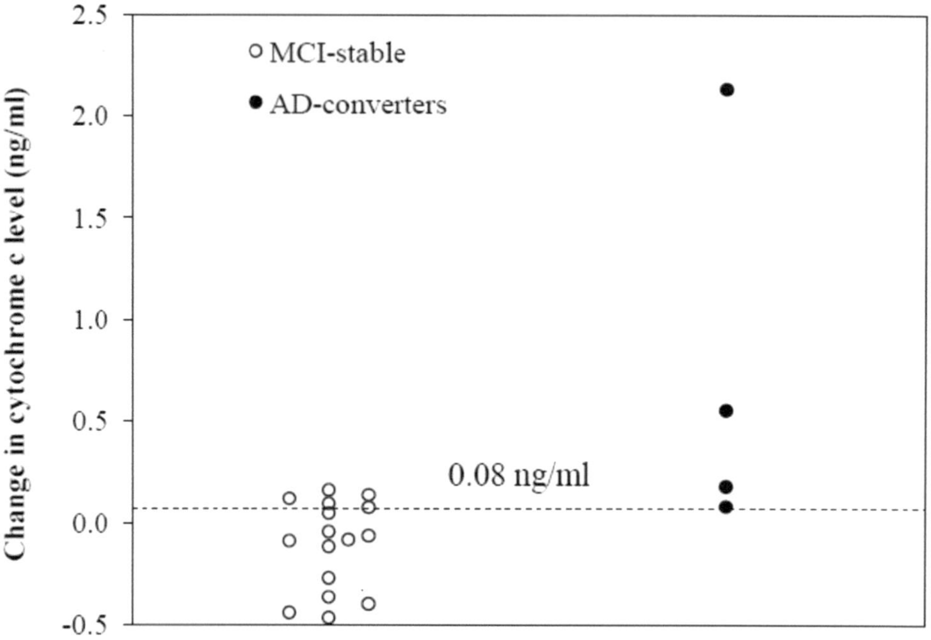

Figure 1: Individual change scores in cytochrome c levels (ng/ml) for MCI stable patients and AD-converters.

AUDITORY EVENT-RELATED POTENTIALS

For the group 1 patients (n=51), amongst investigated variables (N200, P300 and Slow wave latencies, N200 amplitude and P300 amplitude) only N200 amplitude was found to be correlated with CSF cytochrome c levels (r_s=0.310, p=0.03). Significant correlations were observed between N200 and P300 amplitudes (r_s=0.311, p=0.03), N200 and P300 latencies (r_s=0.569, p<0.001), N200 and SW latencies (r_s=0.335, p=0.016) and N200 latency and P300 amplitude (r_s=0.460, p<0.001).

Prolonged latencies and lower amplitudes of ERP components were observed in group 1 patients who converted to AD, compared with those of the MCI-stable patients. However, the only significant difference was that of N200 latency (Mann-Whitney test, Z=-3.549, p<0.001, effect size r=0.50).

A ROC curve analysis of N200 latency baseline measurements was conducted for the discrimination between MCI stable patients (n=46) and AD-converters (n=5), resulted in an AUC of 0.987 (95% CI=0.906-0.995), a cutoff value of 287 ms, a sensitivity of 100% (95% CI=48-100) and a specificity of 91% (95% CI=79.2-97.5). Since these results correspond to baseline measurements, that is before the appearance of the clinical symptoms of AD they highlight any predictive capabilities of N200 latency and suggest that, N200 latency may serve as an independent neurophysiological marker for the discrimination between MCI patients who convert to AD and those who remain stable.

When both N200 latency and cytochrome c increase cut-offs were applied, the prediction of the MCI patients who converted to AD, was 100% (Fig. **2**).

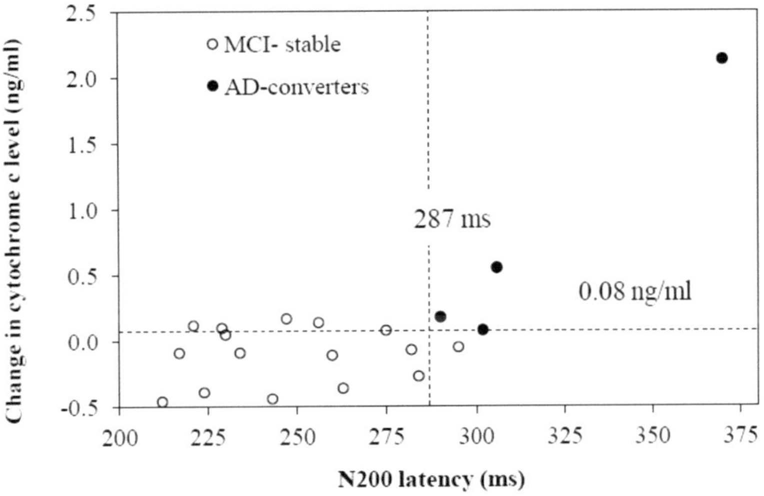

Figure 2: Combination of the change in CSF cytochrome c levels over a period of 11 months and N200 latency at baseline as a discriminating test for MCI and AD. Cut-offs equal to 0.08 ng/ml for cytochrome c change and 287 ms for N200 latency discriminates MCI from AD with sensitivity of 100% and specificity of 100%. (Open dots represent the MCI stable patients and close dots those who later progress to AD).

For the MCI stable patients of group 2 significant increase was observed in P300 and SW latencies between baseline and endpoint examination (Wilcoxon matched-pairs signed-rank test, for P300: Z=-2.415, p=0.01 and for SW: Z=-2.102, p=0.03). The effect sizes for the P300 and SW latency increases were large (r=0.58 and r=0.51 respectively).

No difference over time was found between N200 latencies (Z=-1,610, p>0.05), P300 amplitudes (Z=-1.586, p>0.05) and N200 amplitudes (Z=-0.466, p>0.05).

There were no significant correlations between CSF cytochrome c levels and latencies or amplitudes of the ERP waves. Likewise, there were no significant correlations between cytochrome c levels and age (r_s= 0.154 and 0.048, p=0.55 and 0.85 respectively). Moreover MCI stable and AD converters were age-matched (unpaired t-test t=-1.591, p=0.118>0.05).

The change in cytochrome c levels is not statistically correlated with changes in ERP parameters. The corresponding Spearman correlation coefficients between change in cytochrome c level and change in N200 latency is equal to -0.275 (p=0.240), change in P300 latency =-0.423 (p=0.063), SW latency=0.326 (p=0.161), N200 amplitude=0.043 (p=0.857) and P300 amplitude=-0.167 (p=0.482).

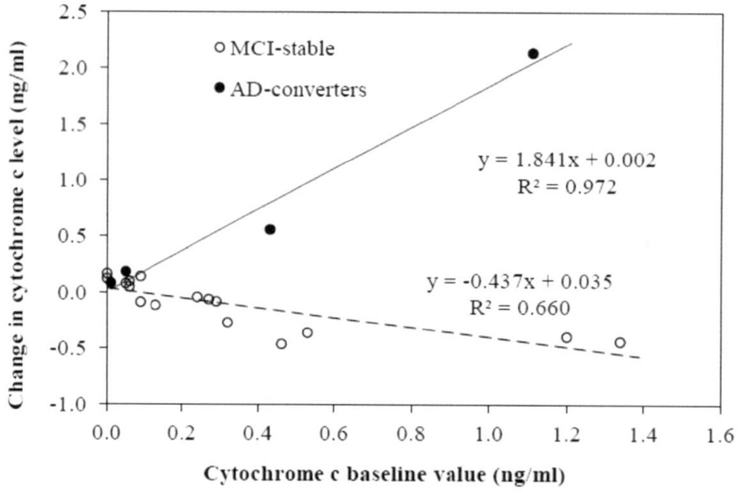

Figure 3: Scatter-plot of n=20 paired cytochrome c measurements showing change (follow-up minus baseline) against baseline. The two lines represent fitted regression lines for the MCI stable patients and the AD-converters.

Fig. (**3**) shows a scatter-plot between changes in cytochrome c levels (follow-up minus baseline values) against baseline for the AD-converters and the MCI stable groups. The slope of the fitted regression line for the AD-converters is positive, whereas for the MCI stable group negative, demonstrating a clear difference between the two groups and a lack of regression to the mean (RTM) effect.

DISCUSSIONS

No significant differences were observed over time in cytochrome c levels in MCI, in a sample that included patients examined twice in a time period ranging from 6 to 22 months. According to the results of the current study, MCI appears to be a stable condition that while it lasts, does not affect the levels of cytochrome c in CSF. Significant difference in P300 and Slow wave latencies were observed between exams, a finding that confirms the results of our previous study [40]. Given that patients with MCI are at high risk for developing AD [37, 41, 42] our results are in a sharp contrast with the view that wants MCI to be the anteroom to AD. The fact that we observed a notable increase in cytochrome c levels in those few MCI patients that developed AD between examinations, agrees with previous studies that suggest that apoptosis is implicated in AD pathophysiology [10, 43, 44, 45] but, in our view, it also suggests that AD and MCI might be two distinct clinical entities. MCI might serve as an aggravating factor for AD development but it is not a causal factor for AD.

The change in cytochrome c levels in the follow-up year may better reflect the ongoing cognitive decline and the conversion from MCI to AD can be predicted by the increase in cytochrome c levels, which may prove to be a useful biomarker for the early diagnosis of AD and predict who may be at risk of converting from MCI to AD. When we used a cytochrome c increase of 0.08 ng/ml as a cut-off, we achieved a sensitivity of 100% and a specificity of 75%. These results support those findings reporting increased levels of apoptotic markers such as Bcl-2, Bax and activated caspases in AD patients compared to healthy subjects [23, 46-53].

N200 latency was elevated at baseline in AD converters, and proved to be an independent single neurophysiological predictor of AD conversion. A cut-off value of 287 ms resulted in a sensitivity of 100% and specificity of 91%. Quite similar results on the capability of N200 latency to predict MCI conversion to AD were also obtained by other researchers using the same or different tasks [54, 55]. No statistical difference was observed in the age of MCI stable patients and AD converters, therefore age is not involved in the cytochrome c and N200 latency differences that were observed between the two groups.

Although our results should be interpreted in caution, given the small size of our sample, they suggest that an increased N200 latency or increase in CSF cytochrome c levels in MCI patients may be clinically useful in AD prediction. It should be noted that, in contrast to the increase in cytochrome c levels, levels of cytochrome c as independent values do not have a predictive value. Therefore N200 latency seems to be a more accurate biomarker than cytochrome c, for early assessment of AD conversion. However, the combination of these two markers is a reliable way of discriminating MCI converters from MCI stable patients in an early stage.

Furthermore, in our opinion, the positive correlations between CSF cytochrome c levels and N200 amplitude (which implies that N200 amplitudes are influenced by the apoptotic processes that take place during the MCI stage), indicate that MCI probably attacks the cells of the human cortex that are involved in lateral inhibition. This comes into agreement with previous studies on N200 wave generation [56]. However, we have to point out that the relatively small number of CSF samples included in our study might be inadequate for supporting such a conclusion and that further and more detailed studies should be performed in order to assess the physiological significance of the stability of cytochrome c levels in MCI and the value of cytochrome c as an AD biomarker.

ACKNOWLEDGEMENT

Declared none.

CONFLICT OF INTEREST

The authors confirm that this chapter content has no conflict of interest.

DISCLOSURE

This chapter is an update of our previous publication in CAR "Prediction of Conversion from Mild Cognitive Impairment to Alzheimer's Disease by CSF Cytochrome c Levels and N200 Latency" published in 'CAR', Volume 6, Number 3, June, pp. 279 to 284.

REFERENCES

[1] Jellinger KA. Challenges in neuronal apoptosis. Curr Alzheimer Res 3:377-391 (2006).

[2] Papaliagkas V, Anogianaki A, Anogianakis G and Ilonidis G. The proteins and the mechanisms of apoptosis: A mini-review of the fundamentals, Hippokratia 11:108-113 (2007).

[3] Braun RJ. Mitochondrion-mediated cell death: dissecting yeast apoptosis for a better understanding of neurodegeneration. Front Oncol.2:182 (2012).

[4] Cribbs DH, Poon WW, Rissman RA, Blurton-Jones M. Caspase-mediated degeneration in Alzheimer's disease. Am J Pathol 165:353-355 (2004).

[5] Rohn TT, Head E, Su JH, Anderson AJ, Bahr BA, Cotman CW *et al.* Correlation between caspase activation and neurofibrillary tangle formation in Alzheimer's disease, Am J Pathol 158:189-198 (2001).

[6] Graham RK, Ehrnhoefer DE, Hayden MR. Caspase-6 and neurodegeneration. Trends Neurosci. 34:646-56 (2011).

[7] Bayir H, Fadeel B, Palladino MJ, Witasp E, Kurnikov IV, Tyurina YY, *et al.* Apoptotic interactions of cytochrome c: redox flirting with anionic phospholipids within and outside of mitochondria, Biochim Biophys Acta 1757:648-659 (2006).

[8] Mavridou DA, Ferguson SJ, Stevens JM. Cytochrome c assembly. IUBMB Life. 65:209-16 (2013).

[9] San Francisco B, Bretsnyder EC, Kranz RG. Human mitochondrial holocytochrome c synthase's heme binding, maturation determinants, and complex formation with cytochrome c. Proc Natl Acad Sci U S A. 110 (2013).

[10] Eckert A, Marques CA, Keil U, Schüssel K and Müller WE. Increased apoptotic cell death in sporadic and genetic Alzheimer's disease, Ann N Y Acad Sci 1010:604-609 (2003).

[11] Bratton SB, Salvesen GS. Regulation of the Apaf-1-caspase-9 apoptosome. J Cell Sci. 123:3209-14 (2010).

[12] Jiang XJ and Wang XD. Cytochrome c-mediated apoptosis, Ann Rev Biochem 73:87-106 (2004).

[13] Marek L. The role of the apoptosome in the activation of procaspase-9. Postepy Hig Med Dosw (Online). 67:54-64 (2013).

[14] Kluck RM, Bossy-Wetzel E, Green DR and Newmeyer DD. The release of cytochrome c from mitochondria: a primary site for Bcl-2 regulation of apoptosis, Science 275:1132–1136 (1997).

[15] Yang J, Liu X, Bhalla K, Kim CN, Ibrado AM, Cai J, *et al.* Prevention of apoptosis by Bcl-2: release of cytochrome c from mitochondria blocked, Science 275:1129–1132 (1997).

[16] Adrain C and Martin SJ. The mitochondrial apoptosome: a killer unleashed by the cytochrome seas, Trends Biochem Sci 26:390-397 (2001).

[17] Woodhouse A, Vickers JC and Dickson TC. Cytoplasmic cytochrome c immunolabelling in dystrophic neuritis in Alzheimer's disease, Acta Neuropathologica 112:429-437 (2006).

[18] Sheng B, Wang X, Su B, Lee HG, Casadesus G, Perry G, *et al.* Impaired mitochondrial biogenesis contributes to mitochondrial dysfunction in Alzheimer's disease. J Neurochem. 120:419-29 (2012).

[19] Zhu X, Perry G, Moreira PI, Aliev G, Cash AD, Hirai K, *et al.* Mitochondrial abnormalities and oxidative imbalance in Alzheimer disease. J Alzheimers Dis. 9:147-53 (2006).

[20] Baloyannis SJ. Mitochondrial alterations in Alzheimer's disease. J Alzheimers Dis. 9:119-26 (2006).
[21] Manczak M, Mao P, Calkins MJ, Cornea A, Reddy AP, Murphy MP, *et al.* Mitochondria-targeted antioxidants protect against amyloid-beta toxicity in Alzheimer's disease neurons. J Alzheimers Dis. 20 Suppl 2:S609-31 (2010).
[22] Hernandez-Zimbron LF, Luna-Muñoz J, Mena R, Vazquez-Ramirez R, Kubli-Garfias C, Cribbs DH, *et al.* Amyloid-β peptide binds to cytochrome C oxidase subunit 1. PLoS One. 7:e42344 (2012).
[23] Blanchard V, Moussaoui S, Czech C, Touchet N, Bonici B, Planche M, *et al.* Time sequence of maturation of dystrophic neurites associated with A deposits in APP/PS1 transgenic mice, Exp Neurol 184:247–263 (2003).
[24] Kim HS, Lee JH and Lee JP. Amyloid [beta] peptide induces cytochrome c release from isolated mitochondria, Neuroreport 13:1989-1993 (2002).
[25] Fossati S, Ghiso J, Rostagno A. Insights into caspase-mediated apoptotic pathways induced by amyloid-β in cerebral microvascular endothelial cells. Neurodegener Dis. 10:324-8 (2012).
[26] Agin V, Chicher R and Chichery MP. Effects of learning on cytochrome oxidase activity in cuttlefish brain, Neuroreport 12:113-116 (2001).
[27] Berndt JD, Callaway NL and Gonzalez-Lima F. Effects of chronic sodium azide on brain and muscle cytochrome oxidase activity: a potential model to investigate environmental contributions to neurodegenerative diseases, J Toxicol Environ Health A 63:67-77 (2001).
[28] Cada A, Gonzalez-Lima F, Rose GM and Bennett MC. Regional brain effects of sodium azide treatment on cytochrome oxidase activity: a quantitative histochemical study, Metab Brain Dis 10:303-320 (1995).
[29] Maurer I, Zierz S, Möller HJ. A selective defect of cytochrome c oxidase is present in brain of Alzheimer disease patients. Neurobiol Aging. 21:455-62 (2000).
[30] Cardoso SM, Proença MT, Santos S, Santana I, Oliveira CR. Cytochrome c oxidase_is decreased in_Alzheimer's_disease_platelets. Neurobiol Aging. 25:105-10 (2004).
[31] Mancuso M, Filosto M, Bosetti F, Ceravolo R, Rocchi A, Tognoni G, *et al.* Decreased platelet cytochrome c oxidase activity is accompanied by increased blood lactate concentration during exercise in patients with Alzheimer disease. Exp Neurol. 182:421-6 (2003).
[32] Woodhouse A, Dickson TC, West AK, McLean CA and Vickers JC. No difference in expression of apoptosis-related proteins and apoptotic morphology in control, pathologically aged and Alzheimer's disease cases, Neurobiol Dis.22:323-33 (2006).
[33] Banquet JP, Guenther W and Smith M. Probability processing in depressed patients. Electroencephalogr Clin Neurophysiol Suppl. 40: 645-650 (1987).
[34] Alho K. Cerebral generators of mismatch negativity (MMN) and its magnetic counterpart (MMNm) elicited by sound changes. Ear Hear.16:38-51 (1995).
[35] Folstein M, Folstein S and McHugh P. `Mini-Mental State' A practical method for grading the cognitive state of patients for the clinician, J Psychiatr Res 12:189-198 (1975).
[36] Fountoulakis K, Tsolaki M, Chantzi H and Kazis A. Mini-Mental State Examination (MMSE): A validation study in the Greek elderly population, Encephalos (Greece) 31:93-102 (1994).
[37] Petersen RC, Smith GE, Waring SC, Ivnik RJ, Tangalos EG and Kokmen E. Mild cognitive impairment: clinical characterization and outcome, Arch Neurol 56:303–308 (1999).

[38] Katsarou Z, Bostantjopoulou S, Kimiskidis V, Rossopoulos E and Kazis A. Auditory event-related potentials in Parkinson's disease in relation to cognitive ability. Percept Mot Skills 98:1441-1448 (2004).

[39] Squires KC, Wickens C, Squires NK and Donchin E. The effect of stimulus sequence on the waveform of the cortical event-related potential, Science 193:1142-1146 (1976).

[40] Papaliagkas VT, Kimiskidis VK, Tsolaki MN and Anogianakis G. Usefulness of event-related potentials in the assessment of mild cognitive impairment. BMC Neurosci 9:107 (2008).

[41] Defrancesco M, Marksteiner J, Deisenhammer E, Kemmler G, Djurdjevic T, Schocke M. Impact of white matter lesions and cognitive deficits on_conversion_from mild cognitive impairment to Alzheimer's_disease. J Alzheimers Dis. 34:665-72 (2013)

[42] Petersen RC. Mild cognitive impairment clinical trials, Nat Rev Drug Discov 2: 646-653 (2003).

[43] de la Monte SM, Sohn YK and Wands JR. Correlates of p53- and Fas (CD95)-mediated apoptosis in Alzheimer's disease, J Neurol Sci 152:73-83 (1997).

[44] Liu X, Kim CN, Yang J, Jemmerson R and Wang X. Induction of apoptotic program in cell-free extracts: requirement for dATP and cytochrome c. Cell 86:147-157 (1996).

[45] Shimohama S. Apoptosis in Alzheimer's disease-an update, Apoptosis 5:9-16 (2000).

[46] Kitamura Y, Shimohama S, Kamoshima W, Ota T, Matsuoka Y, Nomura Y, *et al.* Alteration of proteins regulating apoptosis, Bcl-2, Bcl-x, Bax, Bak, Bad, ICH-1 and CPP32 in Alzheimer's disease, Brain Res 780:260–269 (1998).

[47] Nagy ZS and Esiri MM. Apoptosis-related protein expression in the hippocampus in Alzheimer's disease, Neurobiol Aging 18:565–571 (1997).

[48] Rohn TT, Head E. Caspase activation in Alzheimer's disease: early to rise and late to bed. Rev Neurosci.19:383-93 (2008).

[49] Rohn TT, Rissman RA, Davis MC, Kim YE, Cotman CW and Head E. Caspase-9 activation and caspase cleavage of tau in the Alzheimer's disease brain, Neurobiol Dis 11:341–354 (2002).

[50] Satou T, Cummings BJ and Cotman CW. Immunoreactivity for Bcl-2 protein within neurons in the Alzheimer's disease brain increases with disease severity. Brain Res 697:35–43 (1995).

[51] Stadelmann C, Deckwerth TL, Srinivasan A, Bancher C, Bruck W, Jellinger K, *et al.* Activation of caspase-3 in single neurons and autophagic granules of granulovacular degeneration in Alzheimer's disease, Am J Pathol 155:1459–1466 (1999).

[52] Su JH, Deng G and Cotman CW. Bax protein expression is increased in Alzheimer's brain: correlations with DNA damage, Bcl-2 expression, and brain pathology, J Neuropathol Exp Neurol 56:86–93 (1997).

[53] Zhao M, Su J, Head E and Cotman CW. Accumulation of caspase cleaved amyloid precursor protein represents an early neurodegenerative event in aging and in Alzheimer's disease, Neurobiol Dis 14:391–401 (2003).

[54] Bennys K, Portet F, Touchon J and Rondouin G. Diagnostic value of event-related evoked potentials N200 and P300 subcomponents in early diagnosis of Alzheimer's disease and mild cognitive impairment, J Clin Neurophysiol. 24:405-412 (2007).

[55] Missonnier P, Deiber MP, Gold G, Herrmann FR, Millet P, Michon A, *et al.* Working memory load-related electroencephalographic parameters can differentiate progressive from stable mild cognitive impairment, Neuroscience 150:346-56 (2007).

[56] Allison T, Puce A and McCarthy G. Category-sensitive excitatory and inhibitory processes in human extrastriate cortex, J Neurophysiol 88:2864-2868 (2002).

CHAPTER 7

Cholinesterase Inhibitors and Beyond

Giancarlo Pepeu* and Maria G. Giovannini

Department of Preclinical and Clinical Pharmacology, University of Florence, Viale Pieraccini 6, 50139 Florence, Italy

Abstract: Cholinesterase inhibitors (ChEIs) were introduced in the therapy of Alzheimer Disease (AD) in the nineties with great expectations. The hopes and large interest raised by these drugs are well demonstrated by 12,000 references listed by PubMed under ChEI for 1995-2007. The list is reduced to 2500 if we confine ourselves to ChEIs and dementia. Of them about 500 were published in the last two years. Whereas an increase in brain acetylcholine and an improvement of cognitive deficits have been consistently demonstrated in animal models of AD, from aging rats to transgenic mice, ChEIs clinical effectiveness has been and is still a matter of contrasting opinions. These range from the negative conclusions of the AD2000 trial on donepezil, claiming that it is no cost effective, with benefits below minimally relevant threshold, to the NICE appraisal of 2007 declaring that donepezil, rivastigmine, galantamine are efficacious for mild to moderate AD, irrespective of their different selectivity for AChE and BuChE. The possibility that ChEIs may exert their effects through mechanisms beyond cholinesterase inhibition has been envisaged. However, according to the information presented in this review, the "classical" ChEIs, donepezil, rivastigmine and galantamine, show no pharmacological actions beyond cholinesterase inhibition which may play an important role in their therapeutic efficacy. The diverging opinions on clinical efficacy do not discourage from developing new ChEIs, and the so called multifunctional ChEIs. They represent the future of the cholinergic therapy for AD but other indications for these drugs may be considered, including vascular dementia, mild cognitive impairment, and the ethically sensitive improvement of memory and learning in healthy subjects.

An update of this review carried out four years after its first publication reveals a persistent interest for ChEIs, as demonstrated by the publication of more than 3500 preclinical and clinical papers since 2010. However, no substantial development in the field has come about, namely no novel ChEI effects have been detected beside those caused by inhibition of cholinesterases and the ensuing acetylcholine increase. The only novel indication is the extension of rivastigmine to the treatment of dementia with Lewy bodies and Parkinson' disease dementia, in some countries.

***Corresponding author Giancarlo Pepeu:** Department of Pharmacology, Viale Pieraccini 6, 50139 Florence, Italy; Tel: 39 005 4271274; Fax: 39 005 4271280; E-mail: giancarlo.pepeu@unifi.it

Keywords: Acetylcholine, acetylcholinesterase, alzheimer therapy, β-Amyloid, novel cholinesterase inhibitors.

INTRODUCTION

In a recent paper on the prescription pattern and efficacy of drugs for patients with dementia, Frisoni *et al.* [1] concluded that in 88 Italian Alzheimer Evaluation Units cholinesterase inhibitors (ChEI) were prescribed to 90% of patients with Alzheimer's Disease (AD), 80% with Lewy body dementia and 35-45% with vascular dementia. Moreover, following the outcome of a judicial review in August 2007, NICE [2] amended and reissued its guidance that now states: "Donepezil, galantamine and rivastigmine are recommended as options for the treatment of moderate Alzheimer's disease only".

This is the situation twenty five years after the seminal paper on "The cholinergic hypothesis of geriatric memory dysfunction" by Bartus *et al.* [3] which can be taken as the starting point for the cholinergic therapy of AD. In that paper, many years of preclinical research on the brain cholinergic system in aging were summarized and the limited therapeutic results obtained with physostigmine were described. Physostigmine was the only ChEI that could be administered to man at that time, and the modest cognitive improvement observed after its administration was considered a proof of concept that a therapy based on cholinesterase inhibition could work in AD patients. Twenty five years are a long time and make it possible to look in perspective to the story of ChEI development, their success and failures and to pharmacological effects and clinical applications that may be beyond the primary action of inhibiting acetylcholinesterase (AChE) and butyrylcholinesterase (BuChE). Aim of this paper is to identify whether a "beyond" exists and define what it could be.

Four years after Bartus's paper [3], Summers *et al.* [4] reported striking therapeutic results obtained in a small group of AD patients with tacrine, a more active and longer lasting ChEI than physostigmine, that had been used in man as a decurarizing agent in anaesthesiology. Results obtained with tacrine were considered a breakthrough in AD treatment and the drug was approved in the US in 1993. Its success was short-lasting because of liver toxicity, and it was never licensed in Europe. However, several new drugs, well supported by demonstration of efficacy in animal models of AD, were already on the launching pad at that time. In 1988, in a volume on "Current Research in Alzheimer Therapy", edited by Giacobini and Becker [5], metrifonate, huperzine A and B, galantamine and heptylphysostigmine were presented as potential therapeutic agents for AD. They were overtaken by donepezil (E2020) that was licensed in US in 1996. Its preclinical pharmacology was described by Rogers *et al.* in 1991 [6] and Rogers and Friedhoff [7] reported its clinical efficacy and safety. In the meantime the pharmacology of the carbamate derivative rivastigmine (ENA 713), was reported [8] and the positive results of a large clinical trial on 725 AD patients were published by Rösler *et al.* [9] shortly later. Donepezil is a selective AChE inhibitor while rivastigmine inhibits both AChE and BuChE [10]. This difference appears to have no influence on the clinical efficacy of these drugs [11].

Of the other compounds under preclinical and clinical investigation for many years, the clinical efficacy of heptylphysostigmine (eptastigmine) was demonstrated [12] but adverse hematologic (granulocytopenia) effects reported in two studies resulted in the suspension of further clinical trials [13]. Similarly, clinical trials demonstrated the efficacy of metrifonate in AD patients [14]. Unfortunately, a few cases of muscular weakness occurring in a phase III trial prevented its registration [15]. Eptastigmine and metrifonate are two of the many cases of efficacious drugs failing at the last hurdles before approval because of unexpected side effects. Conversely, galantamine was successful [16] and the drug was approved in 2001. Trials on huperzine A are still in progress but, because of its "herbal" origin, the drug is already used as an "alternative" medicine for dementia [17].

The introduction in AD therapy of tacrine, but particularly of donepezil and rivastigmine, was accompanied and followed by a large number of publications demonstrating the interest and hopes risen by these drugs. For the period between 1991 and the end of 2007 PubMed listed 1299 papers in English for donepezil, of them 272 report clinical trials, rivastigmine has been the subject of 632 papers 131 of which are clinical. Galantamine comes third with 588 papers 93 of which are clinical trials. This is only a small part of the over 22,741 titles, generated by a search on PubMed with the words cholinesterase inhibitors, in the 25 years from

1982 to date. The emotional, social and economic burden of AD and the growing size of the market in the aging developed countries are the main reasons for the large number of publications on the chemistry, pharmacology and therapeutic efficacy of these drugs. Facing these numbers, the present review can not be exhaustive but will quote a fraction of the existing papers only, emphasizing animal and human studies that best document the typical effects resulting from ChE inhibition and the effects resulting from other actions.

CHOLINESTERASE INHIBITION

Acute Effects on AChE and ACh Levels

The loss of forebrain cholinergic neurons and the ensuing reduced synthesis and release of acetylcholine (ACh) is considered a crucial pathogenetic feature of AD since the historical paper of Davies and Maloney [18] (for reviews see Francis *et al.* [19], Francis and Perry [20]). ChEIs have been considered the best tool for restoring an adequate level of ACh in the synaptic gap since they prevent the hydrolysis of the residual ACh in the brain of AD patients. The question arises as to whether ChEIs really increase brain ACh. In the rat an increase in brain ACh extracellular levels, measured by microdialysis, has been consistently demonstrated, as exemplified in Table **1**.

Table 1: Increase of extracellular ACh levels and ChE inhibition following acute administration of different ChEIs

Drug	Dose mg/kg	Brain Region	ACh % Increase#	Duration in Min	% Inhibition AChE	BuChE	Reference
Donepezil	0.5 s.c.	cortex	200	60	15	-	[21]
Donepezil	2.0 s.c.	cortex	2100	180	35	-	[21]
Donepezil	1.0 i.p.	cortex	400	120	22	8	[23]
Donepezil	1.6 i.p.	cortex	80	120	18	-	[91]
Rivastigmine	0.6 i.p.	cortex	400	120	40	18	[23]
Rivastigmine	0.5 i.p.	cortex	78	90	42	-	[91]
Rivastigmine	1.5 os	hippocampus	625	100	-		[35]
Rivastigmine	4.5 os	hippocampus	1157	180	-		[35]
Metrifonate	80 os	frontal cortex	300	80	79	-	[48]
Heptastigmine	5.0 i.p	cortex	700	540	90	-	[92]
PEC*	5.0 i.p.	cortex	250	180	12	37	[23]

*PEC = N^1 phenethyl-norcimserine; # percent increase calculated at the peak increase.

The increase in ACh level is dose-dependent within the same experiment [21]. However, there is a large variability among the results obtained in different laboratories in the percent increase in extracellular ACh levels after the administration of similar ChEI doses, as shown in Table **1**. The differences presumably depend on the placement of the probes, composition and rate of the perfusing medium and other technical details. Nevertheless, within this variability, donepezil and rivastigmine, given at comparable dosages, bring about similar ACh increases even if donepezil is a selective AChE inhibitor and rivastigmine inhibits both AChE and BuChE [22;23]. Moreover, a significant increase in brain ACh occurs not only after AChE inhibition but also after selective BuChE inhibition [23] suggesting a more important role of BuChE in the regulation of AChE extracellular level than commonly believed. From the data presented in Table **1**, no correlation can be drawn between AChE and BuChE inhibition and the increase in extracellular ACh levels. This confirms that a correlation between AChE inhibition and ACh level increase is at the best very approximate, and the information available does not allow one to define which is the minimal ChE inhibition resulting in a significant increase in ACh extracellular levels in the brain [24]. Among the reasons for this lack of correlation, the possibility that the time of the peak increase in ACh level does not necessarily correspond to that of the maximum ChE inhibition, and dilution effects during the determination of enzyme activity. In this regard, it must be kept in mind that donepezil is a reversible, rivastigmine is a pseudo-irreversible and metrifonate is an irreversible ChE inhibitor [25].

Effects of Chronic Treatment on AChE and ACh Levels

Since ChEIs are typically used in long-term therapy, the question has been asked whether tolerance, and consequent decrease in AChE inhibition, develops after repeated administration of the inhibitor. Moreover, whether the persisting high level of ACh results in decreased ACh synthesis and modifications in cholinoceptor function. In Table **2** the extracellular ACh levels and AChE inhibition after 21 days of administration of four different ChEIs are presented.

Table 2: Extracellular ACh levels and AChE inhibition 18 h after the last administration of different cholinesterase inhibitors

Drug	**Dose mg/kg**	**Cortex**		**Hippocampus**	
		ACh fmol/µl±SEM	**AChE % Inhibition**	**ACh fmol/µl±SEM**	**AChE % Inhibition**
Vehicle		1.88±0.3	None	1.4±0.3	none
Tacrine	3	2.6±0.66 (138%)	15±2	1.84±0.4 (126%)	15±2
Donepezil	1.5	3.1± 0.5* (164%)	39±7	n.d	45±5
Rivastigmine	0.75	12.4±1.4* (659%)	52±6	2.7±0.4* (192%)	53±8
Metrifonate	80	25.0 ±5.4* (1330%)	85±3	3.8±0.9* (261%)	80±3

Data were obtained 21 days administration, p.o. twice a day. Number of rats 6-10; n.d. not done; *P< 0.05 at least *vs.* vehicle values. Data taken from Giovannini *et al.* [93] and Scali *et al.* [28]. The numbers in parenthesis are the percent increase.

The table shows that an almost complete AChE inhibition, accompanied by large increase in ACh extracellular level in the cortex and hippocampus, is still present 18 h after the last metrifonate administration. This demonstrates that, using an irreversible inhibitor, AChE inhibition is long-lasting and ACh levels remain high for a long time. In agreement with this finding, after chronic (2 or 5 weeks) metrifonate administration (100 mg/kg daily i.p.), 84 and 68% AChE inhibition was found in the cerebral cortex and hippocampus, respectively [26]. Conversely, AChE activity was largely restored 18 h after the administration of the reversible inhibitors tacrine and donepezil [27], while the increase in ACh level was still present with donepezil only. The pseudo-irreversible inhibitor rivastigmine showed an intermediate position with 50% AChE inhibition 18 h after the last administration [28] and a 6 fold increase in ACh level. Two h after the last administration of rivastigmine (2.75 mg/kg p.o, once per day per 21 days), Enz and Gentsch [29] detected a 27% AChE inhibition.

Whereas in Table **1**, which summarizes acute experiments from different laboratories, no correlation between the increase in ACh and AChE inhibition is shown and a large ACh increase is reported even after a modest 15% inhibition, in Table **2**, reporting long-term experiments from the same laboratory, a rough correlation between AChE inhibition and ACh levels can be observed and about 30% inhibition appears to be sufficient to induce a significant increase in ACh levels.

In rats treated for 1, 4 and 14 days with donepezil, 3 mg/kg s.c., 4 h after the last administration Haug *et al.* [30] found similar level of brain AChE inhibition (about 60%), accompanied by comparable increase in total ACh level (about 35%) and no change in choline acetyltransferase (ChAT) activity, vesicular transporter, choline transporter and the expression of cholinergic genes. No change in ChAT activity also occurred after 2 or 5 week metrifonate administration which caused a 84 and 68 % AChE inhibition in the cerebral cortex and hippocampus, respectively [26].

From the animal experiments investigating the effects of prolonged ChEI treatments here reported, it may be concluded that AChE, ChAT, and the transport mechanisms of choline and ACh do not undergo adaptive changes resulting in reduced AChE inhibition and ACh synthesis and ACh levels remain elevated. Muscarinic M_2 autoreceptors only appear to undergo some adaptation [28].

To which extent AChE and BuChE inhibition and the increase in brain ACh following ChEI administration, demonstrated in preclinical studies, also occur in the brain of AD patients still need to be investigated with appropriate tools. In humans, cholinesterase inhibition has been measured by PET and radiolabeled ACh analogue substrates [31]. Venneri [32], reviewing the existing studies, points out that the degree of AChE inhibition observed after about 6 weeks of donepezil treatment, with standard doses, is around 30%. After 3 to 5 months treatment with typical clinical doses, Kaasinen *et al.* [33] found a 38.5 % inhibition in the frontal cortex with donepezil and 37.1% with rivastigmine and a lower inhibition in other cortical areas. Even these partial inhibitions resulted in cognitive improvement.

Bohnen *et al.* [34] observed that after 12 weeks of donepezil treatment, AChE inhibition was only 19% in the anterior cingulate cortex in patients with mild AD but the degree of enzyme inhibition correlated with improvements in executive and attentional functions.

DIRECT AND INDIRECT ChEI ACTIONS ON OTHER BRAIN NEUROTRANSMITTERS AND ON RECEPTORS

Acute Administration

It has been shown that during the treatment with some ChEIs, levels of neurotransmitters other than ACh are affected. Donepezil at the dose of 0.5 mg/kg s.c. increases the extracellular levels of noradrenaline and, at the dose of 2.0 mg/kg s.c., the levels of noradrenaline and dopamine in the rat cerebral cortex, without affecting those of 5HT [21]. Conversely, a small decrease in noradrenaline and an increase in homovanillic acid extracellular levels were detected in the cerebral cortex of rats after the oral administration of 4.5 mg/kg of rivastigmine [35]. These effects on monoamines could be secondary to ChE inhibition and cholinergic activation or direct on monoaminergic neurones. Trabace *et al.* [36] detected no changes in cortical extracellular levels of noradrenaline, dopamine and serotonin at doses of gangstigmine which caused a dose-dependent increase in ACh extracellular level. The observation that no clear differences exist between the behavioural effects of donepezil and rivastigmine, which, as reported above, have opposite effects on noradrenaline levels suggests that the change in monoamine levels found after large dose of ChEIs have limited functional meanings. Behavioral studies on huperzine A may help clarify this point since this drug, administered systemically or by reverse microdialysis in the cerebral cortex, brings about a dose-dependent increase in extracellular levels of ACh, noradrenaline and dopamine [37].

Some ChEIs bind to cholinoceptors. Galantamine is an allosteric potentiating ligand of the nicotinic ACh receptors (nAChRs) as shown in PC12 cells [38]. It binds allosterically to the α-subunit of nAChR at a site different from that of ACh resulting in a conformational change of the receptor [39]. However, by comparing the effects of galantamine and donepezil on memory performance in rats, Hernandez *et al.* [40] concluded that the allosteric potentiating ligand activity does not afford any advantage over AChE inhibition alone. According to Snape *et al.* [27], tacrine and donepezil show some affinity for muscarinic receptors *in vitro* as indicated by the displacement of [^{3}H]methylscopolamine and the inhibition of carbachol-stimulated [Ca^{2+}] increase, although at concentrations unlikely to have clinical meaning. The same authors demonstrated that tacrine and donepezil have no affinity for monoamine receptors.

Chronic Administration: Effects on Cholinergic and Non-Cholinergic Receptors

ChE inhibition does not develop a significant tolerance and ACh synthesis is not affected by chronic inhibitor treatment, as reported above. This leads to a persisting, large ACh concentration in the synaptic clefts and a long-lasting activation which may result in changes in the number, affinity and function of muscarinic (mAChR) and nicotinic (nAChR) receptors. Scali *et al.* [28] observed that after 21 days of metrifonate treatment, the M_2-M_4 autoreceptors, modulating ACh release, lost their function, as demonstrated by the finding that no increase in ACh release occurred after retrograde perfusion with the M_2-M_4 antagonist AFDX-384. The activity of M_2-M_4 was attenuated after rivastigmine treatment and was not affected by the treatment with donepezil which presumably causes intermittent increases in ACh levels. In agreement with these findings, a decrease in [^{3}H]AFDX binding to M_2-M_4 in several brain areas was observed in rats treated with tacrine for 7 (10 mg/kg i.p.) [41] and 21 days (from 2.5 to 10 mg/kg s.c) [42]. Furthermore, [^{3}H]AFDX binding, was reduced after 15 days of galantamine and donepezil treatment [40]. Repeated administrations of tacrine and donepezil seem to induce different changes in M_1 mAChRs, whose number was quantified by [^{3}H]pirenzepine binding. Decreases in the M_1 receptors were found in cingulate and entorhinal cortex as well as in the putamen caudate after 10 days tacrine injection [41], while increases in the lamina II layer and the olfactory bulb were detected after 15 days of donepezil and galantamine injections [40]. The latter authors found diverging modifications in nAChRs after prolonged treatment with galantamine and donepezil, namely a decrease in the anterior thalamus and an increase in the expression of high affinity nAChRs labelled with [^{125}I]IPH, an epibatidine analogue, in the cingulated cortex and postsubiculum, and no change in the low affinity α7nAChRs identified by [^{125}I]-bungarotoxin binding. In homogenates of hippocampus and cortex of aged rats, an increase in [^{3}H]nicotine binding was observed in animals that received galantamine or donepezil for 33 days *via* osmotic minipumps, compared with saline controls [43]. This finding was not confirmed by Zhang *et al.* [42] who found no significant changes in nAChRs following chronic treatment with tacrine. They had previously shown an increase in nAChR measured by [^{3}H]ACh in rats treated with the same dose of tacrine [44] and by PET in cortical brain regions of AD patients treated with tacrine [45] or rivastigmine (see ref in [42]).

It appears that only the M_2-M_4 autoreceptors are constantly down-regulated in rats treated with ChEIs while other muscarinic receptors, and the nicotinic receptors may undergo contrasting changes presumably depending not so much on the increase in ACh levels but on doses, duration of the treatment, differences in the pharmacological profile of the individual ChEIs, regions investigated, and the receptor ligands used. Therefore, while we may assume that the down-regulation of the M2-M4 autoreceptors, by attenuating an inhibitory control on the release, may contribute in maintaining a high level of extracellular ACh [28], it is difficult to define if the changes in other cholinergic receptors play a role in the therapeutic efficacy of ChEIs.

Few studies investigated whether chronic administration of ChEIs modifies the number and function of non cholinergic receptors, either indirectly through the long-lasting increase in ACh levels or directly by interacting with the receptors. A decrease in AMPA receptor binding throughout the brain was observed by Sihver *et al.* [41] after 7 days of treatment with tacrine (10 mg/kg i.p.) while NMDA, kainate and $GABA_A$ receptor binding were unchanged. A decrease in 5-HT_{2A} receptor density was detected in the midbrain of mice treated with donepezil (0.1 mg/kg i.p.) for 14 days by Hayslett and Tizabi [46]. According to them, this finding may explain the attenuation by donepezil of the head-twitch induced in mice by the administration of DOI, a selective agonist of the 5-$HT_{2A/2C}$ receptors, thus envisaging the possibility to use donepezil in the Tourette's syndrome. Given the small dose of donepezil used in these experiments, it is unlikely that this effect may depend on AChE inhibition.

ChEI EFFECTS ON COGNITIVE PROCESS

Acute Administration

ChEIs are administered with the main purpose of attenuating the cognitive deficits which represent the first and most disturbing symptoms of AD and other dementias. For this reason, the effects of ChEIs on cognitive processes in various models of cognitive deficits have been widely investigated at preclinical levels. An extensive review of the preclinical results obtained with acute and chronic treatment of donepezil, rivastigmine, galantamine and memantine was recently published [47] and we refer the reader to it. Here we present a few examples only, to show the most common models of cognitive impairment in rodents (Tables **3** and **4**) in which different ChEIs have been tested.

Table 3: Improvement of cognitive deficits after acute ChEI administration in animal models of Alzheimer's Disease

Drug	Dose mg/kg	Animal Model	Cognitive Test	Reference
Metrifonate	80 os	Aged rats	Object recognition	[48]
Gangstigmine	3 os	Scopolamine	Object recognition	[36]
Rivastigmine	0.1 – 0.5 ip	Scopolamine	Delayed non-matching to position	[50]
Donepezil	0.3 os	Ibotenic acid	Water maze	[94]
Galantamine	5.0 ip	NBM lesions, mice	Morris Water maze	[95]
PEC	0.25 * 0.5 ip	Aged rats	14 unit T maze	[49]

NBM = nucleus basalis magnocellularis, PEC = (-)-N1-phenetylnorcymserine; * twice per day for 4 days.

In all the examples shown in Table **3**, the increase in ACh extracellular levels following ChE inhibition appears to be the mechanism through which the cognitive impairment was improved. For instance, cortical extracellular ACh levels are lower in aging than in young-adult rats [48] and it is postulated that this is the cause of the impairment in object recognition corrected by metrifonate administration [28]. Similarly, PEC increases ACh level through selective BuChE inhibition [23] and restores the T maze performance in aging rats [49]. Scopolamine causes a cognitive deficit by blocking muscarinic receptors and it is assumed that, following ChEI administration, the ensuing increase in ACh extracellular levels displaces scopolamine from the receptors and attenuates the cognitive deficit [36, 50]. It should be noted that the behavioral tests used in evaluating ChEI activity involve attention, working and spatial memory, processes involving the activation of the forebrain cholinergic system [51].

Effects of Chronic ChEI Administration on Cognitive Processes

Table 4: Improvement of Cognitive Deficits after Chronic Chei Administration in Animal Models of Alzheimer's Disease

Drug	Dose mg/kg	Duration	Animal Model	Cognitive Test	Reference
Donepezil	0.37 - 0.75 sc	15 days	Aged rats	Morris water maze	[40]
Galantamine	3.0 – 6.0 sc	15 days	Aged rats	Morris water maze	[40]
Donepezil	0.1-0.3-1.0	6 weeks	Tg2576 mice	Water T maze, fear conditioning	[60]
Donepezil	0.27 sc Alzet*	2 mo	APP23 mice	Morris water maze	[96]
Rivastigmine	0.5 ip	2 weeks	APP23 mice	Morris water maze	[97]
Rivastigmine	0.2 os	3 weeks	Aged rats	Morris water maze	[98]

*Alzet osmotic minipump.

A few examples of chronic effects are shown in Table **4**. In a long term experiment in APP23 mice, it was found that the dose of 0.27 mg/kg of donepezil was more effective than the higher dose of 0.58 mg/kg in improving the performance in the Morris water maze. This is an example of the inverted U-shaped dose-response curve that characterizes the cognitive effects of ChEIs [52] and, more in general, all the so called "cognition enhancing" drugs [53]. ChEI ability to restore the cognitive deficits after chronic administration, demonstrates that no adaptation develops to these drugs, notwithstanding the receptor binding modifications described in a previous section.

BEYOND CHOLINESTERASE INHIBITION

ChEI Effects on Beta-Amyloid Deposition and Plaques Formation

Modulation of Amyloid Protein Precursor (APP) Metabolism and Aβ Formation and Disposal

The degeneration of the forebrain cholinergic neurons is an important feature of AD, but it is commonly accepted that the main pathogenetic mechanism of AD is the deposition of amyloid beta-protein (Aβ) in the brain, and the neurotoxicity of its peptides [54]. Nitsch *et al.* [55] showed in transfected cultured cells that the stimulation of muscarinic M_1 and M_3 receptors increased the basal secretion of amyloid precursor protein (APP) suggesting the possibility that ChEIs, by restoring ACh levels, may modulate Aβ metabolism and reduce the formation of its deposits. This hypothesis generated many *in vitro* and *in vivo* investigations. They were reviewed by Svensson and Giacobini [56] who concluded that "drugs such ChEIs used with the purpose of increasing cholinergic neurotransmission may improve or correct the APP metabolism imbalance".

Racchi *et al.* [57], reviewing their own work, and the existing experimental evidence on ChEI effect on Aβ deposition, suggested that it depends on multiple complex mechanisms involving either a cholinergic agonistic effect due to the increase in ACh levels or post transcriptional effects, unrelated to ChE inhibition, that modulate the expression of cellular APP.

The importance of the cholinergic neurons in regulating APP processing and Aβ production seems confirmed by the observation that in transgenic Tg2576 mice, a model of AD, treatment with scopolamine for 14 days, suppressing cortical cholinergic transmission by chronic inhibition of the muscarinic ACh receptors, resulted in an increased level of fibrillary $A\beta_{(1-40)}$ and $A\beta_{(1-42)}$, whereas the level of soluble, SDS-extractable Aβ remained unchanged, as compared to vehicle-injected Tg2576 mice. Alpha-Secretase activity determined in cortical tissue from scopolamine-treated Tg2576 mice was lower by about 30% as compared to controls [58]. Although most of the *in vitro* experiments confirmed that ChEIs reduce Aβ accumulation [59], the results of *in vivo* experiments are contrasting. Dong *et al.* [60] found no changes in the deposition of Aβ plaques in transgenic TG2576 mice treated for 6 weeks with donepezil or physostigmine at doses improving the cognitive deficit. Lahiri *et al.* [61] demonstrated in mice that 21 day treatment with phenserine 7.5 and 15 mg/kg ip resulted in a significant decrease in cortical level of $A\beta_{(1-42)}$ but in a non significant decrease of Aβ(1-40). However, the enantiomer (+)-phenserine, posiphen, a weak ChEI, was much more effective than phenserine in reducing Aβ and APP levels, through non cholinergic multiple mechanisms. Daily administration of huperzine A (0.2 mg /kg i.p.) for 12 consecutive days produced significant reversals of the $A\beta_{(1-40)}$-induced down-regulation of secretory APP and protein kinase C in rats. These findings suggest that huperzine A may affect APP processing by up-regulating PKC, especially PKCα [62]. Some clinical studies support the possibility that ChEIs might actually reduce Aβ deposition exerting a "disease modifying" action. Donepezil administered for 30 days in subjects affected by mild to moderate AD induced an increase in the ratio of APP forms with different molecular weights in platelets, a finding suggesting a potential effect of AChE inhibitors on APP trafficking or processing in peripheral cells [63, 64]. In a further investigation in platelets [64] it was demonstrated that donepezil is capable of restoring the balance between α-and β-secretase activity altered in AD patients by increasing α- and reducing β-secretase. In a post-mortem study in 24 patients with dementia with Lewy bodies treated with ChEIs, compared with untreated patients, it was shown that the treated patients had significantly less parenchimal Aβ deposition in the cerebral cortex than untreated patients [65]. Unfortunately, in this study the names of ChEIs administered to the patients were not reported, and further investigations are needed to define if ChEI effect on APP and Aβ metabolism depends on the increase in ACh levels and/or on the chemical structures and peculiar pharmacological properties of the compounds used. Nevertheless, in evaluating the results suggesting a positive effect of ChEIs on Aβ deposition, it should be considered that no changes of $A\beta_{(1-42)}$ levels were found in the CSF of patients with mild AD treated with rivastigmine or tacrine for one year [66]. The same lack of changes in CSF $A\beta_{(1-42)}$ was reported by Parnetti *et al.* [67] after treating patients suffering of mild to moderate AD with donepezil, rivastigmine and galantamine for 6 months.

Neuroprotective Effects

The influence of ChEIs on APP processing and the alteration of the levels of $A\beta_{(1-42)}$ and $A\beta_{(1-40)}$, described in the previous section, leads to an attenuation of Aβ toxicity. For this reason Nordberg [59] attributes a neuroprotective effect to ChEI. Zhang *et al.* [68] investigated the protective effect of huperzine A on Aβ associated neurotoxicity in cultured PC12 cells and cultured primary cortical neurons. They demonstrated that huperzine A exerts antioxidant and antiapoptotic actions. Since the steroisomer (-)-huperzine A is much less potent than (+)-huperzine A as a ChEI but both drugs have similar antioxidant and antiapoptotic actions, these latter effects seem unrelated to ChE inhibition. Unfortunately, there are only few animal experiments confirming the neuroprotective action of ChEI *in vivo*. Zhou and coworkers [69] demonstrated a reduction of the neuronal damage induced by a transient global ischemia in gerbils treated for 14 days with huperzine A (0.1 mg/kg p.o. for 14 days). Neuroprotective actions of galantamine have been demonstrated in cultured cells, in hippocampal slices deprived of oxygen and glucose and in a NGF depleted mice. These actions are attributed mostly to the allosteric nAChR potentiating effect of this drug [70].

Neuroprotective properties are attributed to some of the novel ChEIs, particularly to the so called multifunctional compounds described in the following section.

Multifunctional and Hybrid ChEIs

In AD brain, plaques and tangles, the pathological hallmarks of this disorder, display intense and widespread AChE and BuChE activity [71] and it was demonstrated that these ChEs possess enzymatic properties which are distinctly different from those of neuronal ChE [72] when compared with those associated with normal neurons and axons. The properties of ChEs in plaques and tangles are identical to those found in glial cells [73]. The latter finding lead to the suggestion that the ChEs in plaques and tangles may originate from the glial cells recruited and activated in the AD brain. Recent evidence indicates that ChEs may be involved in the pathogenesis of plaques. Both AChE and BuChE appear to enhance the aggregation of the amyloid-β peptide, a major event in the process of plaque formation [74], and increase the toxicity of Aβ [75]. BuChE seems to play a more important role in plaque pathogenesis since BuChE expression increases as plaques go through the process of maturation from the diffuse type to the pathologic compact variety [76]. AChE interacts with Aβ peptide and promotes amyloid fibril formation by a hydrophobic environment close to the peripheral anionic binding site of the enzyme and the structural motif involved in this reaction has been identified [77]. Therefore, it has been suggested that ChEIs, in addition to ameliorating the cholinergic deficits, may interfere with the process of plaque formation not only acting on APP and Aβ metabolism, as described in the previous section, but also by interfering with Aβ fibril aggregation. Rivastigmine has been shown [78] to inhibit AChE and BuChE in plaque and tangles with the same potency as in normal brain cells. The possibility that this action may modify AD process is supported by preliminary neuropathological observations indicating that brains of AD patients treated with rivastigmine for 3 years or longer contained a significantly lower number of the pathologic compact plaques than the brains of patients who had received no ChE inhibitors [79]. Starting from the observation that the catalytic site for ACh hydrolysis is different from the site promoting Aβ aggregation, new ChEIs have been designed with the purpose of interacting simultaneously with the catalytic and peripheral site of the enzyme. Preliminary *in vivo* studies in transgenic mice overexpressing human APP (hAPP-(751)) suggest that this class of tacrine-indole heterodimers leads to a net reduction of Aβ peptide plaque load in the animals and an improvement in their cognitive functions [80, 81].

Bis(7) tacrine is a dimeric ChEI that reduces the amount of both secreted and intracellular Aβ in transfected cell, through a mechanism involving the activation of alpha-secretase and the inhibition of beta-secretase [82], inhibits nitric oxide synthase *in vitro* [83] and protects rat pheochromocytoma cell from oxidative stress [84]. However, only *in vivo* experiments on animal models of AD will demonstrated whether these interesting properties, beyond ChE inhibition, have therapeutic importance.

Ladostigil is multifunctional or hybrid compound formed by the combination of two pharmacophores, the carbamate moiety of the ChEI inhibitor rivastigmine and the propargilic group of the monoamine oxidase B inhibitor rasagiline [85]. This drug, which is now in Phase 2 clinical trial, inhibits *in vitro* and *in vivo* ChE and monoamine oxidase, reduces apoptosis and stimulates APP processing [86]. The clinical trials will demonstrate the therapeutic value of this drug in AD and other neurodegenerative disease.

The above are the most studied multifunctional ChEIs. Their list could be longer but to describe them is premature since it is not yet clear whether some of their effects depends on actions beyond ChE inhibition.

If the hybrid, multifunctional ChEI represent a novel approach whose usefulness still needs to be proved, the confirmation of a useful, although moderate, clinical efficacy of the available ChEIs, donepezil, rivastigmine and galantamine, and the growing number of patients who need these drugs, are the reasons prompting the development of new "conventional" ChEIs. Among them, the already mentioned phenserine [87] and gangstigmine [88], the selective BuChE inhibitor cymserine [49], new donepezil and galantamine derivatives [86]. Whether these compounds will demonstrate new actions beyond ChE inhibition, it needs to be demonstrated.

THERAPEUTIC INDICATIONS BEYOND AD

Finally if, so far, pharmacological effects depending on ChE inhibition and on actions beyond ChE inhibition have been discussed, possible therapeutic applications beyond the standard ChEI indication of "mild to moderate AD" [11] and recently also severe AD, should be also mentioned. Some of these "off label" indications, listed in Table **5**, are supported by clinical trials, other by preliminary clinical reports only.

Table 5: Proposed "off label" indications for cholinesterase inhibitors

Conditions	Drug	Treatment Duration	Results	Type of Trial	Reference
Lewy bodies dementia	Rivastigmine	20 weeks	Cognitive and neuropsychiatric improvement	Double blind, multicenter	[99]
Vascular dementia	Donepezil, rivastigmine galantamine	6 mo	Small benefits	Metanalysis	[100]
Schizophrenia	Donepezil, rivastigmine, galantamine	> 2 weeks	No clear effect	Metanalysis	[101]
Down syndrome	Donepezil	Up to 16 weeks	Improvement in memory, attention, language	Clinical report	[102]
Narcolepsy	Donepezil	3 mo	Reduced sleepiness	Clinical report	[103]
Healthy subjects (pilots)	Donepezil	30 days	Improvement in flight performance	Clinical investigation	[104]
Students	Huperzine	4 weeks	Improved learning and memory	Clinical investigation	[105]

It is certainly not unexpected that rivastigmine may be efficacious in Lewy body dementia, which is characterized by a cholinergic deficit similar to that of AD

[20]. Conversely, the results obtained with ChEI administration in vascular dementia and schizophrenia are dubious. Single cases seem to respond better than the average but they can not be identified in advance and the situation is reminiscent of the initial period of ChEI therapy in AD, "for the few, but we don't know which few" [89], and justifies further investigations.

The activation of the cholinergic system stimulates the arousal mechanisms, increases alertness, facilitates sustained attention and information acquisition [51]. Presumably, this is the mechanisms through which ChEIs may be active in narcolepsy, in Down syndrome, and improve cognitive processes also in healthy, young subjects. Whether their use as "cognition enhancers" in healthy individuals may be useful and ethically acceptable is a matter of debate.

CONCLUSIONS

Fifteen years after the approval of tacrine by FDA, ChEI preclinical pharmacology has been largely unravelled. ChEIs represent an important group of drugs whose clinical results are, however, not fully satisfactory. According to Franz *et al.* [90] some physicians prescribe them simply to be able to offer "something" to Alzheimer patients and don't expect significant clinical improvements. Nevertheless, ChEIs remain important from a heuristic viewpoint: they are a tool for investigating the role of the cholinergic system in the cognitive processes in health and pathological conditions, may be useful leads for developing new drugs and may have new therapeutic indications. However, according to the information available, the "classical" ChEIs, donepezil, rivastigmine and galantamine, presently widely prescribed, show no pharmacological differences, beyond their inhibitory action on cholinesterase, important enough to result in significant therapeutic differences [11]. Further clinical evidences are needed to prove that ChEI effects on Aβ deposition and plaques formation have disease-modifying efficacy.

UPDATE 2009 – 2013

Four years after the publication of this review, ChEIs are still the most used drugs for the symptomatic treatment of the cognitive deficits of AD [106], in addition to memantine, a NMDA receptor antagonist, administered alone or in association [107]. The development of new treatments acting on the pathogenetic mechanisms of the disease by preventing or removing Aβ load and plaque formation either through the administration of antibodies and vaccines [108] or β and γ secretase inhibitors [109] has met unexpected difficulties due to adverse side effects or lack of efficacy [110]. Of the many new ChEIs under development in 2009, none has been added to the already well established donepezil, rivastigmine and galantamine, and only a new pharmaceutical formulation, rivastigmine transdermal patch [111] was introduced since. Many new multifunctional and hybrid ChEIs have been synthesized but none has yet gone through clinical trials [112]. A clinical trial of phenserine, a ChEI also endowed of modulatory effects on Aβ levels, confirmed some benefits on the cognitive deficits in AD [113], but large phase III trials are still needed to demonstrate its usefulness. Four more years of experience with ChEIs revealed no other pharmacological actions beyond cholinesterase inhibition and the ensuing increase in ACh levels, and no new therapeutic indications beyond AD emerged. Conti *et al.* [114] demonstrated an increase in plasma Aβ antibodies in AD patients treated chronically with ChEIs, irrespective of which ChEI was administered. Nevertheless, it still needs to be demonstrated whether this Aβ antibody increase may be clinically meaningful. The increase in central and peripheral ACh levels following ChEI administration stimulates the cholinergic anti-inflammatory pathway, as repeatedly demonstrated *in vitro* and *in vivo* [115, 116] but there are still no clinical evidences of a therapeutic importance of this ChEI effect.

Of the proposed "off label" indications for ChEIs, listed in Table **5**, rivastigmine has gained a licensed indication in the UK for dementia with Lewy bodies and in mild to moderate Parkinson's disease dementia [106]. ChEI use for treating the cognitive deficits of schizophrenia, as an adjunctive therapy to antipsychotics, has been evaluated in a Cochrane review [117]. The analysis of the clinical trials seems to favor the use of ChEIs in combination with antipsychotics on a few domains of mental state and cognition, but because of various limitations in the studies, the evidence is weak and the indication remains "off label". Although the enhancing effect of ChEIs on attention has been confirmed [118, 119], no adequate studies justify ChEIs use as cognition enhancers in healthy individuals.

ACKNOWLEDGEMENT

Declared none.

CONFLICT OF INTEREST

The authors confirm that this chapter content has no conflict of interest.

DISCLOSURE

This chapter is an update of our previous publication in CAR "Cholinesterase Inhibitors and Beyond" published in 'CAR', Volume 6, Number 2, April, pp. 86 to 96.

REFERENCES

[1] Frisoni GB, Canu E, Geroldi C *et al.* Prescription patterns and efficacy of drugs for patients with dementia: physicians' perspective in Italy. Aging Clin Exp Res 19:349-55 (2007).

[2] National Institute for Health and Clinical Excellence (NICE TA111). Alzheimer's disease - donepezil, galantamine, rivastigmine (review) and memantine for the treatment of Alzheimer's disease. 2007.

[3] Bartus RT, Dean RL, Beer B, Lippa AS. The cholinergic hypothesis of geriatric memory dysfunction. Science 217:408-17 (1982).

[4] Summers WK, Majowski LV, Marsh GM, Kling A. Oral tetrahydroaminoacridine in long term treatment of senile dementia, Alzheime type. New England Journal of Medicine 315:1241-5 (1986).

[5] Giacobini E, Becker R, Eds. Current Research in Alzheimer Therapy. New York: Taylor & Francis (1988).

[6] Rogers SL, Yamanishi Y and Yamatsu K. E2020: the pharmacology of a piperidine cholinesterase inhibitor. In (Eds: Becker R and Giacobini E). *Cholinergic Basis for Alzheimer Therapy.* Boston, MA: *Birkhauser* pp. 314-320 (1991).

[7] Rogers SL, Friedhoff LT. The efficacy and safety of donepezil in patients with Alzheimer's disease: results of a US Multicentre, Randomized, Double-Blind, Placebo-Controlled Trial. The Donepezil Study Group. Dementia 7:293-303 (1996).

[8] Weinstock M, Razin M, Chorev M, Enz A. Pharmacological evaluation of phenyl-carbamates as CNS-selective acetylcholinesterase inhibitors. J Neural Transm Suppl 43:219-25 (1994).

[9] Rosler M, Anand R, Cicin-Sain A *et al.* Efficacy and safety of rivastigmine in patients with Alzheimer's disease: international randomised controlled trial. BMJ 318:633-8 (1999).

[10] Weinstock M. Selectivity of Cholinesterase Inhibition. Clinical Implications for the Treatment of Alzheimer's Disease. CNS Drugs 12:307-23 (1999).

[11] Birks J. Cholinesterase inhibitors for Alzheimer's disease. Cochrane Database Syst Rev CD005593 (2006).

[12] Imbimbo BP, Verdelli G, Martelli P, Marchesini D. Two-year treatment of Alzheimer's disease with eptastigmine. The Eptastigmine Study Group. Dement Geriatr Cogn Disord 10:139-47 (1999]).

[13] Braida D, Sala M. Eptastigmine: ten years of pharmacology, toxicology, pharmacokinetic, and clinical studies. CNS Drug Rev 7:369-86 (2001).

[14] Cummings JL, Cyrus PA, Bieber F *et al.* Metrifonate treatment of the cognitive deficits of Alzheimer's disease. Neurology 50:1214-1221 (1998).

[15] Giacobini E. Cholinesterase in human brain: the effect of cholinesterase inhibitors on Alzheimer's disease and related disorders. In (Eds: Giacobini E and Pepeu G). The brain cholinergic system in health and disease. Abingdon: Informa Healthcare pp. 235-265 (2006).

[16] Scott LJ, Goa KL. Galantamine: a review of its use in Alzheimer's disease. Drugs 60:1095-122 (2000).

[17] Diamond B, Johnson S, Torsney K *et al.* Complementary and alternative medicines in the treatment of dementia: an evidence-based review. Drugs Aging 20:981-98 (2003).

[18] Davies P, Maloney AJR. Selective loss of central cholinergic neurons in Alzheimer's disease. The Lancet 2:1403-5 (1976).

[19] Francis PT, Palmer AM, Snape M, Wilcock GK. The cholinergic hypothesis of Alzheimer's disease: a review of progress. J Neurol Neurosurg Psychiatry 66:137-47 (1999).

[20] Francis PT, Perry EK. Neurochemical pathology of cholinergic system in neurodegenerative and neurodevelopmental disorders. In (Eds: Giacobini E and Pepeu G). The brain cholinergic system in health and disease. Abingdon: Informa Healthcare pp. 59-74 (2006).

[21] Giacobini E, Zhu XD, Williams E, Sherman KA. The effect of the selective reversible acetylcholinesterase inhibitor E2020 on extracellular acetylcholine and biogenic amine levels in rat cortex. Neuropharmacology 35:205-11 (1996).

[22] Giacobini E. Cholinesterase inhibitors: from the Calabar bean to Alzheimer therapy. In (Eds: Giacobini E). Cholinesterases and cholinesterases inhibitors. London: Martin Duniz Ltd pp. 181-226 (2000).

[23] Cerbai F, Giovannini MG, Melani C, Enz A, Pepeu G. N1phenethyl-norcymserine, a selective butyrylcholinesterase inhibitor, increases acetylcholine release in rat cerebral cortex: a comparison with donepezil and rivastigmine. Eur J Pharmacol 572:142-50 (2007).

[24] Pepeu G. Preclinical pharmacology of cholinesterase inhibitors. In (Eds: Giacobini E). *Cholinesterases and cholinesterase inhibitors*. London: Martin Dunitz pp. 145-155 (2000).

[25] Brufani M, Filocamo L. Rational design of cholinesterase inhibitors. In (Eds: Giacobini E). Cholinesterases and cholinesterase inhibitors. London: Martin Dunitz Ltd pp. 27-46 (2000).

[26] Rakonczay Z, Papp H. Effects of chronic metrifonate treatment on cholinergic enzymes and the blood-brain barrier. Neurochem Int 39:19-24 (2001).

[27] Snape MF, Misra A, Murray TK *et al.* A comparative study in rats of the *in vitro* and *in vivo* pharmacology of the acetylcholinesterase inhibitors tacrine, donepezil and NXX-066. Neuropharmacology 38:181-93 (1999).

[28] Scali C, Casamenti F, Bellucci A, Costagli C, Schmidt B, Pepeu G. Effect of subchronic administration of metrifonate, rivastigmine and donepezil on brain acetylcholine in aged F344 rats. J Neural Transm 109:1067-80 (2002).

[29] Enz A, Gentsch C. Co-administration of memantine has no effect on the *in vitro* or *ex vivo* determined acetylcholinesterase inhibition of rivastigmine in the rat brain. Neuropharmacology 47:408-13 (2004).

[30] Haug KH, Bogen IL, Osmundsen H, Walaas I, Fonnum F. Effects on cholinergic markers in rat brain and blood after short and prolonged administration of donepezil. Neurochem Res 30:1511-20 (2005).

[31] Kikuchi T, Okamura T, Fukushi K *et al.* Cerebral acetylcholinesterase imaging: development of the radioprobes. Curr Top Med Chem 7:1790-9 (2007).

[32] Venneri A. Imaging treatment effects in Alzheimer's disease. Magn Reson Imaging 25:953-68 (2007).

[33] Kaasinen V, Nagren K, Jarvenpaa T *et al.* Regional effects of donepezil and rivastigmine on cortical acetylcholinesterase activity in Alzheimer's disease. J Clin Psychopharmacol 22:615-20 (2002).

[34] Bohnen NI, Kaufer DI, Hendrickson R *et al.* Degree of inhibition of cortical acetylcholinesterase activity and cognitive effects by donepezil treatment in Alzheimer's disease. J Neurol Neurosurg Psychiatry 76:315-9 (2005).

[35] Trabace L, Coluccia A, Gaetani S *et al.* *In vivo* neurochemical effects of the acetylcholinesterase inhibitor ENA713 in rat hippocampus. Brain Res 865:268-71 (2000).

[36] Trabace L, Cassano T, Colaianna M *et al.* Neurochemical and neurobehavioral effects of ganstigmine (CHF2819), a novel acetylcholinesterase inhibitor, in rat prefrontal cortex: an *in vivo* study. Pharmacol Res 56:288-94 (2007).

[37] Zhu XD, Giacobini E. Second generation cholinesterase inhibitors: effect of (L)-huperzine-A on cortical biogenic amines. J Neurosci Res 41:828-35 (1995).

[38] Maelicke A, Albuquerque EX. Allosteric modulation of nicotinic acetylcholine receptors as a treatment strategy for Alzheimer's disease. Eur J Pharmacol 393:165-70 (2000).

[39] Pereira EF, Alkondon M, Reinhardt S *et al.* Physostigmine and galanthamine: probes for a novel binding site on the alpha 4 beta 2 subtype of neuronal nicotinic acetylcholine receptors stably expressed in fibroblast cells. J Pharmacol Exp Ther 270:768-78 (1994).

[40] Hernandez CM, Gearhart DA, Parikh V *et al.* Comparison of galantamine and donepezil for effects on nerve growth factor, cholinergic markers, and memory performance in aged rats. J Pharmacol Exp Ther 316:679-94 (2006).

[41] Sihver W, Gunther P, Schliebs R, Bigl V. Repeated administration of tacrine to normal rats: effects on cholinergic, glutamatergic, and GABAergic receptor subtypes in rat brain using receptor autoradiography. Neurochem Int 31:693-703 (1997).

[42] Zhang X, Tian JY, Svensson AL, Gong ZH, Meyerson B, Nordberg A. Chronic treatments with tacrine and (-)-nicotine induce different changes of nicotinic and muscarinic acetylcholine receptors in the brain of aged rat. J Neural Transm 109:377-92 (2002).

[43] Barnes CA, Meltzer J, Houston F, Orr G, McGann K, Wenk GL. Chronic treatment of old rats with donepezil or galantamine: effects on memory, hippocampal plasticity and nicotinic receptors. Neuroscience 99:17-23 (2000).

[44] Nilsson-Hakansson L, Lai Z, Nordberg A. Tetrahydroaminoacridine induces opposite changes in muscarinic and nicotinic receptors in rat brain. Eur J Pharmacol 186:301-5 (1990).

[45] Nordberg A, Lilja A, Lundqvist H *et al.* Tacrine restores cholinergic nicotinic receptors and glucose metabolism in Alzheimer patients as visualized by positron emission tomography. Neurobiol Aging 13:747-58 (1992).

[46] Hayslett RL, Tizabi Y. Effects of donepezil, nicotine and haloperidol on the central serotonergic system in mice: implications for Tourette's syndrome. Pharmacol Biochem Behav 81:879-86 (2005).

[47] Yuede CM, Dong H, Csernansky JG. Anti-dementia drugs and hippocampal-dependent memory in rodents. Behav Pharmacol 18:347-63 (2007).
[48] Scali C, Giovannini MG, Bartolini L *et al.* Effect of metrifonate on extracellular brain acetylcholine levels and object recognition in aged rats. Eur J Pharmacol 325:173-80 (1997).
[49] Greig NH, Utsuki T, Ingram DK *et al.* Selective butyrylcholinesterase inhibition elevates brain acetylcholine, augments learning and lowers Alzheimer beta-amyloid peptide in rodent. Proc Natl Acad Sci U S A 102:17213-8 (2005).
[50] Ballard TM, McAllister KH. The acetylcholinesterase inhibitor, ENA 713 (Exelon), attenuates the working memory impairment induced by scopolamine in an operant DNMTP task in rats. Psychopharmacology (Berl) 146:10-8 (1999).
[51] Pepeu G, Giovannini MG. The role of cholinergic system in cognitive processes. In (Eds: Giacobini E and Pepeu G). Brain Cholinergic Mechanisms. Oxford: Tailor & Francis pp. 221-233 (2006).
[52] Braida D, Paladini E, Griffini P, Lamperti M, Maggi A, Sala M. An inverted U-shaped curve for heptylphysostigmine on radial maze performance in rats: comparison with other cholinesterase inhibitors. Eur J Pharmacol 302:13-20 (1996).
[53] Pepeu G, Spignoli G. Nootropic drugs and brain cholinergic mechanisms. Progress Neuro-psychopharmacology & Biological Psychiatry 13:S77-S88 (1989).
[54] Selkoe DJ. Alzheimer's disease results from the cerebral accumulation and cytotoxicity of amyloid beta-protein. J Alzheimers Dis 3:75-80 (2001).
[55] Nitsch RM, Slack BE, Wurtman RJ, Growdon JH. Release of Alzheimer amyloid precursor derivatives stimulated by activation of muscarinic acetylcholine receptors. Science 258:304-7 (1992).
[56] Svensson AL, Giacobini E. Cholinesterase inhibitors do more than inhibit cholinesterase. In (Eds: Giacobini E). Cholinesterases and cholinesterase inhibitors. London: Martin Dunitz pp. 227-235 (2000).
[57] Racchi M, Mazzucchelli M, Porrello E, Lanni C, Govoni S. Acetylcholinesterase inhibitors: novel activities of old molecules. Pharmacol Res 50:441-51 (2004).
[58] Liskowsky W, Schliebs R. Muscarinic acetylcholine receptor inhibition in transgenic Alzheimer-like Tg2576 mice by scopolamine favours the amyloidogenic route of processing of amyloid precursor protein. Int J Dev Neurosci 24:149-56 (2006).
[59] Nordberg A. Mechanisms behind the neuroprotective actions of cholinesterase inhibitors in Alzheimer disease. Alzheimer Dis Assoc Disord 20:S12-S18 (2006).
[60] Dong H, Csernansky CA, Martin MV, Bertchume A, Vallera D, Csernansky JG. Acetylcholinesterase inhibitors ameliorate behavioral deficits in the Tg2576 mouse model of Alzheimer's disease. Psychopharmacology (Berl) 181:145-52 (2005).
[61] Lahiri DK, Chen D, Maloney B *et al.* The experimental Alzheimer's disease drug posiphen [(+)-phenserine] lowers amyloid-beta peptide levels in cell culture and mice. J Pharmacol Exp Ther 320:386-96 (2007).
[62] Zhang HY, Yan H, Tang XC. Huperzine A enhances the level of secretory amyloid precursor protein and protein kinase C-alpha in intracerebroventricular beta-amyloid-(1-40) infused rats and human embryonic kidney 293 Swedish mutant cells. Neurosci Lett 360:21-4 (2004).
[63] Borroni B, Colciaghi F, Pastorino L *et al.* Amyloid precursor protein in platelets of patients with Alzheimer disease: effect of acetylcholinesterase inhibitor treatment. Arch Neurol 58:442-6 (2001).

[64] Zimmermann M, Borroni B, Cattabeni F, Padovani A, Di Luca M. Cholinesterase inhibitors influence APP metabolism in Alzheimer disease patients. Neurobiol Dis 19:237-42 (2005).

[65] Ballard CG, Chalmers KA, Todd C *et al.* Cholinesterase inhibitors reduce cortical Abeta in dementia with Lewy bodies. Neurology 68:1726-9 (2007).

[66] Stefanova E, Blennow K, Almkvist O, Hellstrom-Lindahl E, Nordberg A. Cerebral glucose metabolism, cerebrospinal fluid-beta-amyloid1-42 (CSF-Abeta42), tau and apolipoprotein E genotype in long-term rivastigmine and tacrine treated Alzheimer disease (AD) patients. Neurosci Lett 338:159-63 (2003).

[67] Parnetti L, Lanari A, Saggese E, Spaccatini C, Gallai V. Cerebrospinal fluid biochemical markers in early detection and in differential diagnosis of dementia disorders in routine clinical practice. Neurol Sci 24:199-200 (2003).

[68] Zhang HY, Yan H, Tang XC. Non-cholinergic Effects of Huperzine A: Beyond Inhibition of Acetylcholinesterase. Cell Mol Neurobiol (2007).

[69] Zhou J, Zhang HY, Tang XC. Huperzine A attenuates cognitive deficits and hippocampal neuronal damage after transient global ischemia in gerbils. Neurosci Lett 313:137-40 (2001).

[70] Geerts H. Indicators of neuroprotection with galantamine. Brain Res Bull 64:519-24 (2005).

[71] Geula C, Mesulam MM. Cholinesterases and the pathology of Alzheimer disease. Alzheimer Dis Assoc Disord 9 Suppl 2:23-8 (1995).

[72] Mesulam MM. Neuroanatomy of cholinesterases in the normal human brain and in Alzheimer's disease. In (Eds: Giacobini E). Cholinesterase and cholinesterase inhibitors. London: Martin Dunitz Ltd pp. 121-137 (2000).

[73] Wright CI, Geula C, Mesulam MM. Neurological cholinesterases in the normal brain and in Alzheimer's disease: relationship to plaques, tangles, and patterns of selective vulnerability. Ann Neurol 34:373-84 (1993).

[74] Inestrosa NC, Alvarez A, Perez CA *et al.* Acetylcholinesterase accelerates assembly of amyloid-beta-peptides into Alzheimer's fibrils: possible role of the peripheral site of the enzyme. Neuron 16:881-91 (1996).

[75] Reyes AE, Chacon MA, Dinamarca MC, Cerpa W, Morgan C, Inestrosa NC. Acetylcholinesterase-Abeta complexes are more toxic than Abeta fibrils in rat hippocampus: effect on rat beta-amyloid aggregation, laminin expression, reactive astrocytosis, and neuronal cell loss. Am J Pathol 164:2163-74 (2004).

[76] Mesulam MM, Geula C. Butyrylcholinesterase reactivity differentiates the amyloid plaques of aging from those of dementia. Ann Neurol 36:722-7 (1994).

[77] De Ferrari GV, Canales MA, Shin I, Weiner LM, Silman I, Inestrosa NC. A structural motif of acetylcholinesterase that promotes amyloid beta-peptide fibril formation. Biochemistry 40:10447-57 (2001).

[78] Eskander MF, Nagykery NG, Leung EY, Khelghati B, Geula C. Rivastigmine is a potent inhibitor of acetyl- and butyrylcholinesterase in Alzheimer's plaques and tangles. Brain Res 1060:144-52 (2005).

[79] Kuljis RO, Farlow M, Grossberg G, Geula C. Long-term exposure to rivastigmine may reduce senile plaque density. Soc.Neurosci.Abstr. 2003;29 (abstr).

[80] Munoz-Ruiz P, Rubio L, Garcia-Palomero E *et al.* Design, synthesis, and biological evaluation of dual binding site acetylcholinesterase inhibitors: new disease-modifying agents for Alzheimer's disease. J Med Chem 48:7223-33 (2005).

[81] Castro A, Martinez A. Targeting beta-amyloid pathogenesis through acetylcholinesterase inhibitors. Curr Pharm Des 12:4377-87 (2006).

[82] Fu H, Li W, Luo J *et al.* Promising anti-Alzheimer's dimer bis(7)-tacrine reduces beta-amyloid generation by directly inhibiting BACE-1 activity. Biochem Biophys Res Commun (2007).

[83] Li W, Lee NT, Fu H *et al.* Neuroprotection *via* inhibition of nitric oxide synthase by bis(7)-tacrine. NeuroReport 17:471-4 (2006).

[84] Xiao XQ, Lee NT, Carlier PR, Pang Y, Han YF. Bis(7)-tacrine, a promising anti-Alzheimer's agent, reduces hydrogen peroxide-induced injury in rat pheochromocytoma cells: comparison with tacrine. Neurosci Lett 290:197-200 (2000).

[85] Weinstock M, Gorodetsky E, Poltyrev T, Gross A, Sagi Y, Youdim M. A novel cholinesterase and brain-selective monoamine oxidase inhibitor for the treatment of dementia comorbid with depression and Parkinson's disease. Prog Neuropsychopharmacol Biol Psychiatry 27:555-61 (2003).

[86] Martinez A, Castro A. Novel cholinesterase inhibitors as future effective drugs for the treatment of Alzheimer's disease. Expert Opin Investig Drugs 15:1-12 (2006).

[87] Klein J. Phenserine. Expert Opin Investig Drugs 16:1087-97 (2007).

[88] Trabace L, Cassano T, Loverre A, Steardo L, Cuomo V. CHF2819: pharmacological profile of a novel acetylcholinesterase inhibitor. CNS Drug Rev 8:53-69 (2002).

[89] Byrne EJ, Arie T. Tetrahydroaminoacridine and Alzheimer's disease. BMJ 308:868-9 (1994).

[90] Franz CE, Barker JC, Kravitz RL, Flores Y, Krishnan S, Hinton L. Nonmedical influences on the use of cholinesterase inhibitors in dementia care. Alzheimer Dis Assoc Disord 21:241-8 (2007).

[91] Liang YQ, Tang XC. Comparative effects of huperzine A, donepezil and rivastigmine on cortical acetylcholine level and acetylcholinesterase activity in rats. Neurosci Lett 361:56-9 (2004).

[92] Messamore E, Warpman U, Ogane N, Giacobini E. Cholinesterase inhibitor effects on extracellular acetylcholine in rat cortex. Neuropharmacology 32:745-50 (1993).

[93] Giovannini MG, Scali C, Bartolini L, Schmidt BH, Pepeu G. Effect of subchronic treatment with metrifonate and tacrine on brain cholinergic function in aged F334 rats. European Journal of Pharmacology 354:17-24 (1998).

[94] Spowart-Manning L, van der Staay FJ. Spatial discrimination deficits by excitotoxic lesions in the Morris water escape task. Behav Brain Res 156:269-76 (2005).

[95] Sweeney JE, Hohmann CF, Moran TH, Coyle JT. A long-acting cholinesterase inhibitor reverses spatial memory deficits in mice. Pharmacol Biochem Behav 31:141-7 (1988).

[96] Van Dam D, Coen K, De Deyn PP. Cognitive evaluation of disease-modifying efficacy of donepezil in the APP23 mouse model for Alzheimer's disease. Psychopharmacology (Berl) (2007).

[97] Van Dam D, Abramowski D, Staufenbiel M, De Deyn PP. Symptomatic effect of donepezil, rivastigmine, galantamine and memantine on cognitive deficits in the APP23 model. Psychopharmacology (Berl) 180:177-90 (2005).

[98] Ohara T, Fukaya H, Itanaka K, Seno N. Ameliorating effects of SDZ ENA 713 on age-associated decreases in learning performance and brain choline acetyltransferase activity in rats. Brain Res Bull 43:39-42 (1997).

[99] Wesnes KA, McKeith IG, Ferrara R *et al.* Effects of rivastigmine on cognitive function in dementia with lewy bodies: a randomised placebo-controlled international study using the cognitive drug research computerised assessment system. Dement Geriatr Cogn Disord 13:183-92 (2002).
[100] Kavirajan H, Schneider LS. Efficacy and adverse effects of cholinesterase inhibitors and memantine in vascular dementia: a meta-analysis of randomised controlled trials. Lancet Neurol 6:782-92 (2007).
[101] Stip E, Sepehry AA, Chouinard S. Add-on therapy with acetylcholinesterase inhibitors for memory dysfunction in schizophrenia: a systematic quantitative review, part 2. Clin Neuropharmacol 30:218-29 (2007).
[102] Spiridigliozzi GA, Heller JH, Crissman BG *et al.* Preliminary study of the safety and efficacy of donepezil hydrochloride in children with Down syndrome: a clinical report series. Am J Med Genet A 143:1408-13 (2007).
[103] Niederhofer H. Donepezil in the treatment of narcolepsy. J Clin Sleep Med 2:71-2 (2006).
[104] Mumenthaler MS, Yesavage JA, Taylor JL *et al.* Psychoactive drugs and pilot performance: a comparison of nicotine, donepezil, and alcohol effects. Neuropsychopharmacology 28:1366-73 (2003).
[105] Sun QQ, Xu SS, Pan JL, Guo HM, Cao WQ. Huperzine-A capsules enhance memory and learning performance in 34 pairs of matched adolescent students. Zhongguo Yao Li Xue Bao 20:601-3 (1999).
[106] Rodda J, Carter J. Cholinesterase inhibitors and memantine for symptomatic treatment of dementia. BMJ 344:e2986 (2012).
[107] Repantis D, Laisney O, Heuser I. Acetylcholinesterase inhibitors and memantine for neuroenhancement in healthy individuals: a systematic review. Pharmacol Res 61:473-81 (2010).
[108] Delrieu J, Ousset PJ, Vellas B. Gantenerumab for the treatment of Alzheimer's disease. Expert Opin Biol Ther 12:1077-86 (2012).
[109] Tayeb HO, Yang HD, Price BH, Tarazi FI. Pharmacotherapies for Alzheimer's disease: beyond cholinesterase inhibitors. Pharmacol Ther 134:8-25 (2012).
[110] Salomone S, Caraci F, Leggio GM, Fedotova J, Drago F. New pharmacological strategies for treatment of Alzheimer's disease: focus on disease modifying drugs. Br J Clin Pharmacol 73:504-17 (2012).
[111] Dhillon S. Spotlight on rivastigmine transdermal patch: in dementia of the Alzheimer's type. Drugs Aging 28:927-30 (2011).
[112] Rampa A, Belluti F, Gobbi S, Bisi A. Hybrid-based multi-target ligands for the treatment of Alzheimer's disease. Curr Top Med Chem 11:2716-30 (2011).
[113] Winblad B, Giacobini E, Frolich L *et al.* Phenserine efficacy in Alzheimer's disease. J Alzheimers Dis 22:1201-8 (2010).
[114] Conti E, Galimberti G, Tremolizzo L *et al.* Cholinesterase inhibitor use is associated with increased plasma levels of anti-Abeta 1-42 antibodies in Alzheimer's disease patients. Neurosci Lett 486:193-6 (2010).
[115] Pavlov VA, Parrish WR, Rosas-Ballina M *et al.* Brain acetylcholinesterase activity controls systemic cytokine levels through the cholinergic anti-inflammatory pathway. Brain Behav Immun 23:41-5 (2009).
[116] Hwang J, Hwang H, Lee HW, Suk K. Microglia signaling as a target of donepezil. Neuropharmacology 58:1122-9 (2010).

[117] Singh J, Kour K, Jayaram MB. Acetylcholinesterase inhibitors for schizophrenia. Cochrane Database Syst Rev Jan 18:1:CD007967 (2012).

[118] Rokem A, Landau AN, Garg D, Prinzmetal W, Silver MA. Cholinergic enhancement increases the effects of voluntary attention but does not affect involuntary attention. Neuropsychopharmacology 35:2538-44 (2010).

[119] Pepeu G, Giovannini MG, Bracco L. Effect of cholinesterase inhibitors on attention. Chem Biol Interact 203:361-4 (2013).

CHAPTER 8

Glial HO-1 Suppression as a Neuroprotective Strategy in Alzheimer's Disease

Hyman M. Schipper[1,*], Ajay Gupta[2] and Walter A. Szarek[3]

[1]Bloomfield Centre for Research in Aging, Lady Davis Institute for Medical Research, Jewish General Hospital, McGill University, Montreal, Quebec, Canada; [2]Osta Biotechnologies Inc., Montreal, Quebec, Canada and [3]Department of Chemistry, Queen's University, Kingston, Ontario, Canada

Abstract: The mechanisms responsible for oxidative damage, pathological brain iron deposition and mitochondrial insufficiency in Alzheimer disease (AD) remain enigmatic. Heme oxygenase-1 (HO-1) is a 32 kDa stress protein that catabolizes heme to biliverdin, free iron and carbon other tissues in various models of disease and trauma. Our laboratory demonstrated that 1) HO-1 protein is significantly over-expressed in AD-affected temporal cortex and hippocampus relative to neurohistologically-normal control preparations, 2) in cultured astrocytes, HO-1 up-regulation by transient transfection of the human *ho-1* gene, or stimulation of endogenous HO-1 expression by exposure to β-amyloid, TNFα or IL-1β, promotes intracellular oxidative stress, opening of the mitochondrial permeability transition pore and accumulation of non-transferrin iron in the mitochondrial compartment, and 3) the glial iron sequestration renders co-cultured neuron-like PC12 cells prone to oxidative injury (reviewed in Schipper HM. *J Neurochem* 110: 469-85, 2009). Induction of the astroglial *ho-1* gene may constitute a 'common pathway' leading to pathological brain iron deposition, intracellular oxidative damage and bioenergetic failure in AD and other human CNS disorders. ***Hypothesis:*** Targeted suppression of glial HO-1 hyperactivity may prove to be a rational and effective neurotherapeutic intervention in AD and related neurodegenerative disorders. To begin testing this hypothesis, studies have been initiated to determine whether systemic administration of a novel, selective and brain-permeable inhibitor of HO-1 activity ameliorates cognitive dysfunction and neuropathology in a transgenic mouse model of AD.

Keywords: Aging, alzheimer disease, astrocyte, heme oxygenase-1, iron, metalloporphyrin, mitochondria, neuroprotection, OB-24, oxidative stress.

***Corresponding author Hyman M. Schipper:** Lady Davis Institute, Jewish General Hospital, 3755 Cote St. Catherine Road, Montreal, Quebec, H3T 1E2 Canada; Tel: 514-340-8260; Fax: 514-340-7502; E-mail: hyman.schipper@mcgill.ca

D.K. Lahiri (Ed)

1. ALZHEIMER DISEASE

1.1. An Unmet Clinical Imperative

Alzheimer disease (AD) is a dementing illness characterized by progressive neuronal degeneration, gliosis, and the accumulation of intracellular inclusions (neurofibrillary tangles) and extracellular deposits of amyloid (senile plaques) in discrete regions of the basal forcbrain, hippocampus, and association cortices [1]. AD is the most common aging-related neurodegenerative disorder, afflicting 5-10% of North Americans over age 65 and 30-40% by the end of ninth decade [2]. Current pharmacotherapy, including acetylcholinesterase inhibitors, NMDA receptor antagonists and neuropsychiatric medications, temporarily ameliorate the symptoms of AD. Unfortunately, no treatment has yet been unequivocally demonstrated to prevent, attenuate or reverse neuronal attrition and clinical decline in this debilitating condition. The advent of effective neuroprotection in AD, a pressing unmet clinical need, presupposes a thorough understanding of the salient etiopathogenetic mechanisms that drive the neurodegenerative process.

1.2. Oxidative Stress, Iron Deposition and Mitochondrial Insufficiency in AD Brain

Oxidative stress and mitochondrial deficits have been consistently implicated in the pathogenesis of sporadic AD. Mitochondrial insufficiency in AD brain is evidenced by: (i) deficits in pyruvate dehydrogenase, α-ketoglutarate dehydrogenase and cytochrome c oxidase protein or activity; (ii) the presence of excessive mtDNA deletion and mis-sense mutations; and (iii) suppressed cerebral metabolism (glucose utilization) in positron emission tomography studies [3-5]. Potential sources of oxidative stress in the AD brain include baseline reactive oxygen species (ROS) generation by senescent mitochondria, accelerated β-amyloid deposition, production of pro-inflammatory cytokines (TNF-α, IL-1β) and nitric oxide (NO) by activated microglia, and excessive sequestration of redox-active iron in the basal forebrain and association cortices [5]. Abnormally high levels of tissue iron have been consistently reported in the cerebral cortex and hippocampus of AD subjects. These pathological iron stores may serve as a key generator of ROS in this condition by reducing H_2O_2 to hydroxyl radical and possibly bioactivating neutral catechols to neurotoxic semiquinone intermediates

[6-11]. The excessive iron appears to be predominantly deposited within astrocytes, microglia, macrophages and microvessels. Increased expression of tissue ferritin, the major intracellular iron storage protein, parallels the distribution of the excess iron and largely implicates non-neuronal (glial) cellular compartments [12, 13]. The extracellular transport of ferric iron and its delivery to virtually all mammalian tissues is mediated by a second iron-binding protein, transferrin. To maintain normal tissue iron homeostasis, plasma membrane transferrin receptor densities and intracellular ferritin concentrations are tightly regulated at transcriptional and post-transcriptional levels by iron bioavailability and intracellular iron stores [14-16]. In the aging and diseased human CNS, there appears to be an overt mismatch between local iron concentrations and the densities of cell surface transferrin binding sites, suggesting alternative mechanisms of iron sequestration in these states. On the basis of evidence adduced from human neuropathological studies, experimental paradigms of aging-associated neurological disorders, and models of astroglial senescence, we hypothesized that *oxidative stress*, *augmented iron deposition* and *mitochondrial insufficiency* in the aging and degenerating CNS constitute a single neuropathological 'lesion', and that the advent of one component of this triad obligates the appearance of the others [5]. Moreover, as discussed below, data were garnered supporting the notion that consolidation of this tripartite lesion in degenerating neural tissues is contingent on the action of the enzyme, heme oxygenase-1.

2. A MODEL FOR PATHOLOGICAL BRAIN IRON DEPOSITION AND MITOCHONDRIAL DAMAGE IN AGING AND AD

2.1. Peroxidase-Positive Astrocytes: A Senescent Glial Phenotype

In aging rats, humans, and other vertebrates, a population of subcortical astrocytes progressively accumulates unique cytoplasmic inclusions that exhibit an affinity for Gomori stains, orange-red autofluorescence, and non-enzymatic (pseudo-) peroxidase activity mediated by ferrous iron [6, 17-19]. Using dissociated fetal or neonatal rat brain cell cultures, we observed that exposure to the sulfhydryl agent, cysteamine (CSH; 2-mercaptoethylamine) promotes the accumulation of peroxidase-positive astrocytic inclusions that are structurally and histochemically identical to those that naturally accumulate in subcortical astroglia of the intact aging brain [20]. Elemental iron was readily detected in the inclusions by electron microprobe analysis, and the presence and concentration of the metal correlated closely with the presence and intensity of DAB (peroxidase) staining [21]. Within 24-72 hours of CSH exposure, many astroglial *mitochondria* exhibited progressive swelling, rearrangement or dissolution of their cristae, subcompartmental sequestration of redox-active iron and fusion with lysosomes or cisternae of the endoplasmic reticulum [22, 23]. In young adult rats, subcutaneous CSH injections (150-300 mg/kg twice weekly for 3 weeks) induced 2-3 fold increases in numbers of peroxidase-positive astrocyte granules in the hippocampus, basal ganglia and other brain regions [24]. As in the case of the CSH-treated cultures, peroxidase-positive glial granules in the intact rat and human brain invariably exhibit mitochondrial epitopes in immunohistochemical preparations [19, 25, 26]. Further studies indicated that intracellular oxidative stress was likely responsible for the transformation of normal astrocyte mitochondria to peroxidase-positive inclusions *in vitro* and in the intact aging brain [5, 27-29].

2.2. Iron Sequestration in 'Stressed' Astroglia

We determined that CSH (880μM), dopamine (0.1-1.0 μM), β-amyloid$_{40/42}$ (15 μM), tumour necrosis factor-α (TNFα; 20 ng/ml)) or interleukin-1β (IL-1β; 20 ng/ml) significantly augmented the incorporation of ^{59}Fe (or ^{55}Fe) into astroglial mitochondria without affecting transfer of the metal into whole-cell and lysosomal compartments [30-33]). These effects were only demonstrable when inorganic $^{59}FeCl_3$, but not ^{59}Fe-diferric transferrin, served as the metal donor (ibid). These *in vitro* data are commensurate with the fact that a) pathological iron accumulation appears to be a transferrin-independent process (see above) and b) mitochondrial insufficiency is an invariant feature of AD brain tissues exhibiting iron overload [34]. In the following sections, evidence is presented implicating *glial heme oxygenase-1 (HO-1) expression* as a 'common pathway' leading to pathological iron deposition and oxidative mitochondrial damage in the brains of AD subjects.

2.3. Heme Oxygenase-1: Regulation and Physiology

The heme oxygenases reside within the endoplasmic reticulum where they function, in association with NADPH cytochrome P450 reductase, to oxidize heme to biliverdin, free ferrous iron and carbon monoxide (CO). Biliverdin is metabolized further to the bile pigment, bilirubin by action of biliverdin reductase [35]. Mammalian cells express at least two isoforms of heme oxygenase, HO-1 (a.k.a. heat shock protein*32*) and HO-2. A third protein, HO-3 [36] appears to be a pseudogene unique to rats [37]. HO-1 and HO-2 are encoded by distinct genes and manifest differences with regard to molecular weight, electrophoretic mobility, susceptibility to proteolysis, tissue distribution, regulation and antigenicity. Substrate and co-factor specificities are, however, identical for the two isoforms [38]. HO-2 protein is widely expressed within the rodent neuraxis [39]. In contrast, basal HO-1 immunoreactivity in the normal brain is limited to small groups of dispersed neurons and neuroglia [40]. In humans, the *ho-1* gene (*HMOX1*) is located on chromosome 22q12 and contains 4 introns and 5 exons. A 500-bp promoter, a proximal enhancer, and two or more distal enhancers are located within the regulatory region of the mammalian *ho-1* gene [38]. The latter contains binding sites for AP-1, AP-2, nuclear factor kappa B (NFκB) and HIF-1, as well as heat shock consensus (HSE) sequences, metal response elements (MtRE, CdRE), and stress response elements (StRE). Nrf2 transcription factor binding to Maf response elements (MARE) in the *HMOX1* promoter and its repression by the heme-regulated protein, Bach1 have emerged as a pivotal control mechanism for HO-1 induction and homeostasis in stressed brain and other organs [41-44]. These response elements render *Hmox1* exquisitely sensitive to induction by a wide range of pro-oxidant and inflammatory stimuli including heme, β-amyloid, dopamine, H_2O_2, hyperoxia, UV light, heavy metals, prostaglandins, nitric oxide, peroxynitrite, TH1 cytokines, oxidized lipid products and lipopolysaccharide, as well as certain growth factors [38, 45, 46]. In addition, susceptibility to transcriptional suppression by glucocorticoids is mediated by a 56bp sequence (STAT-3 acute-phase response factor binding site) residing within the *ho-1* gene promoter [47]. In humans, polymorphisms in the lengths of GT repeats [from 11-40] within the *Hmox1* promoter appear to be an important determinant of HO-1 expression and function. Long GT sequences code for relatively unstable (Z-conformation) DNA with attenuated transcriptional activity and diminished baseline and stimulated HO-1 protein expression profiles [48].

Heme turnover occurs in all mammalian cells and all three products of the heme oxygenase reaction are biologically-active. Oxidative stress may transiently increase the intracellular "free heme pool" by promoting the conformational modification and accelerated degradation of hemoproteins [35, 46]. In the face of oxidative stress, induction of HO-1 may protect cells by enhancing the breakdown of pro-oxidant heme to thc radical-scavenging bile pigments, biliverdin and bilirubin [40, 49-52]. In many tissues, co-induction of ferritin provides a 'sink' for the excess intracellular iron and thereby confers cytoprotection. However, in some tissues and under certain experimental conditions, heme-derived iron and CO may *exacerbate* intracellular oxidative stress and cellular injury by promoting free radical generation within the mitochondrial compartment [53, 54]. While there exists considerable evidence for HO-1-related neuroprotection in various intact animal and tissue culture models of CNS injury and disease, a literature implicating potentially neurodystrophic aspects of HO-1 activity is also at hand [55]. The magnitude and chronicity of HO-1 induction and the chemistry of the local redox microenvironment may determine whether the benefits of a diminished heme:bilirubin ratio or oxidative damage accruing from intracellular mobilization of iron/CO prevail [56, 57].

2.4. Glial HO-1 Expression in AD and MCI

Numbers of neuroglia immunoreactive for HO-1 in cortical and subcortical regions of the normal human brain increase progressively with advancing age [58]. In AD brain, HO-1 protein co-localizes to astrocytes, neurons, neurofibrillary tangles, senile plaques, corpora amylacea, ependymocytes, choroid plexus epithelial cells, and some endothelial and vascular smooth muscle cells [59, 60]. We found that 86% of GFAP-positive astrocytes within the AD hippocampus displayed immunoreactive HO-1, whereas the proportion of hippocampal astroglia expressing HO-1 in normal tissue matched for age and post-mortem interval was a mere 6-7%. Along similar lines, Western blots of protein extracts derived from AD temporal cortex and hippocampus exhibited robust HO-1 bands, whereas the latter were weak or undetectable in normal control preparations [60]. Conceivably, oxidative stress accruing from diverse processes, such as excessive amyloid burden, secretion of pro-inflammatory cytokines and infidelity of electron transport in senescent mitochondria [31, 61], provokes HO-1 expression in the Alzheimer-diseased cerebral cortex and hippocampus. Of note, significant augmentation of astroglial HO-1 expression was also documented in post-mortem brain specimens procured from individuals with mild cognitive impairment (MCI), a frequent harbinger of incipient AD [62]. Glial HO-1 immunoreactivity in the MCI temporal cortex correlated with the burden of neurofibrillary pathology. Furthermore, astroglial HO-1 expression in the temporal cortex was associated with decreased scores for global cognition, episodic memory, semantic memory and working memory; hippocampal astroglial HO-1 expression was associated with lower scores for global cognition, semantic memory and perceptual speed. The results of the MCI study argue strongly that glial HO-1 induction is a relatively early event in the pathogenesis of sporadic AD. In the following sections, we provide evidence that the pathological brain iron deposition and bioenergy deficits complicating AD may arise, at least in part, due to antecedent up-regulation of HO-1 in affected astroglia.

2.5. Glial HO-1 Expression and Mitochondrial Iron Sequestration

Cysteamine, β-amyloid$_{40/42}$, and TH1 cytokines implicated in the pathogenesis of AD, *viz.*, TNFα and IL-1β, up-regulate HO-1 mRNA, protein and/or activity levels in cultured neonatal rat astroglia within 3-12 hours of treatment. Using various pharmacological approaches, we determined that oxidative stress is a likely common mechanism mediating glial *Hmox1* induction under these experimental conditions [33, 63]. Within 3-6 days of exposure to these stimuli, sequestration of ^{59}Fe (or ^{55}Fe) by the mitochondrial compartment is significantly augmented in these cells [6, 32]. As alluded to previously, these effects were only demonstrable when $^{59}FeCl_3$, but not ^{59}Fe-diferric transferrin, served as the metal donor (ibid) commensurate with transferrin-independent pathways of iron mobilization implicated in AD brain (see above). Administration of dexamethasone (DEX), a transcriptional suppressor of *Hmox1*, significantly attenuated mitochondrial iron sequestration in cultured astrocytes exposed to β-amyloid, TNFα or IL-1β [32]. Moreover, administration of tin mesoporphyrin (SnMP), a competitive inhibitor of heme oxygenase activity, abrogated the pathological accumulation of mitochondrial ^{55}Fe in rat astroglia engineered to over-express the human *ho-1* gene by transient transfection [6, 31, 32]. Dynamic secondary ion mass spectrometry recently confirmed the accumulation of iron in mitochondria and autophagic granules of rat astroglia transfected with *HMOX1* [64] and in transgenic mice overexpressing human HO-1 in the astroglial compartment [65]. Collectively, these findings indicate that up-regulation of HO-1 is a key event in the cascade leading to excessive mitochondrial iron deposition in oxidatively-challenged astroglia.

2.6. HO-1, Intracellular Oxidative Stress and the Mitochondrial Permeability Transition Pore

In astrocytes, up-regulation of HO-1 promotes intracellular oxidative stress as evidenced by our observations that a) treatment with SnMP or antioxidants (ascorbate, melatonin or resveratrol) blocked the compensatory induction of the manganese superoxide dismutase gene in astrocytes challenged with dopamine or transiently transfected with human(h) HO-1 cDNA [54] and b) levels of protein carbonyls (protein oxidation), 8-epiPGF2α (lipid peroxidation), 8-OHdG (nucleic acid oxidation) and a synthetic redox reporter molecule were significantly increased in glial mitochondrial fractions after 3-4 days of *HMOX1* transfection relative to sham-transfected controls and HO-1-transfected cells receiving SnMP [66, 67]. Treatment with cyclosporin A and trifluoperazine, potent inhibitors of the mitochondrial permeability transition pore, also curtailed mitochondrial iron trapping in *HMOX1* transfected glia and cells exposed to β-amyloid, TNFα or IL-1β [32, 33]. Conceivably, in astrocytes, intracellular oxidative stress resulting from HO-1 activity promotes pore opening [68, 69] and ingress of cytosolic iron to the mitochondrial matrix. Markers of enhanced oxidative stress (augmented manganese superoxide dismutase and α-synuclein mRNA and protein levels) were recently documented in the brains of transgenic mice overexpressing *HMOX1* in astrocytes [70].

3. HYPOTHESIS

On the basis of the data reviewed above, we hypothesized that targeted suppression of glial HO-1 hyperactivity may prove to be a rational and effective neurotherapeutic intervention in AD and related neurodegenerative disorders.

3.1. Experimental Approach

3.1.1. Objective

To begin testing our *hypothesis*, studies funded by the Institute for the Study of Aging (ISOA; New York) have been initiated to determine whether systemic administration of a novel and selective inhibitor of HO-1 activity ameliorates cognitive dysfunction and neuropathology in a transgenic mouse model of AD.

3.1.2. Metalloporphyrin Inhibitors of Heme Oxygenase Activity

The current pharmacological approach to the suppression of heme oxygenase activity *in vivo* and *in vitro* entails administration of a synthetic metalloporphyrin compound, such as zinc protoporphyrin-IX (ZnPP) or tin mesoporphyrin-IX (SnMP), which competes for heme at the active site of the enzyme. Metalloporphyrin inhibitors have been invaluable in delineating the roles of heme oxygenases under various experimental conditions and have been used clinically in the management of neonatal hyperbilirubinemia (jaundice) and certain adult liver conditions [71, 72]. However, metalloporphyrin suppression of heme oxygenase activity has several important limitations: (i) The compounds are non-selective for HO-1 and HO-2; (ii) they may induce HO-1 gene transcription; (iii) they may inhibit other heme-containing enzymes, such as nitric oxide synthase, soluble guanylyl cyclase and cytochrome P450 enzymes; (iv) they penetrate the blood-brain barrier poorly; and (iv) clinical use is complicated by skin photosensitization [73].

3.1.3. Selective HO-1 Inhibition

To address the concerns related to the use of metalloporphyrins, a novel class of HO-1 inhibitors was developed by Drs. W. Szarek and K. Nakatsu at Queens University [73-75] and licensed to Osta Biotechnologies. A lead compound, OB-24 has been identified which is a specific and potent inhibitor of HO-1 as evidenced by IC_{50} values for HO-1 inhibition (rat spleen) and HO-2 inhibition (rat brain) of 1.9 and >100 μM, respectively. OB-24 is a non-peptidic, small molecule (molecular weight 374) with pKa 7.18 and log P value (octanol/buffer, pH 7.4) 1.7, favorable characteristics for CNS application. As previously shown with SnMP (above), administration of OB-24 (0.8-6.5 μM) dose-dependantly attenuated HO activity and whole cell and mitochondrial oxidative protein damage (carbonyl formation) accruing from *HMOX1* transfection in primary rat astroglial cultures (Schipper, Song and Gupta, unpublished results). In mouse cancer models currently under investigation in our laboratories, OB-24 (30-60 mg/kg b.w.) administered i.p. or i.v. every second day for up to 28 days exhibited potent biological activity without overt toxicity on the basis of fur texture, behavior, body weight and mortality [76]. At 120 mg/kg b.w., there was skin necrosis at the injection sites and body tremors, the latter likely indicative of CNS penetration (Alaoui-Jamali, Gupta and Schipper, unpublished results).

3.1.4. The APPswe/PS1 Mouse Model of Alzheimer Disease

This transgenic mouse model of AD elaborates mutant (Mo/HuAPP695swe) amyloid precursor protein and excessive β-amyloid, accelerated temporally by expression on a mutant presenilin-1 (PS1-dE9) background. These animals exhibit β-amyloid plaques in multiple brain regions and cognitive deficits (impaired spatial learning) by 6-7 months of age [77-79]. Initial studies will be performed in control animals to confirm entry of OB-24 into brain and its pharmacokinetic profile. Starting at 3 months of age, OB-24 (0, 30 or 60 mg/kg b.w.) will be administered i.p. to transgenic and control animals. At 7 and 10 months of age, we will assess cognitive behavior, general and AD neuropathology, brain HO-1 expression, iron deposition, oxidative stress, and mitochondrial status using appropriate behavioral, histochemical, biochemical and morphological techniques.

3.1.5. Anticipated Results

Extensive *in vitro* data summarized above suggest that up-regulation of HO-1 in AD-affected neural tissues (astrocytes) contributes to the pathological brain iron deposition, oxidative stress and bioenergetic failure characteristic of this condition. As such, we anticipate that suppression of glial HO-1 activity with the potent and selective HO-1 inhibitor, OB-24 will mitigate these pathological changes and alleviate associated behavioral impairment in the APPswe/PS1 mouse model of AD.

4. CONCLUDING REMARKS

Attenuation of neuropathology and behavioural toxicity in the APPswe/PS1 mice by treatment with the HO-1 inhibitor, OB-24 would flag HO-1 as a potential therapeutic target in the management of AD and possibly other aging-related human neurodegenerative diseases [80-83]). Positive results in this tier of experiments would help unify several seemingly disparate pathological features of

AD, *viz*., oxidative stress, iron mobilization and mitochondrial insufficiency into a single "lesion" possibly devolving from the action of HO-1 [5]. They would also further attest to the dynamic role astrocytes are increasingly being recognized to play in brain aging, AD and other neurodegenerative conditions [84]. Although we do not regard aberrant HO-1 expression as a 'cause' of AD, we view glial HO-1 over-expression and its cytophysiological consequences as one of several key mechanisms that may render the senescent nervous system vulnerable to AD and other aging-related neurodegenerations. Contemporary pharmacotherapy for AD is almost exclusively symptomatic in nature and effective neuroprotection would be a welcome development. Although oxidative stress has been amply documented in AD-affected neural tissues, and antioxidant therapies widely advocated, an *enzymatic* (HO-1) basis for oxidative mitochondrial injury in this disease may prove considerably more amenable to pharmacological control than free radical damage accruing from unregulated chemical processes [85, 86].

ACKNOWLEDGEMENTS

The work described herein was supported by grants from the Canadian Institutes of Health Research, the Fonds de la Recherche en Santé du Québec, the Alzheimer's Association (US), the Parkinson Foundation of Canada and Osta Biotechnologies Inc. Investigation of the potential neurotherapeutic actions of OB-24 was enabled by generous funding from the ISOA.

CONFLICT OF INTEREST

The authors are co-inventors on a patent protecting OB-24 and related compounds as novel inhibitors of HO-1.

DISCLOSURE

This chapter is an update of our previous publication in CAR "Suppression of Glial HO-1 Activitiy as a Potential Neurotherapeutic Intervention in AD" published in 'CAR', Volume 6, Number 5, October, pp. 424 to 430.

REFERENCES

[1] Selkoe, D.J., *The molecular pathology of Alzheimer's disease.* Neuron, 1991. 6(4): p. 487-98.

[2] Chertkow, H., *et al.*, *Assessment of suspected dementia.* Can J Neurol Sci, 2001. 28 Suppl 1: p. S28-41.

[3] Beal, M.F., *Mitochondria take center stage in aging and neurodegeneration.* Ann Neurol, 2005. 58(4): p. 495-505.

[4] Schapira, A.H. and J.M. Cooper, *Mitochondrial function in neurodegeneration and ageing.* Mutat Res, 1992. 275(3-6): p. 133-43.

[5] Schipper, H.M., *Brain iron deposition and the free radical-mitochondrial theory of ageing.* Ageing Res Rev, 2004. 3: p. 265-301.

[6] Schipper, H.M., *Glial HO-1 expression, iron deposition and oxidative stress in neurodegenerative diseases.* Neurotox Res, 1999. 1(1): p. 57-70.

[7] Perry, G., *et al.*, *The role of iron and copper in the aetiology of neurodegenerative disorders: therapeutic implications.* CNS Drugs, 2002. 16(5): p. 339-52.

[8] Cuajungco, M.P., *et al.*, *Metal chelation as a potential therapy for Alzheimer's disease.* Ann N Y Acad Sci, 2000. 920: p. 292-304.

[9] Smith, M.A., *et al.*, *Abnormal localization of iron regulatory protein in Alzheimer's disease.* Brain Res, 1998. 788(1-2): p. 232-6.

[10] Bartzokis, G., *et al.*, *Brain ferritin iron as a risk factor for age at onset in neurodegenerative diseases.* Ann N Y Acad Sci, 2004. 1012: p. 224-36.

[11] Quintana, C., *et al.*, *Study of the localization of iron, ferritin, and hemosiderin in Alzheimer's disease hippocampus by analytical microscopy at the subcellular level.* J Struct Biol, 2006. 153(1): p. 42-54.

[12] Janetzky, B., *et al.*, *Iron and oxidative damage in neurodegenerative disease.* Mitochondria and Free Radicals in Neurodegenerative Diseases, ed. M.F. Beal, N. Howell, and I. Bodis-Wollner1997, New York: Wiley-Liss. 407-421.

[13] Youdim, M., *Inorganic neurotoxins in neurodegenerative disorders without primary dementia*, in *Neurodegenerative Diseases*, D.B. Calne, Editor 1994, Saunders, W.B: Philadelphia. p. 251-276.

[14] Klausner, R.D., T.A. Rouault, and J.B. Harford, *Regulating the fate of mRNA: the control of cellular iron metabolism.* Cell, 1993. 72(1): p. 19-28.

[15] Richardson, D.R. and P. Ponka, *The molecular mechanisms of the metabolism and transport of iron in normal and neoplastic cells.* Biochim Biophys Acta, 1997. 1331(1): p. 1-40.

[16] Theil, E.C., *Regulation of ferritin and transferrin receptor mRNAs.* J Biol Chem, 1990. 265(9): p. 4771-4.

[17] Schipper, H.M., *Astrocytes, brain aging, and neurodegeneration.* Neurobiol Aging, 1996. 17(3): p. 467-80.

[18] Schipper, H., *et al.*, *Role of the gonads in the histologic aging of the hypothalamic arcuate nucleus.* Biol Reprod, 1981. 25(2): p. 413-9.

[19] Schipper, H.M., *et al.*, *Astrocyte mitochondria: a substrate for iron deposition in the aging rat substantia nigra.* Exp Neurol, 1998. 152(2): p. 188-96.

[20] Schipper, H.M., *et al.*, *Gomori-positive astrocytes in primary culture: effects of in vitro age and cysteamine exposure.* Brain Res Dev Brain Res, 1990. 54(1): p. 71-9.

[21] McLaren, J., J.R. Brawer, and H.M. Schipper, *Iron content correlates with peroxidase activity in cysteamine-induced astroglial organelles.* J Histochem Cytochem, 1992. 40(12): p. 1887-97.

[22] Brawer, J.R., *et al.*, *The origin and composition of peroxidase-positive granules in cysteamine-treated astrocytes in culture.* Brain Res, 1994. 633(1-2): p. 9-20.

[23] Chopra, V.S., *et al.*, *A cellular stress model for the differential expression of glial lysosomal cathepsins in the aging nervous system.* Exp Neurol, 1997. 147(2): p. 221-8.

[24] Schipper, H.M., M.B. Mydlarski, and X. Wang, *Cysteamine gliopathy in situ: a cellular stress model for the biogenesis of astrocytic inclusions.* J Neuropathol Exp Neurol, 1993. 52(4): p. 399-410.

[25] Brawer, J.R., *et al.*, *Composition of Gomori-positive inclusions in astrocytes of the hypothalamic arcuate nucleus.* Anat Rec, 1994. 240(3): p. 407-15.

[26] Schipper, H.M. and S. Cissé, *Mitochondrial constituents of corpora amylacea and autofluorescent astrocytic inclusions in senescent human brain.* Glia, 1995. 14(1): p. 55-64.

[27] Manganaro, F., *et al.*, *Redox perturbations in cysteamine-stressed astroglia: implications for inclusion formation and gliosis in the aging brain.* Free Radic Biol Med, 1995. 19(6): p. 823-35.

[28] Sahlas, D.J., A. Liberman, and H.M. Schipper, *Role of heme oxygenase-1 in the biogenesis of corpora amylacea.* Biogerontology, 2002. 3(4): p. 223-31.

[29] Srebro, Z., *Periventricular Gomori-positive glia in brains of X-irradiated rats.* Brain Res, 1971. 35(2): p. 463-8.

[30] Wang, X., F. Manganaro, and H.M. Schipper, *A cellular stress model for the sequestration of redox-active glial iron in the aging and degenerating nervous system.* J Neurochem, 1995. 64(4): p. 1868-77.

[31] Ham, D. and H.M. Schipper, *Heme oxygenase-1 induction and mitochondrial iron sequestration in astroglia exposed to amyloid peptides.* Cell Mol Biol (Noisy-le-grand), 2000. 46(3): p. 587-96.

[32] Mehindate, K., *et al.*, *Proinflammatory cytokines promote glial heme oxygenase-1 expression and mitochondrial iron deposition: implications for multiple sclerosis.* J Neurochem, 2001. 77(5): p. 1386-95.

[33] Schipper, H.M., *et al.*, *Mitochondrial iron sequestration in dopamine-challenged astroglia: role of heme oxygenase-1 and the permeability transition pore.* J Neurochem, 1999. 72(5): p. 1802-11.

[34] Schipper, H.M., *Chapter 123. Metal accumulation during aging*, in *Encyclopedia of Neuroscience*, L.R. Squire, Editor 2009, Academic Press: Oxford. p. 811-818.

[35] Ryter, S.W. and R.M. Tyrrell, *The heme synthesis and degradation pathways: role in oxidant sensitivity. Heme oxygenase has both pro- and antioxidant properties.* Free Radic Biol Med, 2000. 28(2): p. 289-309.

[36] McCoubrey, W.K., Jr., T.J. Huang, and M.D. Maines, *Isolation and characterization of a cDNA from the rat brain that encodes hemoprotein heme oxygenase-3.* Eur J Biochem, 1997. 247(2): p. 725-32.

[37] Scapagnini, G., *et al.*, *Gene expression profiles of heme oxygenase isoforms in the rat brain.* Brain Res, 2002. 954(1): p. 51-9.

[38] Dennery, P.A., *Regulation and role of heme oxygenase in oxidative injury.* Curr Top Cell Regul, 2000. 36: p. 181-99.

[39] Verma, A., *et al.*, *Carbon monoxide: a putative neural messenger.* Science, 1993. 259(5093): p. 381-4.

[40] Baranano, D.E. and S.H. Snyder, *Neural roles for heme oxygenase: contrasts to nitric oxide synthase.* Proc Natl Acad Sci U S A, 2001. 98(20): p. 10996-1002.

[41] Igarashi, K. and J. Sun, *The heme-Bach1 pathway in the regulation of oxidative stress response and erythroid differentiation.* Antioxid Redox Signal, 2006. 8(1-2): p. 107-18.

[42] Ogawa, K., *[Heme metabolism in stress response].* Nippon Eiseigaku Zasshi, 2002. 56(4): p. 615-21.

[43] Sun, J., *et al.*, *Hemoprotein Bach1 regulates enhancer availability of heme oxygenase-1 gene.* Embo J, 2002. 21(19): p. 5216-24.

[44] Suzuki, H., *et al.*, *Cadmium induces nuclear export of Bach1, a transcriptional repressor of heme oxygenase-1 gene.* J Biol Chem, 2003. 278(49): p. 49246-53.

[45] Schipper, H.M., *Heme oxygenase-1: role in brain aging and neurodegeneration.* Exp Gerontol, 2000. 35(6-7): p. 821-30.

[46] Loboda, A., *et al.*, *Heme oxygenase-1 and the vascular bed: from molecular mechanisms to therapeutic opportunities.* Antioxid Redox Signal, 2008. 10(10): p. 1767-812.

[47] Lavrovsky, Y., G.S. Drummond, and N.G. Abraham, *Downregulation of the human heme oxygenase gene by glucocorticoids and identification of 56b regulatory elements.* Biochem Biophys Res Commun, 1996. 218(3): p. 759-65.

[48] Exner, M., *et al.*, *The role of heme oxygenase-1 promoter polymorphisms in human disease.* Free Radic Biol Med, 2004. 37(8): p. 1097-104.

[49] Stocker, R., *et al.*, *Bilirubin is an antioxidant of possible physiological importance.* Science, 1987. 235(4792): p. 1043-6.

[50] Nakagami, T., *et al.*, *A beneficial role of bile pigments as an endogenous tissue protector: anti-complement effects of biliverdin and conjugated bilirubin.* Biochim Biophys Acta, 1993. 1158(2): p. 189-93.

[51] Llesuy, S.F. and M.L. Tomaro, *Heme oxygenase and oxidative stress. Evidence of involvement of bilirubin as physiological protector against oxidative damage.* Biochim Biophys Acta, 1994. 1223(1): p. 9-14.

[52] Dore, S., *et al.*, *Bilirubin, formed by activation of heme oxygenase-2, protects neurons against oxidative stress injury.* Proc Natl Acad Sci U S A, 1999. 96(5): p. 2445-50.

[53] Zhang, J. and C.A. Piantadosi, *Mitochondrial oxidative stress after carbon monoxide hypoxia in the rat brain.* J Clin Invest, 1992. 90(4): p. 1193-9.

[54] Frankel, D., K. Mehindate, and H.M. Schipper, *Role of heme oxygenase-1 in the regulation of manganese superoxide dismutase gene expression in oxidatively-challenged astroglia.* J Cell Physiol, 2000. 185(1): p. 80-6.

[55] Mawal, Y., *et al.*, *Heme oxygenase-1 and Alzheimer disease*, in *Heme Oxygenase in Biology and Medicine*, A.J. Abraham NG, Nath KA, Editor 2002, Kluwer Academic/Plenum Publishers: New York. p. 145-155.

[56] Galbraith, R., *Heme oxygenase: who needs it?* Proc Soc Exp Biol Med, 1999. 222(3): p. 299-305.

[57] Suttner, D.M. and P.A. Dennery, *Reversal of HO-1 related cytoprotection with increased expression is due to reactive iron.* Faseb J, 1999. 13(13): p. 1800-9.

[58] Hirose, W., K. Ikematsu, and R. Tsuda, *Age-associated increases in heme oxygenase-1 and ferritin immunoreactivity in the autopsied brain.* Leg Med (Tokyo), 2003. 5 Suppl: p. S360-6.

[59] Smith, M.A., *et al.*, *Heme oxygenase-1 is associated with the neurofibrillary pathology of Alzheimer's disease.* Am J Pathol, 1994. 145(1): p. 42-7.

[60] Schipper, H.M., S. Cissé, and *E.G.* Stopa, *Expression of heme oxygenase-1 in the senescent and Alzheimer-diseased brain.* Ann Neurol, 1995. 37(6): p. 758-68.

[61] Butterfield, D.A., *et al.*, *Evidence that amyloid beta-peptide-induced lipid peroxidation and its sequelae in Alzheimer's disease brain contribute to neuronal death.* Neurobiol Aging, 2002. 23(5): p. 655-64.

[62] Schipper, H.M., *et al.*, *Glial heme oxygenase-1 expression in Alzheimer disease and mild cognitive impairment.* Neurobiol Aging, 2006. 27(2): p. 252-261.

[63] Mydlarski, M.B., J.J. Liang, and H.M. Schipper, *Role of the cellular stress response in the biogenesis of cysteamine-induced astrocytic inclusions in primary culture.* J Neurochem, 1993. 61(5): p. 1755-65.

[64] Zukor, H., *et al.*, *HO-1-mediated macroautophagy: a mechanism for unregulated iron deposition in aging and degenerating neural tissues.* J Neurochem, 2009. 109(3): p. 776-91.

[65] Song, W., *et al.*, *Unregulated brain iron deposition in transgenic mice overexpressing HMOX1 in the astrocytic compartment.* J Neurochem, 2012. 123: p. 325-336.

[66] Song, W., *et al.*, *Over-expression of heme oxygenase-1 promotes oxidative mitochondrial damage in rat astroglia.* J Cell Physiol, 2006. 206(3): p. 655-63.

[67] Vaya, J., *et al.*, *Effects of heme oxygenase-1 expression on sterol homeostasis in rat astroglia.* Free Radic Biol Med, 2007. 42(6): p. 864-71.

[68] Petronilli, V., *et al.*, *Physiological effectors modify voltage sensing by the cyclosporin A-sensitive permeability transition pore of mitochondria.* J Biol Chem, 1993. 268(29): p. 21939-45.

[69] Bernardi, P., *The permeability transition pore. Control points of a cyclosporin A-sensitive mitochondrial channel involved in cell death.* Biochim Biophys Acta, 1996. 1275(1-2): p. 5-9.

[70] Song, W., *et al.*, *Schizophrenia-like features in transgenic mice overexpressing human HO-1 in the astrocytic compartment.* J Neurosci, 2012. 32: p. 10841–10853.

[71] Drummond, G.S. and A. Kappas, *Chemoprevention of severe neonatal hyperbilirubinemia.* Semin Perinatol, 2004. 28(5): p. 365-8.

[72] Kappas, A., G.S. Drummond, and R.A. Galbraith, *Prolonged clinical use of a heme oxygenase inhibitor: hematological evidence for an inducible but reversible iron-deficiency state.* Pediatrics, 1993. 91(3): p. 537-9.

[73] Kinobe, R.T., *et al.*, *Selectivity of imidazole-dioxolane compounds for in vitro inhibition of microsomal haem oxygenase isoforms.* Br J Pharmacol, 2006. 147(3): p. 307-15.

[74] Kinobe, R.T., *et al.*, *Effectiveness of novel imidazole-dioxolane heme oxygenase inhibitors in renal proximal tubule epithelial cells.* J Pharmacol Exp Ther, 2007. 323(3): p. 763-70.

[75] Vlahakis, J.Z., *et al.*, *Imidazole-dioxolane compounds as isozyme-selective heme oxygenase inhibitors.* J Med Chem, 2006. 49(14): p. 4437-41.

[76] Alaoui-Jamali, M.A., *et al.*, *A novel experimental heme oxygenase-1-targeted therapy for hormone-refractory prostate cancer.* Cancer Res, 2009. 69(20): p. 8017-24.

[77] Gordon, M.N., *et al.*, *Time course of the development of Alzheimer-like pathology in the doubly transgenic PS1+APP mouse.* Exp Neurol, 2002. 173(2): p. 183-95.

[78] Holcomb, L., *et al.*, *Accelerated Alzheimer-type phenotype in transgenic mice carrying both mutant amyloid precursor protein and presenilin 1 transgenes.* Nat Med, 1998. 4(1): p. 97-100.

[79] Holcomb, L.A., *et al.*, *Behavioral changes in transgenic mice expressing both amyloid precursor protein and presenilin-1 mutations: lack of association with amyloid deposits.* Behav Genet, 1999. 29(3): p. 177-85.

[80] Schipper, H.M., *Heme oxygenase-1: Transducer of pathological brain iron sequestration under oxidative stress*, in *Redox-active Metals in Neurological Disorders*, S. LeVine, J.R. Connor, and H.M. Schipper, Editors. 2004, Ann NY Acad Sci 1012: New York. p. 84-93.

[81] Schipper, H.M., *Heme oxygenase expression in human central nervous system disorders.* Free Radic Biol Med, 2004. 37(12): p. 1995-2011.

[82] Schipper, H.M., *Heme oxygenase-1 in Alzheimer disease: a tribute to Moussa Youdim.* J Neural Transm, 2011. 118(3): p. 381-7.

[83] Schipper, H.M., *et al.*, *Heme oxygenase-1 and neurodegeneration: expanding frontiers of engagement.* J Neurochem, 2009. 110(2): p. 469-85.

[84] Schipper, H.M., *Astrocytes in Brain Aging and Neurodegeneration*1998, Austin: R.G. Landes Co. 256.

[85] Droge, W., *Free radicals in the physiological control of cell function.* Physiol Rev, 2002. 82(1): p. 47-95.

[86] Droge, W. and H.M. Schipper, *Oxidative stress and aberrant signaling in aging and cognitive decline.* Aging Cell, 2007. 6(3): p. 361-70.

CHAPTER 9

Music Therapy for Individuals with Dementia: Areas of Intervention and Research Perspectives

Alfredo Raglio[1,*] and Maria V. Gianelli[2]

[1]Sospiro Foundation, Cremona, Italy and INTERDEM Group, (Psycho-Social Interventions in Dementia), EU and [2]University of Genova, Italy and INTERDEM Group, (Psycho-Social Interventions in Dementia), EU

Abstract: This contribution focuses on the definition of music therapy as a specific applicative context to be seen as distinct from the generic use of music in a variety of pathologies. Music therapy is presented as a discipline grounded upon both relationship and the theoretical-methodological principles peculiar to each applicative model. The therapeutic nature proper to music therapy is highlighted with specific reference to the domain of the dementias. Music therapy facilitates expression, communication and relationship in the non-verbal context. Such an opportunity allows persons with dementia to establish contact, to express, and even contrive an organisation/regulation of their emotions, through the sonorous-musical relationship with the music therapist. With reference to a brief analysis of the relevant literature, attention is drawn to the importance of both evidence–based clinical practice and music therapy evaluations, aimed at proving the effectiveness of music therapy, while promoting its correct application.

Keywords: Music, music therapy, outcomes - scientific basis, relationship, theoretical/methodological aspects.

INTRODUCTION

The use of music and of the sonorous-musical element in the context of dementia has gradually become quite widespread over the last few decades, although its experimental applications appear to be differentially connotated as are the finalities of its varied contents [1].

In the literature these activities fall under the heading "music therapy", thus being included in scientific databases whenever a study conforms to adequate

***Corresponding author Alfredo Raglio:** Sospiro Foundation, Piazza Libertà, 2 – 26048 Sospiro, Cremona, Italy; Tel: +390372620264; E-mails: raglioa@tin.it; musicoterapia@fondazionesospiro.it

D.K. Lahiri (Ed)

methodological criteria. The following introductory notes, therefore, highlight two caveats that we consider important – and that we believe should be given greater attention:

a) the need – and recommendation - not to include under the heading "music therapy" any and every musical initiative addressed to persons with dementia;

b) the need for assessing the music therapeutic process, while also clearly expressing and illustrating its contents (quoting theoretical and applicative references) along with the related methodological aspects.

We believe that such premises should, on the one hand, contribute to help identify an adequate definition of the term "music therapy" and, on the other, promote its correct application. The authors of this study firmly believe that a serious attempt at answering these queries might represent a significant starting point for the creation of a scientific basis for music therapy.

This would substantially modify the structure and approach to music therapeutic interventions.

The article presents some reflections regarding music and music therapy applications in the field of dementia.

Table **1** summarizes the principal topics and hypotheses concerning these applications.

COMPARISONS BETWEEN MUSIC AND MUSIC THERAPY IN DEMENTIA

A large number of psycho-social interventions in dementia care are based upon musical activities, their main objective being to create a situation of temporary well-being in a socializing context, whose content consists of a variety of musical initiatives (rhythmic use of instruments, singing, movement associated to music, *etc.*).

Table 1: Principal points and hypotheses of the present chapter

- A large number of psycho-social interventions in dementia care is based upon musical and music therapy activities. - It is possible to define specific characteristics of the musical and music therapeutic interventions in relation to the aims, the applicative modalities and the contents of the proposals. - Active music therapy approach (interaction through sonorous-musical instruments) is the most adequate in music therapeutic treatments for individuals with dementia. - Music therapy improves Behavioral and Psychological Symptoms of Dementia. - Music therapy induces a better organization and/or (co)regulation of the emotional components of the personality in individuals with dementia. - Music therapy, based on non verbal communication techniques, enhances expressive and relational components. - Music therapy stimulates cognitive functions in dementia. - Music therapy requires clear theoretical and applicative bases along with methodological and scientific rigour in research design (Clinical Controlled Trials and Randomized Controlled Trials) and in the process and outcomes assessment.

Listening to music is another type of experience, again oriented to a variety of goals:

a) the evocative potentialities of music can stimulate memories or frames of mind by means of verbalizing activities immediately following a listening activity;

b) music can be used to facilitate the recognition of specific parts of the physical environment or of structured periods of the day;

c) listening to music as a "generic" activity (classical music, favourite music, *etc.*) is employed in the conviction that it can be effective in reducing challenging behavior, improving mood and promoting socialization.

d) different effects are produced by listening to preferred or individualized music: the literature has showed significant effects obtained by these experiences on some behavioral problems, such as agitation and anxiety [2-4].

Although it is no doubt highly plausible that music harbours beneficial potentialities, it is also very important to stress how often these are elicited in no specific relation with the concept of therapy. The outcome of the latter should always be connected to the possibility of obtaining both symptom attenuation and the prevention/stabilization of complications deriving from the symptoms themselves (secondary and tertiary prevention), with the predictable repercussions on the general quality of life of the persons concerned. It is obvious that the benefits deriving from therapy should be systematically replicable, should last over time and be explicitly based upon an explicative theory [5]. Nor must one overlook the importance of understanding - through in-depth clinical/ observational approaches – which subjects are more liable to respond effectively. Along with the generic beneficial potentialities of music, often defined "music therapy activities", although in absence of the above-mentioned characterizing elements, there exists a specific definition of "music therapy" acknowledged and supported by the international music therapy community. In this definition music therapy is described as the use of music and/or of its components (sound, rhythm, melody and harmony) by a qualified music therapist, in individual or group relationships, in the context of a formally defined process, with the aim of facilitating and promoting communication, relationships, learning, mobilization, expression, organization and other relevant therapeutic goals intended to meet physical, emotional, mental, social and cognitive needs. The main finality of music therapy is that of developing potentialities and/or rehabilitating an individual's functions so that he/she might achieve an improved integration on the intra- and interpersonal levels and therefore an ameliorated quality of life through prevention, rehabilitation or therapy (World Federation of Music Therapy, 8th World Conference on Music Therapy, Hamburg, 1996).

The definition identifies a number of components that are to be considered crucial if an intervention employing sonorous-musical elements is to be considered potentially therapeutic:

- the presence of a qualified care-worker (the music therapist).
- a music therapeutic referential model grounded on theoretical and methodological criteria.
- the presence of a structured setting.

- aims (aspiring to become stable and long-lasting over time) linked to changes occurring in the person, or in parts of his/her functions.

- constant reference to an intrapersonal and/or interpersonal plan or project to be made during the therapeutic action.

Each of these elements is clearly identifiable and definable in the context of whatsoever music therapy intervention; the confusion generally derive either from the lack of adequate knowledge in the field of music therapy, or from the attribution of a presumed greater "dignity" or "efficacy" to those interventions which can be defined "music therapeutic" rather than "musical" tout court.

The training of music therapists is another issue that deserves consideration: the acquisition of the musical and relational competences that characterize those who work in this field takes place through specific training courses which in many countries are university-based (Bachelor, Master of Arts and PhD programs) structured according to widely consolidated and shared criteria.

The choice of a music therapeutic model is a fundamental element which should characterize any intervention based upon a therapeutic relationship. Although the definition of the current range of music therapeutic approaches is in progress, and therefore presents a rich and articulated scenario, the World Federation of Music Therapy – during The 9th World Conference of Music Therapy, held in Washington in 1999 – acknowledged and defined five important music therapy models: the creative music therapy model (Nordoff-Robbins) [6], based upon creative improvisation and linked to humanistic psychology, the behaviorist model (Madsen) [7], the Jungian and humanistic receptive psycho-therapeutic model (Bonny) [8], the Freudian analytic model (Priestley) [9], the psycho-dynamic improvisational model (Benenzon) [10].

Another important issue in music therapy is the definition of a temporal-spatial structure, along with the set of rules defining the therapeutic setting: these two elements, acting together, acquire a fundamental importance as facilitators of therapeutic actions, and as a consequence, of changes for the better.

We also believe that the above – as for any other therapeutic treatment – implies a codified praxis, applicable to any treatment. This is in line with the general concept of "Evidence Based Practice", expressed by Mace [11] and quoted by Vink [12]. Such a practice should involve reflections and applicative implications, which can be summarized as follows:

- clinical criteria for admission to treatment.
- music therapeutic assessment (finalized to inclusion in/ exclusion from treatment).
- definition of therapeutic goals.
- therapeutic contract.
- treatment.
- evaluation.
- conclusion.

Music therapy is therefore on its way towards a systematisation process intended to strengthen the scientific basis of the discipline.

This should involve in-depth reflections linking practice to theoretical and methodological/applicative elements by way of rigorous efforts towards the achievement of a greater coherence in the theory-praxis relationship, and should also involve the establishment of evidence-based research as the fundamental and mandatory grounding of the discipline.

Music therapy in fact is easier to define as practice rather than as theory – in common with most knowledge domains of more recent application; *i.e.*, it is generally described as an empirically-based intervention applied to various pathological contexts, through the use of sound and music. Though placing therapeutic relationships at the centre of its interest, music therapy is as yet characterized by a series of gaps and inconsistencies, both of a theoretical nature, and in the accomplishing of interventions which often appear to be devoid of actual therapeutic contents.

The mere juxtaposition of "music" and "pathology" (dementia, in our case) induces one to employ the term "music therapy", with no consideration for the therapeutic specificity of the intervention, which should on the contrary be related to:

a) a theoretical basis;

b) applicative aspects;

c) specific contents;

d) verifiability of outcomes [13].

Table **2** summarizes the main differences between "music" and "music therapy" (Table **2**).

Table 2: Differences between "music" and "music therapy" interventions in dementia

Music	**Music Therapy**
Presence of a professional of the music area	Presence of a professional of the music-therapeutic area with specific relational and musical competences
Absence of a specific therapeutic setting	Presence of a structured therapeutic setting
Absence of a specific intervention model	Presence of a music-therapeutic referential model grounded on theoretical and methodological criteria
Aims: temporary well-being, improving mood, promoting socialization, memories and stimulation of frames of mind, relaxation, *etc.*	Aims (aspiring to become stable and long-lasting over time): attenuation of behavioral and psychiatric symptoms and prevention/stabilization of complications; increase in communication and relationship skills; improving cognitive functions
Contents: structured musical initiatives (rhythmic use of instruments, singing, movement associated to music, *etc.*) and listening to music (classical music, favourite music, *etc.*)	Contents: sonorous-musical improvisation; listening activities that involve verbal and elaborative competences (preferably at initial stages of dementia)

THE THERAPEUTIC PERSPECTIVES OF MUSIC THERAPY IN THE DEMENTIAS

With reference to the above illustrated concepts, we believe that in dementia – as in other pathologies characterized by the impairment of those communicative functions which are most recent in human ontogenetic evolution - one may hypothesize the possibility of re-activating and broadening those archaic expressive and relational abilities which persist along the whole life-span of each human being, as forms of interpersonal experience, alternative to the verbal one. It is within this context that we envisage the possibility of music therapy building a communicative bridge for people with dementia. Music therapy being a pre-verbal, non-verbal communication technique - subsisting without need either for symbolic representations of reality, abstractive abilities or culture-bound learning processes - we believe that relational and expressive modalities, archaic in origin and nature and therefore more likely to be still present in persons with cognitive impairment, can be activated by means of its potential. Music therapy can promote the preservation of recognition of the external environment, of a sense of identity, of personhood even, in individuals with dementia.

In psychological terms a regression, shared and guided by the therapist, takes place, helping the person with dementia to achieve an improved adaptation, through new and more harmonious inner frames of reference *vs.* the impairment induced by neurological damage [14]. Music therapy can also induce an improved organization of the emotional components of the personality [15] while simultaneously stimulating, in a natural fashion, cognitive functions such as memory, attention, executive functions, sensory-motor co-ordination, abilities of stimulus discrimination [1, 16] – since music is also a mental activity. In the dementias, music therapy can influence mental and behavioral disorders, and possibly promote new learning strategies, while improving relational and social aspects, and therefore the overall quality of life of the sufferer.

Music therapy constantly refers both to a relational process, to an "affect attunement" [17] between two sonorous-musical identities – that of the therapist and that of the patient - and to an empathetic listening which produces the therapeutic character of the intervention, whatever the referential model or the contents of the activity might be.

We believe, furthermore, that the above might be pursued more adequately through an active approach (sonorous-musical improvisation), which implies the prevalence of non-verbal sonorous-musical aspects in the direct patient/music therapist relationship. It is our informed opinion, in fact, that the interaction based upon the use of sonorous-musical instruments can facilitate organizational processes and the (co-)regulation of emotional components [17-20]. Receptive techniques (those based upon listening skills) in music therapy involve verbal and elaborative competences such as a person with moderate-severe dementia might unfortunately have lost. In this case in fact, listening to music might trigger emotions that the person may not be able to manage and control, thus creating states of ill-being and even distress.

CONTROLLED AND RANDOMIZED CONTROLLED TRIALS IN THE FIELD OF MUSIC THERAPY

In this section we have considered articles found in PubMed and in other relevant websites by using the following key words: "music", "music therapy" and "dementia" (up to May 2012). We have therefore selected those studies which attribute specific attention to experimentations most correctly corresponding to the criteria of evidence-based research and which employ strictly music therapeutic techniques, or those closest possible to them.

The first significant review on the subject is contributed by Koger & Brotons [21], who comment on the lack of rigour and methodological design which characterizes studies (randomized and controlled) carried out to date upon the effectiveness of music therapy in dementias. The Authors, however, stress the emergence of important, documented data concerning potential effects of music therapy, recommending further in-depth research projects on the subject. In this article the need to systematize clinical practice in music therapy and to adequately construct research designs is stressed.

The updating of the review by Vink *et al.* [22] includes 10 randomized, controlled studies that will be summarized below. Clark *et al.* [23] describe an intervention based upon listening to favorite music during bathing (10 bathing sessions) by patients (n = 18) with dementia and aggressive behavior during routine care. Significant improvements were reported especially in the reduction of aggressive behavior. This intervention involved a limited number of patients for a short period of time (two weeks) and it does not contemplate a direct music therapist/patient interaction: the music employed was chosen on the grounds of a-specific presuppositions, therefore as such, not generalizable. A study carried out by Gerdner [2] reports the outcomes of a music intervention on agitation. A comparison is established between the short- and long-term effects of "individualized" music and those of music proposals considered to be "relaxing". Thirty-nine subjects with severe cognitive impairment were recruited, divided into two groups and exposed first to the listening of individualized music for 6 weeks and successively, after a two-week interval, to six listening sessions of classical music defined "relaxing". The meetings took place twice a week and lasted 30 minutes each. Both conditions resulted more effective as against baseline. Moreover, the use of the Cohen-Mansfield Agitation Inventory revealed a more relevant decrease in agitation states during and after listening sessions of music chosen by the subjects themselves. In this intervention also, the use of music is rather a-specific and is employed for listening sessions in the absence of any identifiable therapeutic connotation whatsoever. The sessions are devoid of any element relating the listening modalities to precise therapeutic modalities (*e.g.* precise criteria for the choice of music to be made, moments of introspection and/or elaboration, etc). The difference between the above and authentic music therapy approaches based upon listening activities is very evident, since the latter focus upon providing opportunities for the verbal re-elaboration of emotional-affective reactions, stemming from the experience. Groene [24] analyses the effects of music therapy upon wandering behavior in patients with a diagnosis of moderate-severe Alzheimer's disease. The 30 subjects taking part in the study were exposed to two different treatment approaches: a music therapy activity, and a listening session of readings. Each subject took part in a daily session of 15 minutes' duration for seven days. The experimental group attended 5 music sessions, followed by two reading sessions, whereas the control group took part in 5 reading sessions and 2 music sessions. The music therapy treatment approach consisted in listening initiatives, music productions with percussion instruments, singing and movement. Both activities were guided by a music therapist. The materials presented to the two groups were selected, whenever possible, according to the requests of the participants themselves. Although no statistically significant differences were reported between the two groups, either concerning cognitive aspects or the reduction of wandering behavior, the participants appeared to spend more time in the music therapeutic setting rather than in the reading room. The same evidence was encountered in a study by Rosswurm *et al.*, centred upon the observation of persons with wandering behavior during multi-sensorial sessions, including a music activity [25]. This result is also confirmed by another work by Scruggs *et al.*, comparing patients' permanence in a room during music activities *vs.* time spent in the absence of activities [26]. From the clinical point of view, we believe that the sessions were too brief for a therapeutic relationship to be established, and that the duration of the intervention appeared to be definitely too limited for an authentic change to be therapeutically induced. Moreover, neither in this intervention was any reference to a music therapeutic model to be found. All these reasons induce us to define the intervention as an experiment in "stimulation" *via* musical activities, movement and dancing, rather than as a music therapy activity proper. The experimentation conducted by Brotons *et al.* [27] compared the efficacy of group music therapy with that produced by a verbal intervention (conversational interaction) with reference to cognitive and linguistic abilities. The subjects with dementia (n = 26), divided into small groups, took part in twice-weekly sessions for a total of 8 meetings (4 in music therapy and 4 in conversation or vice-versa). The preliminary assessments were carried out during the week prior to the onset of the study by means of the Mini Mental State Examination, for the evaluation of cognitive function and the Western Aphasia Battery for the assessment of linguistic abilities. The latter were re-assessed every two weeks, *i.e.* every 4 sessions. The results revealed a significant improvement in language performance after music therapy, both with regard to contents and to expressive abilities in spontaneous speech. Neither cognitive function nor verbal comprehension showed relevant differences between the two treatment groups. As in the previously described study, we are here in the presence of a rather brief intervention (4 sessions) based upon songs with a guitar accompaniment, followed by questions intended to stimulate a conversation related to the song themes (animals, flowers, Spring, St Patrick's Day, the United States). The music therapy sessions are preceded by a welcoming song, that is repeated at the end of the session by way of leave-taking. The setting does not appear to be defined according to specific therapeutic criteria in this case either, and music is employed in a generic singing session. Lord *et al.* [28] have studied the effects of music therapy in relation to improvements in social and emotional functions. Sixty patients with a diagnosis of dementia of the Alzheimer's type were divided into 3 groups: the first was invited to listen to "big band" music of the '20's and '30's, that the patients were allowed to accompany by playing simple musical instruments; the second was asked to perform a series of "puzzle exercises", while the third took part in standard drawing and painting activities. A follow-up was carried out after 6 months. Outcomes and statistical analyses referring to the 3 groups are not reported. Data analysis identified positive effects upon mood, ability to remember personal history and social interaction in the persons included in group one (listening to music). No music therapeutic model is present in this study, which can be identified very clearly as 'musical experience'.

Svansdottir *et al.* [29] have examined the effects of music therapy upon challenging behavior (Behavioral and Psychiatric Symptoms of Dementia) in patients with moderate-severe dementia. Forty-seven subjects with moderate or severe dementia were included in the study. The drop-out percentage was statistically significant: only 38 patients (20 participants and 18 controls) eventually took part in all sessions. Assessment was performed using the Behavioral Pathology in Alzheimer's Disease Rating Scale, administered in blind modality by nursing staff before the intervention, at conclusion, and 4 months after conclusion. The experimental group took part in music therapy sessions, lasting 30 minutes, 3 times a week, over a period of 6 weeks. The control group was exposed to standard therapies. The study was conducted by a qualified music therapist who, at the beginning of the study, had presented a number of Icelandic songs, from which the participants themselves chose the ones to be performed. At the end of each performance the participants had the possibility of talking both with the therapist and with the other group members. Music instruments were also available to be played in free or thematic improvisations. Patients were allowed to move about, following the rhythm of the music. At the end of the intervention, the experimental group showed a relevant decrease in aggressiveness, anxiety and other disorders displayed during the activity, while these outcomes were not identified in the control group. The follow-up at 4 weeks after conclusion highlighted symptom recurrence. The total Behavioral Pathology in Alzheimer's Disease Rating Scale score did not show significant variations in either group. Despite the brevity of this intervention, the contents proposed were in greater agreement with the concept of music therapy proposed in this study. Reference is made, in fact, both to improvisation techniques and to a use of sonorous-musical materials referring to broader relational implications. A clear music therapeutic typology of approach, however, is not explicitly mentioned. The duration of intervention is more significant with respect to that proposed in previously described studies, and presents, in our opinion, greater potential for the development of a therapeutic relationship with patients suffering from dementia.

Sung *et al.* [30] assessed the effects of music upon agitation in 36 older adults with moderate and severe dementia. The patients were divided into two groups of 18 subjects each. The experimental group was exposed to music listening (familiar pieces, pleasant and with a moderate rhythmic course) during a motor stimulation activity. Behavioural evaluation revealed that agitated behaviour had significantly decreased in the experimental group after 4 weeks' sessions.

Guetin *et al.* [31] enrolled 30 mild-moderate AD patients. The experimental group underwent 16 weekly sessions of individual receptive music therapy, while controls had the same number of reading sessions. The treated group showed a statistically significant improvement in anxiety and depression disorders, starting from the fourth week and continuing up to follow-up (2 months after conclusion of treatment).

The three following studies aim on the one hand at defining the criteria for a specific therapeutic application employing music, and on the other, at identifying rigorous modalities for the assessment of music therapy efficacy on behavioral disturbances and of the therapeutic process and its outcomes. The first study [32] is part of the ministerial research project titled "Valutazione e Sviluppo della Rete Integrata per la Malattia di Alzheimer", d.g.r. n. VII/6437, 12/10/2001, UO n.5. Its main focus was to draw attention both upon the observation/evaluation criteria of the therapeutic process, and upon the outcomes of a music therapeutic intervention of a relational type. The 16 patients selected for the study, affected by moderate-severe dementia assessed by means of the Clinical Dementia Rating, took part in twice-weekly music therapy sessions lasting 30 minutes each. The use of sonorous-musical material in a prevalently non-verbal context, along with all aspects of analogic and pre-verbal communication finalized to "affect attunement" [17], represented the nucleus around which the experimentation developed, in the attempt to demonstrate a decrease in behavioral and mental disorders. The conceptual frame of reference is that which characterizes inter-subjective psychology [33]. The sessions were video-recorded with a fixed camcorder and the video-tapes were then analysed by an observational coding scheme, by a music-therapist not involved in the process. Three possible modalities of sonorous-musical interaction were identified: exploration, listening and sonorous-musical interaction with communicative-relational finalities (the latter characterized by elements implying emotional involvement, such as syntonic movement and countenance congruent with the sonorous-musical context, with the patient/therapist relationship or with the musical variations). The second part of the protocols analysed both the number of acceptance/involvement signals (smiles, body movements attuned to sonorous-musical context, singing, positive verbalisations) and the non-acceptance/distress expressed by the patient (negative verbalisations, difficulties in remaining within the music therapy setting, irritability, wandering) directly observable from the video-recording analysis. A number of scales were used for the extra-setting letto assessment (administered before the sessions and after 4 months' treatment): the Mini Mental State Examination for cognitive function; the Barthel Index for functional assessment, the Neuropsychiatric Inventory for behavioral assessment. The control group was analogously assessed and monitored. During music therapeutic treatment no significant variations were made to current pharmacological treatment (neuroleptic and/or sedative). The definitely most relevant outcome was the statistically significant decrease of behavioral disorders in the experimental group *vs.* a worsening in cognitive and functional states. The control group displayed similar results, with a more relevant worsening of the functional and cognitive profile, and a mild – though not significant – improvement in behavioral disorders. The study presents a few limitations, such as for example, the small-scale sample, and the absence of a randomization modality. Such limitations were overcome in a further study [34], which included the above mentioned criteria. The project involved 59 subjects (30 making up the experimental group and 29 the control group) and presented similar characteristics to the previous one, with results confirming the findings of the latter. The treated group, in fact, displayed a statistically significant decrease in mental and behavioral disorders, both from a severity and a frequency point of view – with special attention being paid to irritability, agitation, apathy, aberrant motor activity, delusions and night-time disturbances. From a music therapy point of view, the empathetic relationship and the patients' active participation in the music therapy approach, also improved in the experimental group. As to the positive answers expressed by the patients during sessions, an increase in acceptance/involvement signals - such as smiles, syntonic movement and singing – was expressed.

The third study by Raglio *et al.* [35] aimed at evaluating the efficacy of MT (Three 12-session cycles alternating with one-month intervals in absence of treatment) upon BPSDs in patients with moderate-severe dementia. All patients (n=60) received standard care (educational and occupational activities) while the experimental group was additionally exposed to an MT intervention (inter-subjective, improvisational approach) three times a week. Results show that MT was more effective than standard of care in the reduction of BPSDs (NPI global scores).

The research data suggest the potential efficacy of music therapeutic interventions, although emphasizing how complex the task of checking results is, especially due to the lack of formalised and standardized assessment tools and outcome indicators for this purpose. In addition, one must take into account the difficulties encountered in selecting homogeneous samples from a clinical point of view, besides the inevitable psycho-physical impairment of the person with dementia. Finally, another consideration might be related to the difficulties inherent in monitoring general alterations occurring in the life of these patients: the scales in use do not in fact appear to be adequate in analytically identifying the behavioral and mental aspects which respond more sensitively to possible variations brought about by the music therapy intervention.

Research in music therapy, besides studying the effects of sound upon psychological and behavioral aspects, has attempted to investigate possible correlations with some biological and physiological parameters [36, 37].

More recently, Suzuki *et al.* [38] investigated the variations in levels of chromogranin A from an endocrinological point of view. Ten subjects with moderate-severe dementia were assessed before and after a cycle of 16 twice-weekly music therapy sessions. Evaluations also concerned cognitive and behavioral levels. No significant changes emerged from the administration of the Mini Mental State Examination, with the exception of language abilities, whilst the Multidimensional Observation Scale For Elderly Subjects revealed a decrease in irritability. The study showed a decrease in these proteins at the end of the intervention. From a music therapy point of view, Japanese songs were proposed, often chosen by the patients themselves, who were also stimulated both to use (especially percussion) instruments and to sing. Each session started and ended with a song including names of all patients. The goal of these sessions was to stimulate physical function and encourage social interaction. A successive, analogous study [39] confirms the decrease in chromogranin A levels after a music therapeutic treatment lasting 3 months with twice-weekly sessions.

The long-term effects of music therapy were investigated according to both psychological and physiological criteria, by T. Takahashi *et al.* [40]. The Authors studied a group of older adults with dementia who were submitted to a series of tests, examining blood pressure, levels of cortisol (adrenocortical hormone whose level increases with stress) through a saliva sample. The 43 subjects – 24 being treated and 19 making up the control group – fulfilled homogeneity criteria with respect to dementia severity, physical conditions and life style. The saliva samples were obtained from all components of both groups before and after initiation of therapy, taking place once a week, and successively at 6 months, 1 and 2 years after conclusion of the first music therapy session. The same modality was used for measuring blood pressure and for cognitive assessment, by means of the Revised Hasegawa Dementia Scale. The music therapy intervention, conducted by a specialized care-worker and a collaborator who accompanied him at the piano, presented a five-step articulation: exchange of greetings, exercises (performable also from a sitting position), vocalisations, singing, instrumental group performance. The singing repertoire included songs learned at school, familiar or favourite songs, *e.g.* because linked to reminders of patients' youth, Japanese ballads and folk-songs. Percussion instruments were employed, Japanese drums in particular. The choice of repertoire was subordinated to the finality of the intervention, designed to encourage and promote verbal exchanges between subjects on topics related to their reminiscences. Data analysis led to the conclusion that music therapy produces a homeostatic effect, *i.e.* of blood pressure regulation. It can therefore be considered a prevention therapy for cardio-circulatory and cerebral pathologies. With reference to cortisol levels, no statistically significant differences were found between the pre-therapy stage and at follow-up after six months, 1 year and 2 years from conclusion of therapy. The cognitive evaluation, over the 2-year period of treatment, shows that the Revised Hasegawa Dementia Scale scores were maintained in the music therapy group, whereas the scores decreased in the control group. The difference between the two groups was not statistically significant.

Recently Raglio *et al.* [35] evaluated the effects of active music therapy approach upon behavioral disturbances in Alzheimer's disease and vascular dementia patients when associated to changes in physiological parameters such as heart rate and its variability 20 subjects were randomized and exposed either to music therapy or to standard care. In patients exposed to music a reduction in depressive symptoms was recorded (50% of patients) and in Cardiac Frequency, along with an increase in Variability.

A more recent review by Raglio *et al.* [1] describes also other significant studies regarding the effects of music and music therapy techniques on behavioral, cognitive, motor and physiological outcomes in dementia.

Table **3** reports characteristics of the main studies described in the present paper (Table **3**).

Table 3: Music therapeutic or musical contents and characteristics of main studies described in this Review

Studies	Research Designs*	No. of Patients	Diagnosis	No. of Sessions	Activity**	Assessment	Results
Gerdner, 2000 [2]	RCT	39	Mild to severe dementia	24	Listening to individualized and classical music; B	Behavioral evaluation	Agitation reduction
Clark *et al.*, 1998 [23]	RCT	18	Severe dementia	10	Listening to music (hymns, familiar songs, big band and classical music) while bathing;	Behavioral evaluation	Reduction of aggressive behaviors

Studies	Research Designs*	No. of Patients	Diagnosis	No. of Sessions	Activity**	Assessment	Results
					A		
Groene, 1993 [24]	RCT	30	Moderate-severe Alzheimer's Disease	5 daily sessions for 5 days	Stimulation by listening to music, playing percussion instruments, singing and dancing; A	Behavioral evaluation	Wandering reduction
Brotons *et al.*, 2000 [27]	RCT	26	Alzheimer's Disease and related disorders	4	Singing songs and verbal interaction; A	Cognitive and speech evaluation	Speech abilities improvement
Lord *et al.*, 1993 [28]	RCT	60	Alzheimer's Disease	6	Listening to music (Big band of '20s and '30s) and playing instruments; A	Evaluation of social and emotional functions	Mood improvement
Svansdottir *et al.*, 2006 [29]	RCT	38	Moderate-severe Alzheimer's Disease	18	Active music therapy (familiar songs with guitar accompaniment use of instruments, improvisation); A	Behavioral evaluation	Reduction of activity disturbances, aggressiveness and anxiety
Sung *et al.*, 2006 [30]	RCT	36	Moderate-severe dementia	8	Group music program with movement intervention A	Behavioral evaluation (agitation)	Significant reduction of agitated behaviors
Guetin *et al.*, 2009 [31]	RCT	30	Mild-to-moderate Alzheimer-type dementia	16	Receptive music therapy B	Behavioral evaluation (anxiety and depression)	Significant reduction of anxiety and depression
Raglio *et al.*, 2006 [32]	CCT	16	Moderate-severe dementia	30	Improvisational music therapy; B	Cognitive, functional behavioral and music therapy process evaluation	Reduction of behavior disorders and improvement of communication and relationship skills
Raglio *et al.*, 2008 [34]	RCT	60	Moderate-severe dementia	30	Improvisational Music therapy; B	Cognitive, functional behavioral and music therapy	Reduction of behavior disorders and improvement of

Studies	Research Designs*	No. of Patients	Diagnosis	No. of Sessions	Activity**	Assessment	Results
						process evaluation	communication and relationship skills
Raglio *et al.*, 2010 [35]	RCT	60	Moderate-severe dementia	36	Improvisational Music therapy; B	Cognitive, functional behavioral and music therapy process evaluation	Reduction of behavior disorders
Suzuki *et al.*, 2004 [38]	CCT	23	Alzheimer's Disease and Vascular dementia	16	Singing songs, playing percussion instruments; A	Cognitive, behavioral and endocrinological evaluation	Irritability and stress reduction, language improvement
Takahashi *et al.*, 2006 [40]	CCT	43	Moderate-severe dementia	Weekly music therapy session (2 years)	Active reminiscence music therapy (familiar and seasonal songs with piano accompaniment, use of percussion instruments in a concert); A	Physiological and cognitive evaluation	Homeostatic effect in blood pressure regulation and maintenance of physical and mental states
Raglio *et al.*, 2010 [41]	RCT	20	Moderate-severe dementia	30	Improvisational Music therapy; B	Physiological (heart rate, heart rate variability) and psychological evaluation	Significant reduction of depression and improvement of PNN50 in music therapy group

* RCT= Randomized Controlled Trial; CCT= Clinical Controlled Trial.
** A= theoretical and methodological criteria of music therapeutic referential model not quoted.
B= theoretical and methodological criteria of music therapeutic referential model are present.

DISCUSSIONS

The present study aims principally at drawing attention to the contents of interventions defined as 'music therapeutic'. Therefore, our considerations do not so much concern the methodological aspects of research as, rather, the typology of the interventions proposed, and their relevance for those approaches that place *relationship* at the centre of their interest. The studies we have analysed demonstrate how the term 'music therapy' is often employed in the absence either of a therapeutic setting or of the related contents and finalities. Generic musical activities are often proposed for brief periods and in the absence of any therapeutic structure whatsoever. Moreover, no reference is made to conceptual frameworks, and omissions abound both with reference to the applicative techniques employed and to grounding criteria for the therapeutic process assessment measures. The above is especially evident in the quoted reviews and consequently in the studies they describe. The work by Svansdottir *et al.* [29] and the three Italian studies [32, 34, 35] display much greater detail. The two latter in particular aim to better define the music therapeutic approach and address the problem of context-bound assessments, by outlining a possible testing instrument: the results obtained in the music therapeutic relationship are, in fact, compared with external outcomes of treatment. The congruence of such results corroborates in our opinion the effectiveness of music therapeutic interventions. We believe that the idea of introducing biological indicators as confirming evidence of treatment effectiveness [38-41] might be seen as a crucial supporter both of the scientific value of these procedures, and of their non-invasiveness – which vouches for their employment. Generally speaking, the numerical limitation of samples, as well as their scant clinical definition, the short duration of treatments, the frequent absence of theoretical models and of explicit, codified assessment criteria are issues that remain unsolved – or only partially addressed. A much clearer documentation of the evidence, within a more rigorous methodological design is required in future studies on music therapy.

This paper presents the recent studies that have been considered the most significant and rigorous with respect to research methodology. Special attention has also been devoted to those studies that propose activities with an, at least partial, therapeutic connotation. The limitations are evident in this context. We therefore believe it necessary for music therapy to make a greater effort at defining its applicative models (conceptual frames of reference, techniques and assessment criteria for music therapy interventions) aimed at producing and incrementing "Evidence Based Practice" [11, 12, 42]. It also appears evident that corrections still need to be made concerning methodological design of research, *e.g.* the limitations both in sample magnitude and clinical definition, along with limited duration of interventions and absence of standardized, validated measures for the assessment of the therapeutic process. The number of randomized, controlled studies is still insufficient: it is the increase and improvement of such designs that might lead to an "evidence based music therapy" whilst at the same time attributing greater significance and scientific dignity to the therapeutic function of music therapy. We also believe that when assessing intervention outcomes, additional strategies should be developed allowing to perceive in a more adequate and subtle way any changes occurring in the relational and emotional/affective domains – also *via* observational techniques possibly structured outside the actual music therapy setting. The instrument/process that immediately comes to mind is Tom Kitwood's Dementia Care Mapping method (DCM) [43, 44]. DCM is a validated observational instrument with high inter-rater and test-retest reliability. During a six-hour period a DCM mapper keeps track of 26 activities or states in which 5-8 residents engage (Behavior Category Coding - BCC) in the communal area of a residential facility, as well as the (positive or negative) level of mood and engagement (ME) which accompanies them. The latter is rated on a six-level Likert scale (+5, +3, +1, -1, -3, -5) indicating that the person is experiencing emotions which range from the extreme well-being scored as +5 (through self-expression, highly satisfactory engagement and social interaction) to the opposite extreme of apathy, withdrawal, anxiety, grief or despair, scored as –5.

We are planning to employ DCM in a randomized, controlled study, video-recording the reactions of the subjects during and after music therapy sessions. We believe that such a type of study may add strength to what has been advocated in this paper, *i.e.* the necessity for well-organized music therapy programs according to evidence-based-practice criteria.

One final consideration concerns the use of biological evaluations as effectiveness indicators. Since they can be obtained through absolutely non-invasive methods and are compatible with a music therapy context, they can easily be employed in addition to more traditional assessments also for persons with dementia. The elements of objectivity and measurability they bring to the detection of change, enhance the extremely important potential they can contribute to enforcing the conceptual background of the present study.

To conclude as we began: in drawing attention to the authentic meaning of the word "music therapy", we wish to find the correct answer to the following question: is the term related to the application of musical techniques in a pathological context, or should it be specifically referred to the presence of those elements that therapeutically characterize the intervention (see the section "Comparisons between music and music therapy in dementia" in this paper)?

If we start off from the distinction between music and music therapy, we shall find it easier to set up randomized placebo-controlled trials where comparisons might be established between the experimental group, exposed to proper music therapeutic interventions, *vs.* a control group performing generic musical activities. This is the type of methodological design most suitable for enforcing the concept of the potential specificity of music therapy and its related evidence-based effectiveness.

We trust that these considerations might become a stimulus for future studies, with the finality of proving the curative potentialities and beneficial effects of music therapy, through the empirical quantification and clinical documentation of the evidence.

ACKNOWLEDGEMENT

Declared none.

CONFLICT OF INTEREST

The authors confirm that this chapter content has no conflict of interest.

DISCLOSURE

This chapter is an update of our previous publication in CAR "Music Therapy for Individuals with Dementia: Areas of Interventions and Research Perspectives" published in 'CAR', Volume 6, Number 3, June, pp. 293 to 301.

REFERENCES

[1] Raglio A, Bellelli G, Mazzola P, Bellandi D, Giovagnoli AR, Farina E, Stramba-Badiale M, Gentile S, Gianelli MV, Ubezio MC, Zanetti O and Trabucchi M. 'Music, music

therapy and dementia: a review of literature and the recommendations of the Italian Psychogeriatric Association'. Maturitas 72: 305-310 (2012).

[2] Gerdner LA. 'Effects of individualized *vs.* classical "relaxation" music on the frequency of agitation in elderly persons with Alzheimer's disease and related disorders'. Int Psychogeriatr.12 (1): 49-65 (2000).

[3] Sung HC, Chang AM, Lee WL. 'A preferred music listening intervention to reduce anxiety in older adults with dementia in nursing homes'. J Clin Nurs. 19:1056-64 (2010).

[4] Raglio A, Bellandi D, Baiardi P, Gianotti M, Ubezio MC and Granieri E. 'Listening to music and active music therapy in behavioral disturbances in dementia: a crossover study'. J Am Geriatr Soc, 61(4):645-647 (2013).

[5] Schön D, Akiva-Kabiri L and Vecchi T. In: 'Psicologia della Musica'. Carocci, Roma (2007).

[6] Nordoff P and Robbins C. In: 'Creative Music Therapy'. Harper and Row, New York (1977).

[7] Madsen CK, Cotter V and Madsen CH. 'A Behavioral Approach to Music Therapy'. J Music Ther. 15 (2): 69-71 (1968).

[8] Bonny H. 'Sound and Symbol: Guided Imagery and Music in Clinical Practice'. Music Therapy Perspectives. 6: 7-11 (1989).

[9] Priestley M. In: 'Essays on Analytical Music Therapy'. Barcelona Publishers, Phoenixville (2004).

[10] Benenzon RO. In: 'Manual de Musicoterapia'. Editorial Paidos Iberica, Barcelona (1981).

[11] Mace C, Moorey S and Roberts B. In: 'Evidence in the psychological therapies: a critical guide for practitioners.' Brunner-Routledge, New York (2001).

[12] Vink AC and Bruinsma M. 'Evidence Based Music Therapy'. Music Therapy Today (online, http://musictherapyworld.net) 4:5 (2003).

[13] Raglio A and Villani D. 'Musicoterapia e Demenze: Teoria, Applicazione e Ricerca'. G Gerontol. 53 (5): 528-532 (2005).

[14] Raglio A, Manarolo G and Villani D. In: 'Musicoterapia e Malattia di Alzheimer: proposte applicative e ipotesi di ricerca'. Cosmopolis, Torino, 2001.

[15] Benenzon RO. In: 'La Nuova Musicoterapia'. Phoenix, Roma (1997).

[16] Alridge D. 'Alzheimer's disease: rhythm, timing and music as therapy'. Biomed Pharmacother. 48 (7): 275-281 (1994).

[17] Stern D. In: 'The Interpersonal World of the Infant'. Basic Books, New York (1985).

[18] Stern D. In: 'The Present Moment in Psychotherapy and Everyday Life'. Norton & Company Ltd, London (2004).

[19] Fogel A. In: 'Developing through relationships: origins of communication, self and culture'. University of Chicago Press, Chicago (1993).

[20] Tronick EZ. 'Interventions that effect change in psychotherapy: a model based on infant research'. Infant Ment Health J. 19 (3): 277-279 (1998).

[21] Koger SM and Brotons M. 'Music therapy for dementia symptoms'. Cochrane Database Syst Rev. [database online] (2-3):CD001121 (2000).

[22] Vink AC, Birks JS, Bruinsma MS and Scholten RJS. 'Music Therapy for people with Dementia'. Cochrane Database Syst Rev. [database online] 4: CD003477 (2004).

[23] Clark ME, Lipe AW and Bilbrey M. 'Use of music to decrease aggressive behaviors in people with dementia'. J Gerontol Nurs. 24 (7):10-17 (1998).

[24] Groene RW. 'Effectiveness of music therapy 1:1 intervention with individuals having senile Dementia of the Alzheimer's type'. J Music Ther. 30 (3): 138-157 (1993).

[25] Rosswurm MA, Zimmermann SL, Schwartz-Fulton J and Normann GA. 'Can we manage wandering behavior?'. J Long Term Care Adm. 14 (3): 5-8 (1986).

[26] Scruggs SD. 'The effects of structured music activities *vs.* contingent music listening with verbal prompt on Wandering behavior and cognition in geriatric patients with Alzheimer's disease'. The Florida State University. Unpublished Master's Thesis (1991).

[27] Brotons M and Koger SM. 'The impact of Music Therapy on language functioning in Dementia'. J Music Ther. 37 (3): 183-95 (2000).

[28] Lord TR and Garner JE. 'Effects of music on Alzheimer patients'. Percept Mot Skills. 76 (2): 451-455 (1993).

[29] Svansdottir HB and Snaedal J. 'Music therapy in moderate and severe dementia of Alzheimer's type: a case-control study'. Int Psychogeriatr. 18 (4): 613-21 (2006).

[30] Sung HC, Chang SM, Lee WL and Lee MS. 'The effects of group music with movement intervention on agitated behaviours of institutionalized elders with dementia in Taiwan'.Complement Ther Med. 14:113-9 (2006).

[31] Guetin S, Portet F, Picot MC, Pommié C, Messaoudi M, Djabelkir L, Olsen AL, Cano MM, Lecourt E and Touchon J. 'Effect of music therapy on anxiety and depression in patients with Alzheimer's type dementia: randomised, controlled study'. Dement Geriatr Cogn Disord 28:36-46 (2009).

[32] Raglio A, Ubezio MC, Puerari F, Gianotti M, Bellelli G, Trabucchi M and Villani D. 'L'efficacia del trattamento musicoterapico in pazienti con demenza di grado moderato-severo'. G Gerontol. 54: 164-169 (2006).

[33] Raglio A and Oasi O. 'La musicoterapia in una prospettiva intersoggettiva'. Quaderni di Gestalt. XXIII/42-43: 9-20 (2009).

[34] Raglio A, Bellelli G, Traficante D, Gianotti M, Ubezio MC, Villani D and Trabucchi M. 'Efficacy of music therapy in the treatment of behavioral and psychiatric symptoms of dementia'. Alzheimer Dis Assoc Disord. 22 (2): 158-162 (2008).

[35] Raglio A, Bellelli G, Traficante D, Gianotti M, Ubezio MC, Gentile S, Villani D and Trabucchi M. 'Efficacy of music therapy treatment based on cycles of sessions: a randomised controlled trial'. Aging Ment Health. 14:900-904 (2010).

[36] Kubota N and Hasegawa Y. 'Change in NK cell activity in the elderly through music therapy'. The Journal of Japan Biomusic Association. 17 (2): 183-187 (1999).

[37] Kumar AM, Tims F, Cruess DC, Mintzer MJ, Ironson G, Loewenstein D, Cattan R, Fernandez JB, Eisdorfer C and Kumar M. 'Music Therapy increases serum melatonin levels in patients with Alzeheimer's disease'. Alternative Therapeutic Health Medicine. 5 (6): 49-57 (1999).

[38] Suzuki M, Kanamori M, Watanabe M, Nagasawa S, Kojima E and Ooshiro H. 'Behavioral and endocrinological evaluation of music therapy for elderly patients with dementia'. Nurs Health Sci. 6 (1): 11-18 (2004).

[39] Suzuki M, Kanamori M, Nagasawa S and Saruhara T. 'Behavioral, stress and immunological evaluation methods of music therapy in elderly patients with senile dementia'. Nippon Ronen Igakkai Zasshi. 42(1):74-82 (2005).

[40] Takahashi T and Matsushita H. 'Long- Term Effect of Music Therapy on Elderly with Moderate/Severe Dementia'. J Music Ther. 43 (4): 317-333 (2006).

[41] Raglio A, Oasi O, Gianotti M, Manzoni V, Bolis S, Ubezio MC, Gentile S, Villani D and Stramba-Badiale M. 'Effects of Music Therapy on Psychological Symptoms and Heart Rate Variability in Patients with Dementia. A Pilot Study'. Curr Aging Sci. 3:242-246 (2010).

[42] Raglio A. In: 'Musicoterapia e scientificità: dalla clinica alla ricerca'. Franco Angeli, Milano, 2008.

[43] Kitwood T. In: 'Dementia Reconsidered: The Person Comes First'. Open University Press-McGraw Hill, Berkshire, 1997.

[44] Brooker D and Surr C. In: 'Dementia Care Mapping - DCM 8: Principles and Practice'. Bradford Dementia Group, University of Bradford Division of Dementia Studies, Bradford, 2005.

CHAPTER 10

Natural Non-Transgenic Animal Models for Research in Alzheimer's Disease

Manuel Sarasa* **and Pedro Pesini**

Araclon Biotech S.L., 50009 Zaragoza, Spain

Abstract: The most common animal models currently used for Alzheimer disease (AD) research are transgenic mice that express a mutant form of human Aβ precursor protein (APP) and/or some of the enzymes implicated in their metabolic processing. However, these transgenic mice carry their own APP and APP-processing enzymes, which may interfere in the production of different amyloid-beta (Aβ) peptides encoded by the human transgenes. Additionally, the genetic backgrounds of the different transgenic mice are a possible confounding factor with regard to crucial aspects of AD that they may (or may not) reproduce. Thus, although the usefulness of transgenic mice is undisputed, we hypothesized that additional relevant information on the physiopathology of AD could be obtained from other natural non-transgenic models. We have analyzed the chick embryo and the dog, which may be better experimental models because their enzymatic machinery for processing APP is almost identical to that of humans. The chick embryo is extremely easy to access and manipulate. It could be an advantageous natural model in which to study the cell biology and developmental function of APP and a potential assay system for drugs that regulate APP processing. The dog suffers from an age-related syndrome of cognitive dysfunction that naturally reproduces key aspects of AD including Aβ cortical pathology, neuronal degeneration and learning and memory disabilities. However, dense core neuritic plaques and neurofibrillary tangles have not been consistently demonstrated in the dog. Thus, these species may be natural models with which to study the biology of AD, and could also serve as assay systems for Aβ-targeted drugs or new therapeutic strategies against this devastating disease.

Keywords: Aβ, APP, Chick embryo, dog, dolphin, rabbit, rat.

INTRODUCTION

The ethics of scientific research obliges to reduce the use of laboratory animals to the minimum possible. Nevertheless, studies in animal models are still necessary

***Corresponding author Manuel Sarasa:** Araclon Biotech S.L., 50009 Zaragoza, Spain; Tel: 34 876 241 666; Fax: 34 976 020 011; E-mail: msarasa@araclon.com

D.K. Lahiri (Ed)

to understand the mechanisms of many human diseases and to try new therapeutic strategies. In any case, experiments with animals must always be approved by ethical committees and to enforce general and local normatives (see for example European and Spanish legislations on animal handling 86/609/EU and Real Decreto 1201/2005, respectively).

Rodents in general, and the rat and the mouse in particular, are the animals most frequently used as experimental model organisms for a great variety of human diseases. The short reproductive cycle of these small mammals (21 days of gestation), their high birth rate, and their small size make them relatively easy to maintain and manage. Recent developments in genetic engineering and biotechnology have led to the production of a diverse selection of transgenic animals, mainly mice. These transgenic animals (bearing an exogenous gene, usually from human origin), together with other agenics or knockouts (in which a particular gene has been blocked or eliminated) have been very useful in studying the presumptive roles and mechanisms involving the proteins coded by the transgene or the knockout gene of interest. Translational research has brought these technologies to the field of clinical investigation with the production of inbred animal lines that serve as models for human diseases. Numerous knockout and transgenic animal models have been developed to explore particular aspects of Alzheimer's disease.

Suppression of genes that encode proteins involved in Alzheimer's, such as APP, apolipoprotein E (ApoE), β-secretase, or presenilins, has helped us to anticipate the effects of presumptive new molecules designed to regulate these proteins. For example, presenilin knockout mice develop striking neurodegeneration of the cerebral cortex and worsening impairments of memory and synaptic function with increasing age, which call for caution in the therapeutic use of γ-secretase inhibitors [1]. In contrast, β-secretase knockout mice are perfectly viable [2]. The absence of lethal phenotypes for β-secretase knockouts, which cannot generate Aβ peptide, feeds the hope of success for therapeutic strategies based on the use of β-secretase inhibitors or aimed directly at the blockade or elimination of Aβ peptide. Nevertheless, APP knockout mice present overt neurological deficiencies which can be reverted if the endogenous APP locus is replaced by a gene-targeted allele (knock-in mice) that exclusively express the secreted APP ectodomain [3, 4]. In addition, functional redundancy between APP and other APP-like proteins has been reported [5]. The development of transgenic mice lines with mutated human APP genes has been particularly enlightening, since these animals develop Aβ deposits in their brains and reproduce some of the neurological symptoms of AD (for a recent review see supplementary reference SR [1]). However, most of these species lack essential features of AD despite the increasingly complex genotypes that are being engineered to approach a more complete disease phenotype [6-14]. The heterogeneity of different transgenics should be considered a possible confounding factor that seeds doubts when observations made in humans must be interpreted in the light of results obtained in these models. Uncertainty is also unavoidable when the efficacy of new AD therapies must be forecasted from trials in transgenic mice.

Thus, although the usefulness of transgenic mice is undisputed, we hypothesized that additional relevant information regarding the pathological mechanisms of AD could be obtained from natural non-transgenic models. In line with this, it has been recently reported that studying the effects of environmental enrichment in wild-type mice exposed to human Aβ oligomers can better model the early developmentof Aβ-mediated neurotoxicity in the majority of humans without a deterministic genetic predisposition to AD SR [2]. In the following pages we will refer to some of the results obtained in our laboratory that led us to propose new wild type animal models for the analysis of relevant aspects of AD. We have designed and produced highly specific and sensitive antibodies against the two major isoforms of the Aβ amyloid to aid in this research, and are currently exploring the use of these Aβ immunogens in the search for premorbid biomarkers and immunotherapeutic strategies.

THE RAT

The rat is the most frequently utilized experimental animal in neuroscience, although with regard to AD the use of transgenic mice has been increasing. Nevertheless, an enormous amount of work has been produced in the rat, and important advances in the understanding of APP processing- including the studies central to the discovery of neprilysin [15] and insulin degrading enzyme (IDE) [16] as the main proteases implicated in Aβ degradation- have been obtained from experiments conducted in rats. The rat has also been used to study the effects of induced cortical Aβ accumulation on the cholinergic, noradrenergic, and serotonergic systems [17], as well as the influence of diet and age on the effects of intracerebral beta-amyloid injection [18]. However, it should be emphasized that the primary structures of the Aβ peptide in rats (and mice) differ from their human counterpart at three amino acid residues, and that the complete Aβ-peptide profile produced by the processing of APP in these rodents also reveals major differences compared to that of humans [19].

In our laboratory, the rat was chosen to study the kinetics of the expression of the different APP isoforms in response to axotomy [20]. We found increased levels of APP 695, 714, 751, and 770 mRNAs after facial or hypoglossal nerve axotomy of the parent ipsilateral motor neurons. The increase was gradual, reaching maximal values 7 days after axotomy, and returning to normal values by 60 days after the lesion. Increased APP immunostaining was also detected in the chromatolytic motor neurons, but not in the reactive astrocytes surrounding axotomized neurons. These results suggested a possible neuroprotective role for APP that could also be involved in a variety of cell processes that remain poorly understood [21-23]. In particular, APP has been implicated in neurotrophic, synaptogenic, and growth promoting mechanisms which led us to investigate the expression of this protein during the rat embryogenesis [24]. Using oligonucleotides recognizing each of the four major APP (APP-695, APP-714, APP-751, and APP-770) mRNAs, we found that each APP displays a specific temporal and spatial expression pattern. The prototype isoform APP-695 appears early in embryogenesis within cells actively implicated in morphogenetic events, such as the mesodermal cells that invaginate at the level of the primitive streak, and is later restricted to the neurectodermal derivatives (neural tube, neural crests, and neurogenic placodes). By contrast, expression of the longest isoform, APP-770, occurs later and is restricted to mesodermal and endodermal derivatives. The isoforms of 714 and 751 amino acids are expressed still later in the course of prenatal development, and appear to be distributed ubiquitously.

Another wild type rodent used for research in AD is the guinea pig [25]. Beta-amyloid peptide sequence expressed by guinea pigs is identical to the human sequence, and appears to represent a more physiological model with which to examine *in vivo* the long-term effects of experimental manipulations on APP processing. Additionally, APP processing in guinea pig primary neuronal cultures is demonstrably similar to analogous cultures of human origin [25]. However, the use of these animals is limited because they do not develop the pathological features of the disease (senile plaques and neurofibrillary tangles) and there are not well-established behavioral tests for this species.

THE RABBIT

As in guinea pigs, the rabbit Aβ peptide sequence is identical to human [26] and does not present AD pathology spontaneously. However, when copper is added to the diet of cholesterol-fed rabbits, they develop cortical amyloid deposits and up to twelve other pathological markers seen in AD, including retardation of the ability to learn a difficult task [27]. This finding suggests that copper (but apparently not other heavy metals like aluminum or zinc) may influence the progression of Alzheimer's disease by reducing clearance of Aβ from the brain [28, 29]. This finding also emphasized the usefulness of the rabbit model, whose validity is being extended even to treatment modalities [30-32].

THE CHICK EMBRYO

Our studies regarding the prenatal expression of different APPs in the rat embryo [24] were coincident in time with the publication of reports on the lack of substantial phenotypic differences in APP knockout mice [5]. This led us to explore the chick embryo as a possible model for the investigation of presumptive APP functions during prenatal development. The chick embryo is readily available and easy to work with, and our laboratory has extensive experience with this model. Before engaging in experiments on the functional blocking of APP, we first needed to know the sequence of the APP gene in the chicken. We isolated the total RNA from the chick embryo and cloned the cDNA [33]. We found two of the major APP isoforms, APP-751, which contains the KPI domain, and APP-695. The APP-770 isoform, which is the longest isoform and contains the OX-2 domain, was absent or minimally expressed. Interestingly, the chick and human gene sequences are almost identical, with 93% amino acid identity and 96% similarity. The KPI domain of APP-751 has 52 identical residues out of 56 (93%

identity), and three of the four different residues belong to the same group of amino acids (98% similarity). The 40–42 amino acid residues of the Aβ domain are identical, as are the last 101 C-terminal amino acids of the APP sequence (corresponding to the Aβ, transmembrane and intracytoplasmic domains). We also established through whole-mount *in situ* hybridization histochemistry and immunohistochemistry[1] that chicken APP expression parallels mammalian APP expression both temporally and topographically [32]. After the 3rd day of embryonic development, APP-695 mRNA expression levels were much higher than APP-751 expression levels in the neuroectodermal derivatives, including the neural tube; the sensory, autonomic and cranial ganglia; the retina; and the otic vesicle. Furthermore, the chick embryo expresses the genes that encode the main proteases implicated in the production of beta-amyloid protein, including BACE-1, BACE-2, presenilin-1, presenilin-2, and nicastrin; Aβ1-42 is the major Aβ peptide produced during chick embryogenesis [33]. Neprilysin, the main Aβ-degrading enzyme, and ADAM-17, a protease implicated in the non-amyloidogenic processing of APP, are also expressed in chick embryos. Thus, we propose the chick embryo as a suitable natural model in which to study the cell biology and developmental function of beta-amyloid precursor protein, and a potential assay system for drugs that regulate beta-amyloid precursor protein processing. But do chicks suffer any Alzheimer-like pathology? We have explored whether relatively aged chickens might develop brain amyloid pathology, and have obtained negative results. However, our access has been limited to the brains of chicken up to 10 years old; these individuals appear to be too young to develop amyloid deposits, since the chicken lifespan reaches approximately 30 years [34]. In fact, the brains of 10-year-old chickens do not appear to differ from the brains of chickens between 2 and 14 months old.

THE DOG

The dog has been pointed out as an especially appropriate model for the study of human brain aging and neurodegenerative diseases. The numerous domestic dog breeds exhibit greater diversity in body size than any other terrestrial vertebrate, and geneticists are taking advantage of this diversity to investigate the genetic basis of size and its relationship to lifespan [35-37]. Canines have evolved phylogenetically in close proximity to humans, making them unusually skilled at reading human social and communicative behavior- even more so than our nearest primate relatives [38, 39]. Provided that ethical normative is enforced, individuals of every age are available for study among the immense population of pet dogs. Canine neurology, including behavioral medicine, is state of the art among veterinary clinical sciences, and access to longitudinal records is already possible in many cases [40, 41]. Dogs are frequently used for the preclinical development of a wide variety of drugs (see for example [42, 43]). Regarding AD, almost every current treatment strategy has been tried out in the dog, from cholinergic agonists to antioxidant and mitochondrial enzymatic cofactors [44-49]. Increasing interest in this model is based on the fact that the dog may naturally develop an age-related cognitive dysfunction that reproduces several aspects of AD [47, 50-53]. Thus, numerous studies with dog cohorts that were submitted to several behavioral paradigms have revealed subsets of aged dogs that had learning and memory impairments [46, 54-57]. This cognitive damage correlated with the extent of Aβ deposits in the cerebral cortex [58-60]. Interestingly, a similar correlation has been reported in domestic pet dogs, based on cognitive status evaluated from questionnaires that were answered by their caregivers [61-63]. Furthermore, we have recently reported that the plasma levels of Aβ1-42 and the Aβ 42/40 ratio were significantly higher in aged dogs with mild cognitive impairment than in either aged matched cognitively unimpaired or severely affected dogs. These results suggest that increased plasma Aβ1-42 levels and Aβ42/40 ratio could be a biomarker for canine cognitive dysfunction, as has been suggested for AD SR [3]. Most of these tests for evaluation of the cognitive status assess four main behavioural categories: disorientation (on daily walks or at home), interaction with owners (lost of interest in greeting or playing; lost of response to incitation), sleep/awake cycle (wander and/or bark during night) and lost of the house training habits. Interestingly, we have found that the severity of cognitive dysfunction (but not age), as assessed by owner-based observational questionnaire, influenced the spontaneous activity in pet dogs. In particular, we found that the more severe the impairment, the higher the locomotor activity and frequency of corner-directed (aimless) behaviours, and the lower the frequency of door-aimed activities SR [4]. In addition, the severity of the cognitive dysfunction was also associated with a decreased response to social isolation and human interaction in these dogs SR [5]. Thus these results may serve as an indirect validation of our owner-based questionnaire for the diagnosis of canine cognitive dysfunction syndrome, although further research should be carried out to achieve a complete validation of these psychometric owner-based questionnaires. It has been reported that 28% of 11-12 year old dogs present impairments in one or more of these categories, of which 10% have impairments in two or more categories and are considered severely impaired. Among 15-16 year old dogs, 68% have impairment in one or more category, of which 35% have impairments in two or more categories [64, 65].

Histopathological studies on this putative canine model of AD showed that the earliest and more consistently affected areas were in the prefrontal cortex, including the gyrus proreus and the hippocampus [59, 66, 67]. Deposition of Aβ in the dog appears to progress from deep to superficial cortical layers, and from diffuse patches to denser and better-delimited plaques [68]. However, dense core neuritic plaques and neurofibrillary tangles have not been consistently demonstrated in the dog [69-72]. Aβ deposits do not appear in every aged dog, as might be expected if they were merely a consequence of normal aging (Fig. **1A-C**). Instead, as occurs in humans, exogenous and/or genetic factors may determine the susceptibility of individual dogs toward developing amyloid pathology at a given age [73, 74]. Nevertheless, in a recent study we have found Aβ angiopathy and a moderate to heavy Aβ burden in two aged dogs, although they have no apparent cognitive symptoms. This finding is reminiscent of similar reports of extensive Aβ deposits in human brains that had not been diagnosed with dementia (reviewed by [75]). It poses the possibility that, as occurs in AD, the development of neuropathological lesions may precede apparent clinical symptoms by a long period of time in the dog. The availability of biomarkers and more refined neuropsychological tests in veterinary clinics may enable the definition of a canine model for mild cognitive impairment in the near future.

We have recently found that the canine is also a suitable AD model from the molecular point of view, because APP and most of the enzymatic machinery for its processing bear extensive homology between dogs and humans SR [6]. In particular, the amino acid sequence of Aβ1-42 is identical in dogs and humans, whereas in rats

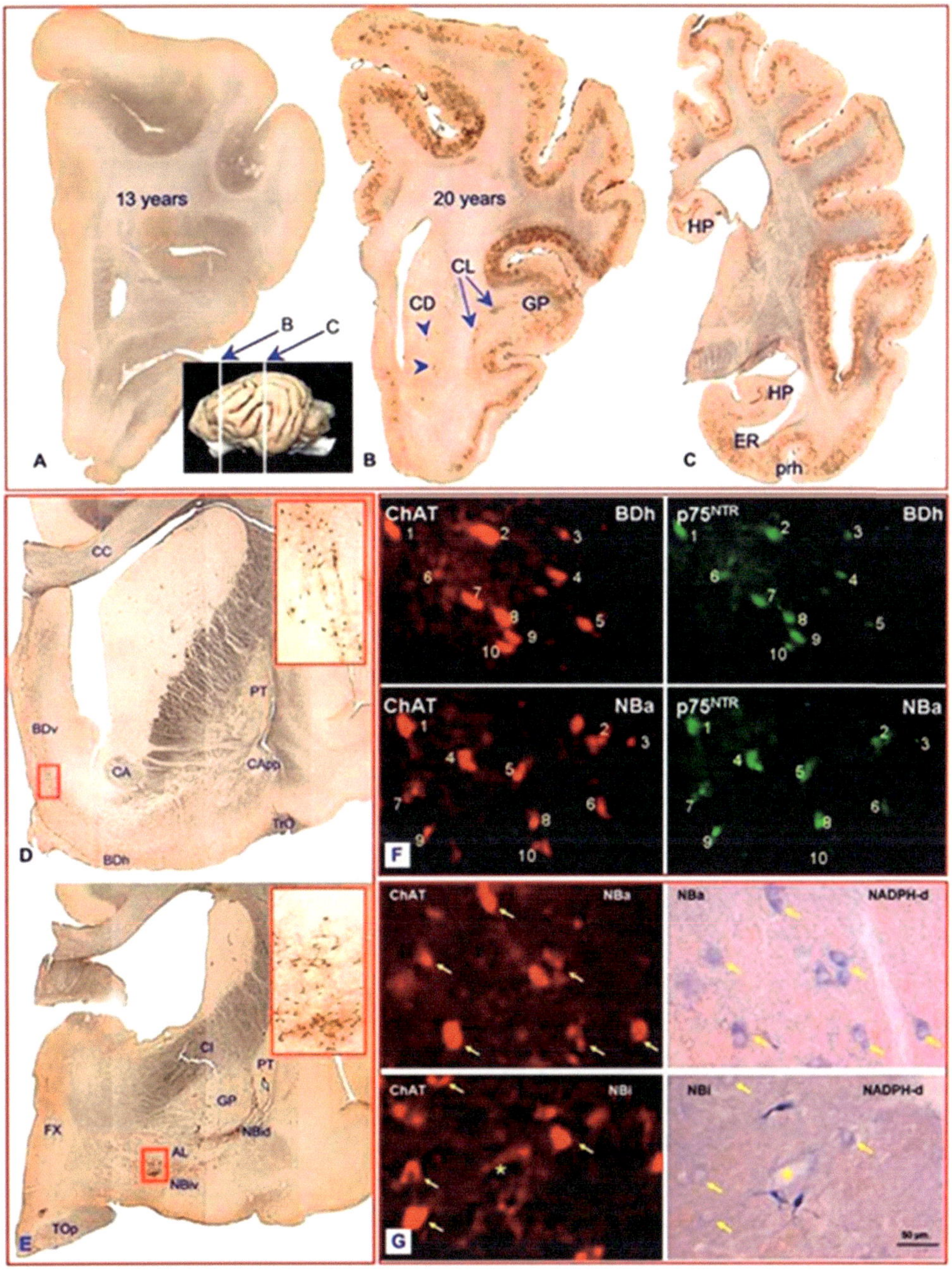

Fig. (1A-G). The canine model of Alzheimer's disease. (A-C) Cortical Aβ pathology in the dog. (A) Brain section from a 13 years old Pekinese dog without Aβ deposits and (B-C) from a 20 years old individual of the same breed with extensive Aβ deposits. The three sections were stained in the same batch with 6E10 monoclonal antibody (Signet Lab. Dedham, USA). The level of B and C section is marked over the lateral view of the brain (inset). The earliest and more consistently affected areas in the dog were the prefrontal cortex, including the gyrus proreus (GP), the entorhinal cortex (ER) and the hippocampus (HP). However in severe cases as the one shown here (B and C), amyloid deposits spread throughout the cortex and can be found also in the caudate (arrowheads) and the claustrum (CL). (D-E) the anatomical distribution of the neurons expressing the low affinity nerve growth factor receptor (p75NTR) in the basal forebrain of the dog. Section in D is at the level of the vertical and horizontal diagonal band (BDv and BDh, respectively); section in E is at the level of the dorsal and ventral subdivision of the intermediate part of nucleus basalis of Meynert (NBid and NBiv, respectively). Framed area in D and E are enlarged in the corresponding inset. (F) Double immunofluorescence staining showing that practically all magnocellular cholinergic neurons (red staining) in the basal forebrain co-express p75NTR (green staining). (G) Co-expression of choline acetyl transferase (ChAT, red immunofluorescence) and NADPH-D (blue staining, bright field illumination) in most (~80%) of the basal magnocellular neurons in the anterior and intermediate parts of the dog (NBa and NBi respectively; yellow arrows). These images were presented at the 17th ECVIM-CA congress and 9th ESVCP congress. Budapest, September 2007. (Suárez M-L, Insua D, Corredoira A, Bernedo V, Santamarina G, and Pesini P. The basal forebrain cholinergic neurons in aged dogs with and without cortical amyloid pathology).

and mice it differs from the human sequence by three amino acids [26]. Moreover, the pattern of expression of these proteins in the dog is congruent with data previously reported in human beings SR [6]. Furthermore, the profile of the various shorter Aβ peptides found by mass spectrometry in the canine LCR is almost identical to that found in humans, and both present substantial differences when compared to rats and mice [19] SR [7]. Thus, the study of both APP and Aβ peptide processing in the dog could help us to understand their biological function and relevance to AD, contributing results more reliably translatable to humans than those obtained using transgenic mice. The dog has also been used in immunotherapeutic assays against fibrillar Aβ, and to confirm observational data in humans that combining an antioxidant-enriched diet and behavioral enrichment (including social, physical, and cognitive components) can lead to substantial improvements in cognition and reduced brain pathology [47, 76].

However, a pitfall for a more extended use of the dog is the dearth of neuroanatomical data regarding the organization, normal aging process, and response to pathological aging of the main neurotransmitter systems implicated in AD. We have begun to study this issue and have made a number of relevant findings. The cytoarchitectural characteristics of the basal forebrain cholinergic neurons in the dog are similar to those of humans, as are several relevant phenotypic characteristics of these neurons, including their expression of NOS, calbindin D-28K, and $p75^{NTR}$ nerve growth factor receptor (Fig. **1D-G**) [77]. As has been found in AD brains, the number of A6-A7 noradrenergic neurons in the dog shows a negative correlation with the extension of cortical Aβ deposits as measured in the gyrus proreus [78]. Recently, we have extended these studies to show that, as occurred in AD, both serotonergic and cholinergic systems are affected in aged dogs suffering cognitive dysfunction syndrome. In particular, we found that cognitively-impairedaged dogs showed an approximately 20% decrement (p = 0.009) in p75NTR positive neurons (considered a marker for basal forebrain cholinergic neurons) compared to both the young and the aged cognitively-unimpaired animals SR [8]. Furthermore, aged dogs with Aβ cortical pathology had 33% fewer serotonergic neurons in the dorsal and median raphe nucleithan than aged dogs without Aβ cortical deposits (108,043 +/- 18,800 *vs.* 162,242 +/- 39,942, respectively; P = 0.01). In contrast, no significant variations were found between young and aged dogs without Aβ cortical deposits SR [9].

The investigation of brain aging in the dog also deserves attention from a veterinary point of view. As in the case of human medical technologies, improvements in veterinary medicine and husbandry have contributed to lengthening the lifespan of our domestic animals, with the unwanted side effect of a greater incidence of age-related neurodegenerative diseases [44]. The modern society requires more attention to the welfare of pet animals, increasingly considered as actual "family members", and there is a growing demand for attention and treatment of these pet dogs' age related diseases.

PRIMATES AND DOLPHINS

Primates, like dogs, are among the few animal species demonstrating age-dependent brain pathologies resembling AD [79-82]. An important advantage of several primate models, but not all [80], is that they show AD-like tau-pathology accounting for a more complete disease model. More over, some of these species have relatively short life span as for example the mouse lemur (*Microcebus murinus*) which is considered to be elderly over 5 years of age. Interestingly, among elderly mouse lemurs approximately 20% develop massive brain atrophy, abundant amyloid plaques, cytoskeletal tau pathology and loss of cholinergic neurons [83]. Furthermore, recently it has been documented the first case of tauopathy with paired helical filaments, ultrastructurally indistinguishable from those seen in Alzheimer's disease, in an aged chimpanzee (Pan troglodytes) [84]. Pathologic forms of tau were histologically identified in neuronal somata, neuropil threads, and plaque-like clusters of neurites throughout the neocortex of this animal. Nevertheless, accumulation of the abnormally phosphorylated tau protein in the brains of animals has been less study than the formation of Aβ deposits. Age-related neurofibrillary changes were described in sheep and goat in the absence of Aβ [85-87] and in wolverine (*Gulo gulo*) [88], polar bear [89] and dog [72] in the presence of Aβ. Thus, non-primate species develop age-related cytoskeletal abnormalities similar to those occurring in humans. However to define an operative model from these species is hampered by which appear to be species specific variations in the process of phosphorylation and cleavage of tau protein. This, together with their phylogenetic proximity to humans, would make primates ideal experimental models (for example, leading studies in immunotherapy are currently being carried out in these species) [90, 91]. However, their use is extremely limited for most laboratories because of high price, restricted availability, maintenance requirements, and ethical considerations.

Other animals that may suffer brain pathology resembling AD are cetaceans. Some cetacean species like dolphins have extended life spans, could be accessible in determined circumstances, and might be useful models to analyze some aspects of the disease. We recently hypothesized that the coastal beaching of these animals could be related to cognitive impairments of the aged individuals (occasionally followed by herds of younger specimens) that might present with Aβ deposits or other AD like neuropathological features. In tissue samples from stranded dolphins, we have found extensive Congo red positive Aβ-immunolabeled deposits throughout the brain, including the cerebellum and the medulla oblongata [2] where such deposits have only been reported in the more severe AD cases . In addition, we have found high amino acidic homology between the APP, BACE, presenilin-1, and presenilin-2 in various dolphin species and their corresponding human counterpart (GenBank entries: AY926583, AY926588, AY926589, AY926584, AY926586 and AY926585); in particular, the Aβ1-42 peptide in the three dolphin species that have been studied so far (*Grampus griseus, Stenella coeruleoalba* and *Tursiops truncatus*) was 100% identical to the human peptide.

CONCLUDING REMARKS

There are a variety of species that can serve as experimental models for AD research. In addition to numerous transgenic mouse lines, which have proven to be powerful tools to aid in understanding various aspects of the disease, there are other species that can serve as 'natural' wild-type models to shed light on different psychopathological mechanisms or even to try new therapeutic strategies. Among these natural models we emphasize the chick embryo to assay molecules that act on APP metabolism, and the canine model specifically to study the first phase of the disease and to test new therapies. Dogs have a relatively long lifespan (12-20 years depending on the breed), share our environment, and their behavior and clinical state are easier to explore than those of other species. Furthermore, canine APP is identical (98%) to the human counterpart, and dogs are the most accessible among the few animal species demonstrating age-dependent brain pathology and clinical correlates resembling AD.

ACKNOWLEDGEMENTS

The works included in this review have been financed by the Spanish Ministerio de Ciencia y Tecnología and FEDER (project #. SAF2003-08444; SAF2003-08444-C02-02; SAF 2006-13332), by the Xunta de Galicia (project # PGIDIT04PXIC26105PN), by the Diputación General de Aragón (project # PM040) and FIS (PI04/0620).

CONFLICT OF INTEREST

The authors declare no actual or potential conflicts of interest. Araclon Biotech S.L. is a start-up biotechnology company aiming to develop biomarkers and therapeutics for Alzheimer's disease and other disorders. Manuel Sarasa is the scientific founder and program director for Araclon Biotech S.L., and he owns shares in the company. Pedro Pesini is head of laboratory in Araclon Biotech S.L.

DISCLOSURE

This chapter is an update of our previous publication in CAR "Natural Non-Trasgenic Animal Models for Research in Alzheimer's Disease" published in ''CAR', Volume 6, Number 2, April, 2009, pp. 171 to 178.

REFERENCES

[1] Saura CA, Choi SY, Beglopoulos V, Malkani S, Zhang D, ShankaranarayanaRao BS, *et al.* Loss of presenilin function causes impairments of memory and synaptic plasticity followed by agedependent neurodegeneration. Neuron 42: 23-36 (2004).

[2] Luo Y, Bolon B, Kahn S, Bennett BD, Babu-Khan S, Denis P, *et al.* Mice deficient in BACE1, the Alzheimer's beta-secretase, have normal phenotype and abolished beta-amyloid generation. Nat Neurosci 4: 231-2 (2001).

[3] Muller U, Cristina N, Li ZW, Wolfer DP, Lipp HP, Rulicke T, *et al.* Behavioral and anatomical deficits in mice homozygous for a modified beta-amyloid precursor protein gene. Cell 79: 755-65 (1994).

[4] Ring S, Weyer SW, Kilian SB, Waldron E, Pietrzik CU, Filippov MA, *et al.* The secreted beta-amyloid precursor protein ectodomain APPs alpha is sufficient to rescue the anatomical, behavioral, and electrophysiological abnormalities of APP-deficient mice. J Neurosci 27: 7817-26 (2007).

[5] Heber S, Herms J, Gajic V, Hainfellner J, Aguzzi A, Rulicke T, *et al.* Mice with combined gene knock-outs reveal essential and partially redundant functions of amyloid precursor protein family members. J Neurosci 20: 7951-63 (2000).

[6] Gómez-Isla T and Irizarry MC. Alzheimer's disease and transgenic mouse models. In: Handbook of neuropsychology (Boller F, Kappa S. Eds). Elsevier, Amsterdam, pp. 23-37 (2001).

[7] Mudher A and Lovestone S. Alzheimer's disease-do tauists and baptists finally shake hands? Trends Neurosci 25: 22-6 (2002).

[8] Price DL and Sisodia SS. Mutant genes in familial Alzheimer's disease and transgenic models. Annu Rev Neurosci 21: 479-505 (1998).

[9] Lannfelt L, Folkesson R, Mohammed AH, Winblad B, Hellgren D, Duff K, *et al.* Alzheimer's disease: molecular genetics and transgenic animal models. Behav Brain Res 57: 207-13 (1993).

[10] Price DL and Sisodia SS. Cellular and molecular biology of Alzheimer's disease and animal models.Annu Rev Med 45: 435-46 (1994).

[11] Bayer TA and Wirths O. Review on the APP/PS1KI mouse model: intraneuronalAbeta accumulation triggers axonopathy, neuron loss and working memory impairment. Genes Brain Behav 7 (Suppl 1): 6-11 (2008).

[12] Higgins GA and Jacobsen H. Transgenic mouse models of Alzheimer's disease: phenotype and application. BehavPharmacol 14: 419-38 (2003).

[13] Dodart JC, Mathis C, Bales KR and Paul SM. Does my mouse have Alzheimer's disease? Genes Brain Behav 1: 142-55 (2002).

[14] vanDooren T, Dewachter I, Borghgraef P and van Leuven F. Transgenic mouse models for APP processing and Alzheimer's disease: early and late defects. SubcellBiochem 38: 45-63 (2005).

[15] Iwata N, Tsubuki S, Takaki Y, Watanabe K, Sekiguchi M, Hosoki E, *et al.* Identification of the major Abeta1-42-degrading catabolic pathway in brain parenchyma: suppression leads to biochemical and pathological deposition. Nat Med 6: 143-50 (2000).

[16] Vekrellis K, Ye Z, Qiu WQ, Walsh D, Hartley D, Chesneau V, *et al.* Neurons regulate extracellular levels of amyloid beta-protein *via* proteolysis by insulin-degrading enzyme. J Neurosci 20: 1657-65 (2000).

[17] Gonzalo-Ruiz A, Gonzalez I and Sanz-Anquela JM. Effects of beta-amyloid protein on serotoninergic, noradrenergic, and cholinergic markers in neurons of the pontomesencephalictegmentum in the rat. J ChemNeuroanat 26: 153-69 (2003).
[18] Gonzalo-Ruiz A, Sanz JM, Arevalo J, Geula C and Gonzalo P. Amyloid beta peptide-induced cholinergic fibres loss in the cerebral cortex of the rat is modified by diet high in lipids and by age. J ChemNeuroanat 29: 31-48 (2005).
[19] Du P, Wood KM, Rosner MH, Cunningham D, Tate B and Geoghegan KF. Dominance of amyloid precursor protein sequence over host cell secretases in determining beta-amyloid profiles studies of interspecies variation and drug action by internally standardized immunoprecipitation/mass spectrometry. J PharmacolExpTher 320: 1144-52 (2007).
[20] Sola C, Garcia-Ladona FJ, Sarasa M, Mengod G, Probst A, Palacios G, *et al.*Beta APP gene expression is increased in the rat brain after motor neuron axotomy. Eur J Neurosci 5: 795-808 (1993).
[21] Wang P, Yang G, Mosier DR, Chang P, Zaidi T, Gong YD, *et al.* Defective neuromuscular synapses in mice lacking amyloid precursor protein (APP) and APP-Like protein 2. J Neurosci 25: 1219-25 (2005).
[22] Anliker B and Muller U. The functions of mammalian amyloid precursor protein and related amyloid precursor-like proteins. Neurodegener Dis 3: 239-46 (2006).
[23] Koo EH. The beta-amyloid precursor protein (APP) and Alzheimer's disease: does the tail wag the dog? Traffic 3: 763-70 (2002).
[24] Sarasa M, Sorribas V, Terradoal J, Climent S, Palacios JM and Mengod G. Alzheimer beta-amyloid precursor proteins display specific patterns of expression during embryogenesis. Mech Dev 94: 233-6 (2000).
[25] Beck M, Bigl V and Rossner S. Guinea pigs as a nontransgenic model for APP processing *in vitro* and *in vivo*. Neurochem Res 28: 637-44 (2003).
[26] Johnstone EM, Chaney MO, Norris FH, Pascual R and Little SP. Conservation of the sequence of the Alzheimer's disease amyloid peptide in dog, polar bear and five other mammals by cross-species polymerase chain reaction analysis. Brain Res Mol Brain Res 10: 299-305 (1991).
[27] Sparks DL and Schreurs BG. Trace amounts of copper in water induce beta-amyloid plaques and learning deficits in a rabbit model of Alzheimer's disease. Proc NatlAcadSci USA 100: 11065-9 (2003).
[28] Sparks DL. Cholesterol metabolism and brain amyloidosis: evidence for a role of copper in the clearance of Abeta through the liver. Curr Alzheimer Res 4: 165-9 (2007).
[29] Sparks DL, Friedland R, Petanceska S, Schreurs BG, Shi J, Perry G, *et al.* Trace copper levels in the drinking water, but not zinc or aluminum influence CNS Alzheimer-like pathology. J Nutr Health Aging 10: 247-54 (2006).
[30] Ghribi O, Golovko MY, Larsen B, Schrag M and Murphy EJ. Deposition of iron and beta-amyloid plaques is associated with cortical cellular damage in rabbits fed with long-term cholesterolenriched diets. J Neurochem 99: 438-49 (2006).
[31] Ghribi O, Larsen B, Schrag M and Herman MM. High cholesterol content in neurons increases BACE, beta-amyloid, and phosphorylated tau levels in rabbit hippocampus. Exp Neurol 200: 460-7 (2006).
[32] Woodruff-Pak DS, Agelan A and Del Valle L. A rabbit model of Alzheimer's disease: valid at neuropathological, cognitive, and therapeutic levels. J AlzheimersDis 11: 371-83 (2007).

[33] Carrodeguas JA, Rodolosse A, Garza MV, Sanz-Clemente A, Perez-Pé R, Lacosta AM, *et al.*The chick embryo appears as a natural model for research in beta-amyloid precursor protein processing. Neuroscience 134: 1285-300 (2005).

[34] Dani SU. Mechanisms of aging: A survey. In: (Dani SU. Hori A and Walter GF. Eds.). Principles of Neural Aging Elsevier, Amsterdam, pp. 5-18 (1997)

[35] Speakman JR. Body size, energy metabolism and lifespan. J Exp Biol 208: 1717-30 (2005).

[36] Speakman JR, van Acker A and Harper EJ. Age-related changes in the metabolism and body composition of three dog breeds and their relationship to life expectancy. Aging cell 2: 265-75 (2003).

[37] Sutter NB, Bustamante CD, Chase K, Gray MM, Zhao K, Zhu L, *et al.* A single IGF1 allele is a major determinant of small size in dogs. Science 316: 112-5 (2007).

[38] Hare B, Brown M, Williamson C and Tomasello M. The domestication of social cognition in dogs. Science 298: 1634-6 (2002).

[39] Hare B and Tomasello M. Human-like social skills in dogs? Trends CognSci 9: 439-44 (2005).

[40] Overall KL. Clinical behavioral medicine for small animals.St. Louis. Missouri: Mosby (1997).

[41] Pageat P. Patología del comportamiento del perro. 2nd ed. Barcelona: Pulso (2000).

[42] Hu J, Chen H and Li Y. Development of a gas chromatographytime-of-flight mass spectrometry method for the determination of buagafuran, a promising antianxiety drug in dog blood. J Pharm Biomed Anal 47: 383-7 (2008).

[43] Cuyckens F, Balcaen LI, De Wolf K, De Samber B, Van Looveren C, Hurkmans R, *et al.* Use of the bromine isotope ratio in HPLCICP-MS and HPLC-ESI-MS analysis of a new drug in development. Anal BioanalChem 390: 1717-29 (2008).

[44] Landsberg G. Therapeutic agents for the treatment of cognitive dysfunction syndrome in senior dogs.ProgNeuropsychopharmacolBiol Psychiatry 29: 471-9 (2005).

[45] Milgram NW, Zicker SC, Head E, Muggenburg BA, Murphey H, Ikeda-Douglas CJ, *et al.* Dietary enrichment counteracts ageassociated cognitive dysfunction in canines. Neurobiol Aging 23: 737-45 (2002).

[46] Siwak CT, Tapp PD, Head E, Zicker SC, Murphey HL, Muggenburg BA, *et al.* Chronic antioxidant and mitochondrial cofactor administration improves discrimination learning in aged but not young dogs. ProgNeuropsychopharmacolBiol Psychiatry 29: 4619 (2005).

[47] Head E. Combining an antioxidant-fortified diet with behavioral enrichment leads to cognitive improvement and reduced brain pathology in aging canines: strategies for healthy aging. Ann N Y AcadSci 1114: 398-406 (2007).

[48] Araujo JA, Studzinski CM and Milgram NW. Further evidence for the cholinergic hypothesis of aging and dementia from the canine model of aging.ProgNeuropsychopharmacolBiol Psychiatry 29: 411-22 (2005).

[49] Siwak CT, Gruet P, Woehrle F, Muggenburg BA, Murphey HL and Milgram NW. Comparison of the effects of adrafinil, propentofylline, and nicergoline on behavior in aged dogs. Am J Vet Res 61: 1410-4 (2000).

[50] Siwak-Tapp CT, Head E, Muggenburg BA, Milgram NW and Cotman CW. Region specific neuron loss in the aged canine hippocampus is reduced by enrichment. Neurobiol Aging 29: 39-50 (2008).

[51] Opii WO, Joshi G, Head E, Milgram NW, Muggenburg BA, Klein JB, *et al.* Proteomic identification of brain proteins in the canine model of human aging following a long-term

treatment with antioxidants and a program of behavioral enrichment: Relevance to Alzheimer's disease. Neurobiol Aging 29: 51-70 (2008).

[52] Head E, Liu J, Hagen TM, Muggenburg BA, Milgram NW, Ames BN, *et al.* Oxidative damage increases with age in a canine model of human brain aging. J Neurochem 82: 375-81 (2002).

[53] Cummings BJ, Head E, Ruehl W, Milgram NW and Cotman CW. The canine as an animal model of human aging and dementia.Neurobiol Aging 17: 259-68 (1996).

[54] Tapp PD, Siwak CT, Estrada J, Holowachuk D and Milgram NW. Effects of age on measures of complex working memory span in the beagle dog (Canisfamiliaris) using two versions of a spatial list learning paradigm. Learn Mem 10: 148-60 (2003).

[55] Adams B, Chan A, Callahan H, Siwak C, Tapp D, Ikeda-Douglas C, *et al.* Use of a delayed non-matching to position task to model age-dependent cognitive decline in the dog. Behav Brain Res 108: 47-56 (2000).

[56] Head E, Mehta R, Hartley J, Kameka M, Cummings BJ, Cotman CW, *et al.* Spatial learning and memory as a function of age in the dog. BehavNeurosci 109: 851-8 (1995).

[57] Siwak CT, Tapp PD and Milgram NW. Effect of age and level of cognitive function on spontaneous and exploratory behaviors in the beagle dog. Learn Mem 8: 317-25 (2001).

[58] Head E, Callahan H, Muggenburg BA, Cotman CW and Milgram NW. Visual-discrimination learning ability and beta-amyloid accumulation in the dog.Neurobiol Aging 19: 415-25 (1998).

[59] Head E, McCleary R, Hahn FF, Milgram NW and Cotman CW. Region-specific age at onset of beta-amyloid in dogs. Neurobiol Aging 21: 89-96 (2000).

[60] Cummings BJ, Head E, Afagh AJ, Milgram NW and Cotman CW. Beta-amyloid accumulation correlates with cognitive dysfunction in the aged canine. Neurobiol Learn Mem 66: 11-23 (1996).

[61] Colle M-A, Hauw J-J, Crespeau F, Uchihara T, Akiyama H, Checler F, *et al.* Vascular and parenchymal Abeta deposition in the aging dog: correlation with behavior. Neurobiol Aging 21: 695-704 (2000).

[62] Pugliese M, Geloso MC, Carrasco JL, Mascort J, Michetti F and Mahy N. Canine cognitive deficit correlates with diffuse plaque maturation and S100beta (-) astrocytosis but not with insulin cerebrospinal fluid level. ActaNeuropathol (Berl) 111: 519-28 (2006).

[63] Rofina JE, van Ederen AM, Toussaint MJ, Secreve M, van der Spek A, van der Meer I, *et al.* Cognitive disturbances in old dogs suffering from the canine counterpart of Alzheimer's disease. Brain Res 1069: 216-26 (2006).

[64] Neilson JC, Hart BL, Cliff KD and Ruehl WW. Prevalence of behavioral changes associated with age-related cognitive impairment in dogs. J Am Vet Med Assoc 218: 1787-91 (2001).

[65] Bain MJ, Hart BL, Cliff KD and Ruehl WW. Predicting behavioral changes associated with age-related cognitive impairment in dogs. J Am Vet Med Assoc 218: 1792-5 (2001).

[66] Hou Y, White RG, Bobik M, Marks JS and Russell MJ. Distribution of beta-amyloid in the canine brain.Neuroreport 8: 1009-12 (1997).

[67] Yoshino T, Uchida K, Tateyama S, Yamaguchi I, Nakayama H and Goto N. A retrospective study of canine senile plaques and cerebral amyloid angiopathy. Vet Pathol 33: 230-4 (1996).

[68] Satou T, Cummings BJ, Head E, Nielson KA, Hahn FF, Milgram NW, *et al.* The progression of beta-amyloid deposition in the frontal cortex of the aged canine. Brain Res 774: 35-43 (1997).

[69] Papaioannou N, Tooten PC, van Ederen AM, Bohl JR, Rofina J, Tsangaris T, *et al.*Immunohistochemical investigation of the brain of aged dogs. I. Detection of neurofibrillary tangles and of 4hydroxynonenal protein, an oxidative damage product, in senile plaques. Amyloid 8: 11-21 (2001).

[70] Wisniewski T, Lalowski M, Bobik M, Russell M, Strosznajder J and Frangione B. Amyloid beta 1-42 deposits do not lead to Alzheimer's neuritic plaques in aged dogs. Biochem J 313(Pt 2): 57580 (1996).

[71] Pugliese M, Mascort J, Mahy N and Ferrer I. Diffuse beta-amyloid plaques and hyperphosphorylated tau are unrelated processes in aged dogs with behavioral deficits. ActaNeuropathol (Berl) 112: 175-83 (2006).

[72] Wegiel J, Wisniewski HM and Soltysiak Z. Region- and cell-typespecific pattern of tau phosphorylation in dog brain. Brain Res 802: 259-66 (1998).

[73] Wegiel J, Wisniewski HM, Dziewiatkowski J, Tarnawski M, Dziewiatkowska A, Morys J, *et al.* Subpopulation of dogs with severe brain parenchymal beta amyloidosis distinguished with cluster analysis. Brain Res 728: 20-6 (1996).

[74] Russell MJ, White R, Patel E, Markesbery WR, Watson CR and Geddes JW. Familial influence on plaque formation in the beagle brain.Neuroreport 3: 1093-6 (1992).

[75] Swerdlow RH. Is aging part of Alzheimer's disease, or is Alzheimer's disease part of aging? Neurobiol Aging 28: 1465-80 (2007).

[76] Head E, Barrett EG, Murphy MP, Das P, Nistor M, Sarsoza F, *et al.* Immunization with fibrillar Abeta(1-42) in young and aged canines: Antibody generation and characteristics, and effects on CSF and brain Abeta. Vaccine 24: 2824-34 (2006).

[77] Menéndez L, Insua D, Rois JL, Santamarina G, Suárez ML and Pesini P. The immunohistochemical localization of neuronal nitric oxide synthase in the basal forebrain of the dog. J ChemNeuroanat31: 200-9 (2006).

[78] Insua D, Suárez M-L, Santamarina G, Sarasa M and Pesini P. Dogs with canine counterpart of Alzheimer's disease lose noradrenergic neurons. Neurobiol Aging (2008). In press.

[79] Martin LJ, Pardo CA, Cork LC and Price DL. Synaptic pathology and glial responses to neuronal injury precede the formation of senile plaques and amyloid deposits in the aging cerebral cortex. Am J Pathol 145: 1358-81 (1994).

[80] Lemere CA, Oh J, Stanish HA, Peng Y, Pepivani I, Fagan AM, *et al.* Cerebral amyloid-Beta protein accumulation with aging in cotton-top tamarins: a model of early Alzheimer's disease? Rejuvenation Res 11: 321-32 (2008).

[81] Gearing M, Tigges J, Mori H and Mirra SS. beta-Amyloid (A beta) deposition in the brains of aged orangutans. Neurobiol Aging 18: 139-46 (1997).

[82] Schultz C, Hubbard GB, Rub U, Braak E and Braak H. Age-related progression of tau pathology in brains of baboons. Neurobiol Aging 21: 905-12 (2000).

[83] Bons N, Rieger F, Prudhomme D, Fisher A and Krause KH. Microcebusmurinus: a useful primate model for human cerebral aging and Alzheimer's disease? Genes Brain Behav 5: 120-130 (2006).

[84] Rosen RF, Farberg AS, Gearing M, Dooyema J, LongPM, Anderson DC, *et al.* Tauopathy with paired helical filaments in an aged chimpanzee. J Comp Neurol 509: 259-270 (2008).

[85] Braak H, Braak E and Strothjohann M. Abnormally phosphorylated tau protein related to the formation of neurofibrillary tangles and neuropil threads in the cerebral cortex of sheep and goat. NeurosciLett 171: 1-4 (1994).
[86] Nelson PT, Greenberg SG and Saper CB. Neurofibrillary tangles in the cerebral cortex of sheep. NeurosciLett 170: 187-90 (1994).
[87] Nelson PT and Saper CB. Ultrastructure of neurofibrillary tangles in the cerebral cortex of sheep. Neurobiol Aging 16: 315-23 (1995).
[88] Roertgen KE, Parisi JE, Clark HB, Barnes DL, O'Brien TD and Johnson KH.A beta-associated cerebral angiopathy and senile plaques with neurofibrillary tangles and cerebral hemorrhage in an aged wolverine (*Gulogulo*).Neurobiol Aging 17: 243-7 (1996).
[89] Cork LC, Powers RE, Selkoe DJ, Davies P, Geyer JJ and Price DL. Neurofibrillary tangles and senile plaques in aged bears. J Neuropathol Exp Neurol 47: 629-41 (1988).
[90] Lemere CA, Beierschmitt A, Iglesias M, Spooner ET, Bloom JK, Leverone JF, *et al.* Alzheimer's disease abeta vaccine reduces central nervous system abeta levels in a non-human primate, the Caribbean vervet. Am J Pathol 165: 283-97 (2004).
[91] Gandy S, DeMattos RB, Lemere CA, Heppner FL, Leverone J, Aguzzi A, *et al.* Alzheimer's Abeta vaccination of rhesus monkeys (Macacamulatta). Mech Ageing Dev 125: 149-51 (2004).

SUPPLEMENTARY REFERENCES (SR)

SR[1] Kitazawa M, Medeiros R, Laferla FM. Transgenic mouse models of Alzheimer disease: developing a better model as a tool for therapeutic interventions. Curr Pharm Des 18: 1131-1147 (2012).

SR[2] Li S, Jin M, Zhang D, Yang T, Koeglsperger T, Fu H, Selkoe DJ. Environmental Novelty Activates beta2-Adrenergic Signaling to Prevent the Impairment of Hippocampal LTP by Abeta Oligomers. Neuron 77: 929-941 (2013).

SR[3] González-Martínez A, Rosado B, Pesini P, Suárez M-L, Santamarina G, García-Belenguer S, Villegas A, Monleón I, Sarasa M. Plasma beta-amyloid peptides in canine aging and cognitive dysfunction as a model of Alzheimer's disease. Exp Gerontol 46: 590-596 (2011).

SR[4] Rosado B, Gonzalez-Martinez A, Pesini P, Garcia-Belenguer S, Palacio J, Villegas A, Suarez ML, Santamarina G, Sarasa M. Effect of age and severity of cognitive dysfunction on spontaneous activity in pet dogs - Part 1: Locomotor and exploratory behaviour. Vet J 194: 189-195 (2012).

SR[5] Rosado B, Gonzalez-Martinez A, Pesini P, Garcia-Belenguer S, Palacio J, Villegas A, Suarez ML, Santamarina G, Sarasa M (2012) Effect of age and severity of cognitive dysfunction on spontaneous activity in pet dogs - Part 2: Social responsiveness. Vet J 194: 196-201 (2012).

SR[6] Sarasa, L., Gallego, C., Monleón, I., Olvera, A., Canudas, J., Montañés, M., Pesini, P., Sarasa, M., Cloning, sequencing and expression in the dog of the main APP isoforms and some of the enzymes related with their processing, Neuroscience 171: 1091-1101 (2010).

SR[7] Sarasa L, Allué J, Pesini P, Sarasa M. Identification of beta-amyloid species in canine CSF by mass spectrometry. Neurobiol Aging 34: 2125-2132 (2013).

SR[8] Insua D, Corredoira A, Gonzalez-Martinez A, Suarez ML, Santamarina G, Sarasa M, Pesini P. Expression of p75NTR, a Marker for Basal Forebrain Cholinergic Neurons, in Young and Aged Dogs with or without Cognitive Dysfunction Syndrome. J Alzheimers Dis **28**, 291-296 (2012).

SR[9] Bernedo V, Insua D, Suarez ML, Santamarina G, Sarasa M, Pesini P. Beta-amyloid cortical deposits are accompanied by the loss of serotonergic neurons in the dog. J Comp Neurol **513**; 417-429 (2009).

Advances in Alzheimer's Research, Vol. 2, 2014, 275-290

CHAPTER 11

Detection and Quantitation of Amyloid-β Aggregates in Body Fluids may be Suitable for Early Diagnosis of Alzheimer's Disease

Susanne A. Funke[1,2], Eva Birkmann[1,3] and Dieter Willbold[1,3,*]

[1]Forschungszentrum Jülich, ICS-6, 52425 Jülich, Germany; [2]Hochschule für Angewandte Wissenschaften, Bioanalytik, 96450 Coburg and [3]Institut für Physikalische Biologie, Heinrich-Heine-Universität, 40225 Düsseldorf, Germany

Abstract: The *post mortem* identification of amyloid plaques, consisting of the amyloid-β (Aβ) peptide, and neurofibrillary tangles in the brains of patients still leads to the most reliable diagnosis for Alzheimer's disease (AD). Substantial efforts have been made to identify reliable biomarkers for AD that can be used for early diagnosis of AD. Body fluids of AD patients have been investigated for their content of total or soluble Aβ(1-40) or Aβ(1-42), either using classical ELISA procedures, or non-classical assays with more innovative read-out signals, or a combination of both. The concentration of total soluble Aβ(1-42) in cerebrospinal fluid (CSF) is reduced by 40 to 50 % in AD patients compared to age-matched healthy controls, as confirmed in more than 30 studies, with both sensitivity and specificity exceeding 80 to 90 %. Thus, it was suggested that detection of low levels of Aβ(1-42) in CSF might help preclinical diagnosis. The achievable sensitivity using such CSF biomarkers, however, is 85 % or less. Therefore, these assays cannot deliver any increase in the diagnostic outcome as compared to existing algorithms based on neuropsychological and imaging modalities. Regarding the amyloid cascade hypothesis, Aβ oligomers and aggregates are directly involved in the pathologic process. The presence of Aβ aggregates in CSF could thus be the most direct and most reliable biomarker for AD and increasing efforts are undertaken to develop methods that are suitable to quantify and characterize Aβ aggregate species present in body fluids, especially in CSF. Here, we present an overview of the current status of the development of methods for Aβ aggregate specific detection and quantitation, which is an update of a previous review.

Keywords: Alzheimer's disease, amyloid-β aggregates, biomarker, early diagnosis, prognosis, protein misfolding diseases, therapy monitoring.

***Corresponding author Dieter Willbold:** Forschungszentrum Jülich, ICS-6, D-52425 Jülich, Germany; Tel: +49 2461 612100; Fax: +49 2461 612023; E-mail: dieter.willbold@uni-duesseldorf.de

D.K. Lahiri (Ed)

INTRODUCTION

Alzheimer´s disease (AD) is a progressive neurodegenerative disorder, which is characterized by memory loss, confusion and a variety of cognitive disabilities [1]. AD is the most prevalent dementia, affecting nearly 2 % of the population in the western world, where the incidence of AD increases dramatically in individuals beyond the age of 70. Thus, AD has a great impact on modern societies, leading to disastrous influence on the patient's and the relative's life and enormous economic costs [2]. Neither a causal therapy for recovery, nor a reliable method for early diagnosis, which could improve the evaluation of present therapeutical or preventional clinical studies, is available. Currently, only symptomatic treatment of AD is approved. The majority of scientists in the field agree that therapy of AD will be most effective in early stages [3], and as soon as compounds for causative treatment are available, a method for reliable early diagnosis is essential.

Today, the most reliable diagnosis of AD is the *post mortem* identification of amyloid plaques and neurofibrillary tangles in brain tissue of the deceased patient. The major component of the amyloid plaques is the amyloid-β (Aβ) peptide, consisting of 38 to 43 amino acid residues, predominantly $A\beta_{(1-42)}$. Aβ is derived from the amyloid precursor protein (APP) by two different proteolytic activities, called β- and γ-secretases [4-6]. As originally suggested by the amyloid cascade hypothesis [7], it appears likely that Aβ peptides and their aggregates initiate cellular events leading to the pathologic effects of AD. During recent years, the opinion that soluble Aβ oligomers instead of amyloid plaques mediate toxicity in AD evolved more and more mature [8-10].

Great efforts are undertaken to identify reliable biomarkers for AD, being suitable for minimal invasive early diagnosis and prognosis of AD. During recent years, body fluids of AD patients were investigated for their content of total or monomeric $A\beta_{(1-40)}$ or $A\beta_{(1-42)}$ concentrations using classical ELISA or related methods with additional signal amplification. Cerebrospinal fluid (CSF) concentrations of monomeric $A\beta_{(1-42)}$ are reduced by 40 to 50 % in AD patients compared to age-matched healthy controls as confirmed in over 30 studies, with both sensitivity and specificity exceeding 80 to 90 % in most of the studies (for a review, see [11,12]). Decrease of $A\beta_{(1-42)}$ in the CSF has also been observed during stages of mild cognitive impairment, the earliest clinical manifestation of AD [13]. Thus, it was suggested that detection of low levels of CSF Aβ(1-42) might be useful for preclinical diagnosis. Because the current average sensitivity of AD biomarker detection in the CSF is approximately 85 %, these assays do not offer a considerable increase in predictive value over existing algorithms based on standard neuropsychological and imaging modalities [14]. However, the monomeric form of Aβ is not thought to be responsible for neurotoxicity and neurodegeneration. The opposite seems to be the case, as in recent studies Aβ monomers are found to be beneficial and neuroprotective [15]. Aβ aggregates, such as soluble Aβ oligomer species, have potential to be a more suitable biomarker for disease severity and progression than currently measured monomeric CSF $A\beta_{(1-42)}$. Recent evidence from animal models and AD patients suggest that such soluble oligomers may be the synaptotoxic species and may even proceed insoluble amyloid plaque deposition as a cause for cognitive deficits [16-19]. Therefore, methods for sensitive and specific detection of aggregated Aβ species during lifetime are highly desired. Those methods need to be able to clearly distinguish aggregated Aβ from monomeric species, as monomeric Aβ is also present in healthy humans [20]. The development of such techniques, however, was severely hampered by the low abundance and the metastable nature of Aβ oligomers. This review gives an overview about the recent development of methods for specific detection and quantification of aggregated Aβ-species in CSF, methods which will hopefully leading to the elucidation of a correlation between Aβ aggregate content of body fluids and the progress of AD. All methods discussed here are summarized in Table **1**. In the following text, we will use the term "aggregates" to describe all kinds of non monomeric Aβ species, including protofibrils and fibrils. In contrast, Aβ oligomers are defined as non fibrillar, soluble low-molecular weight oligomers. Other denotations describing certain oligomeric/aggregated Aβ species are used as by the authors of the reviewed methods and explained in the respective paragraphs.

Table 1: Overview of available methods that claim to yield Aβ aggregate quantitation. Definitions of different Aβ species: ADDLs: Aβ derived diffusible ligands: small soluble Aβ oligomers with molecular weights between 17and 42 kDa [21]. Protofibrils: ≥ 100 nm curved linear structures with a diameter of ~ 5 nm and a length up to 200 nm which remain soluble upon centrifugation at 16 000-18000 g [22]. Aggregates: all kinds of diffusible, non monomeric Aβ including prefibrils and fibrils. Aβ oligomers: non fibrillar, soluble low-molecular weight oligomers. Phrases describing certain Aβ species are used as by the authors of the reviewed methods. FCS: fluorescence correlation sprectroscopy. sFIDA: surface fluorescence intensity distribution analysis. MMSE: Mini-Mental Status Exam.

Method	Detected Aβ species as described by the authors	Diagnostic potential in CSF	Reference
Nanoparticle based detection	ADDLs	Higher aggregate content in 15 AD-patient derived CSF samples compared to 15 controls	[23]
Nanoscale optical biosensor method	ADDLs	Higher aggregate content in AD-patient derived CSF (one sample each)	[24]
Misfolded protein assay	Aβ aggregates	Higher concentration of Aβ(1-40) aggregates in 26 samples of AD patients than in 10 controls	[25]
ELISA	High molecular weight Aβ oligomers	Significantly higher signals in 18 AD or 7 MCI samples than in 25 controls, inverse correlation to MMSE scores	[26]
ELISA	Aβ oligomers	No oligomers in CSF detected	[27]
Principle of seeded polymerization in combination with FCS	Aβ aggregates	Higher aggregate content in AD-patient derived CSF	[28]
Principle of seeded polymerization in combination with confocal spectroscopy	Aβ binding particles (LAPs)	No correlation found	[29]
Dual colour FRET detection with flow cytometry in solution	Aβ oligomers	CSF samples of 15 AD patients had higher concentrations than samples of 12 non-demented controls, negative correlation with MMSE score	[30,31]
sFIDA	Aβ aggregates	Higher aggregate content in 14 AD-patient derived CSF samples compared to 10 control samples	[32-34]

Nanotechnology and ELISA-Type Assays for Aβ Aggregate Quantitation

In 2005, Georganopoulou and coworkers described a nanoparticle-based detection method for so called amyloid-β-derived diffusible ligands (ADDLs). ADDLs are described as small soluble Aβ oligomers with molecular weights between 17 and

42 kDa [23]. The oligonucleotide barcode assay, developed by Nam *et al.* for the detection of cancer marker prostate specific antigen in serum [35], can detect protein levels in the attomolar concentration range, six orders of magnitude lower than concentrations detected by ELISA. In the assay, goldnanoparticles with hundreds of copies of a DNA barcode attached and magnetic beads are functionalized with ADDL specific antibodies. Both are mixed with a sample (CSF or synthetically prepared ADDLs), resulting in a DNA-ADDL-magnet sandwich complex which can be extracted from the sample using a magnet. After some washing steps, the total number of DNA barcodes can be determined by a scanometric method. As several hundred copies of the barcode are attached to each gold particle, amplification enables the detection of even tiny amounts of ADDLs. The detection limit of the semiquantitative assay was determined to be at 100 aM. The assay was linear up to concentrations of 500 fM. 10 μl CSF of 30 subjects were sampled in the procedure, 15 of them having a diagnosis of probable AD. Those subjects had higher ADDL concentrations in their CSF compared to the controls, except for 2 patients. For both, there were hints that they could have false-positive diagnoses. One non-demented control subject had a moderate number of plaques in the brain but no ADDLs in CSF, supporting the theory that ADDLs provoke neurodegeneration more than plaques in the brain [23].

The assay, although very sensitive as described by the authors, might be limited for widespread utility in multiple laboratories for technological reasons. The reported protocol contains several critical steps, involving incubation of Aβ at 37 °C under shaking, possibly leading to artificial oligomerization, which could limit the reproducibility and robustness of the assay.

Also in 2005, Haes *et al.* published a nanoscale optical biosensor method based on localized surface plasmon resonance (LSPR) spectroscopy, able to determine the ADDL concentration in brain samples and CSF. In short, ADDL-specific antibodies are attached to surface-confined silver (Ag) nanoparticles. Then, samples containing ADDLs or control samples were incubated. To finally enhance the LSPR shift response, the samples were again incubated with ADDL antibodies (sandwich principle). Transmission UV-vis spectroscopy was used to monitor the optical properties (LSPR) of the Ag nanoparticles. In a preliminary study, the CSF of an AD patient had a higher concentration of ADDLs than the CSF of a control. Nevertheless, the authors stated that the assay had to be optimized, as the suggested binding model was not able to perfectly fit the data, leading to an underestimation of the observed response at low concentrations [24].

In 2010, Gao and coworkers described peptides binding to Aβ aggregates, and used those as a bait for Aβ aggregates in CSF to perform the so-called "misfolded protein assay" (MPA). The aggregates were bound to aggregate specific beads, and subsequently the immobilized Aβ was denatured and the concentration thereof determined using Aβ(1-40) and Aβ(1-42) monomer specific ELISAs. In CSF samples of 26 AD patients higher amounts of Aβ(1-40) aggregates could be detected than in the samples of 10 age-matched controls. Interestingly, a similar result was not found for Aβ(1-42) aggregates [25]. The size and form of the aggregates detected in the assay remained unclear, as the aggregates specific beads were described to bind higher order aggregates as well as Aβ oligomers, and Aβ was denatured for concentration determination as conventional ELISA for Aβ monomers were used. Information on the nature of the detected aggregates, however, might be helpful for characterization of AD pathology and development of diagnostic approaches.

In 2010, Fukumoto and coworkers described an ELISA tool for the specific detection of high molecular weight (HMW) Aβ oligomers. One antibody, BAN50 [36], which binds to Aβ1-16, was used for antigen capture as well as for detection. To characterize the oligomer species characterized by the assay, different synthetic Aβ(1-42) oligomers were prepared and investigated by size exclusion chromatography. The size of the detected Aβ oligomers were determined to be between 40 to 200 kDa, mainly fractionating at 45 to 90 kDa, corresponding to 10 to 20 mers. Monomers and smaller oligomer species were not detected. The detection limit of HMW oligomers was 10 pM (expressed as the equivalent concentration of Aβ monomers). As the HMW oligomers were estimated to be only 1 percent of the whole preparation, the sensitivity of the assay was estimated to be finally 0.1 pM. Why low molecular weight oligomers are not detected by the ELISA was not clarified, but might relay on sterical hindrance. The scientists detected significantly increased amounts of HMW Aβ oligomers in CSF samples derived from AD and MCI patients, as compared to age matched control samples.

Additionally, the authors demonstrated a negative correlation of oligomer readout with MMSE (mini-mental-status examination) scores in the AD/MCI group [26].

Very recently, the group of Selkoe published an article on novel ELISAs with high specificity for soluble Aβ oligomers. Two different assays employing a highly sensitive elektrochemoluminescence detection system were developed and validated, whereas in one of them an aggregated Aβ specific monoclonal antibody was used for capture in combination with an monoclonal antibody binding to the N-terminal of Aβ for detection, in the other the latter antibody was used for both. Both set-ups did not detect Aβ monomers, but Aβ oligomers prepared from synthetic Aβ were detected over a wide range of concentrations, ranging from dimers crosslinked by a disulfide bridge to larger assemblies with lower detection limits of approximately 10 pg/ml for synthetic Aβ dimers. Excellent reproduceability combined with low standard errors were demonstrated by the authors. Nevertheless, in extracts of AD brains, Aβ oligomers were detected in a wide range of sizes, but surprisingly, the assays failed to detect Aβ oligomers in 89 human CSF samples. Abundant Aβ monomers could be detected in the same samples by conventional ELISA systems for Aβ(1-40) or Aβ(1-42). The authors themselves discussed that the hydrophobicity of Aβ oligomers might result in a low concentration below the detection limits of the ELISA systems, or even the absence of Aβ oligomers in the CSF samples. Blotting studies verified the fact that the concentration of Aβ oligomers might be low in comparison to Aβ monomers. Another possible explanation was the epitope masking of Aβ oligomers by other proteins, but this possibility was excluded after spiking Aβ oligomers in human CSF after serial dilution [27].

Several of the assays described in this part of the review are based on the binding of certain Aβ species to Aβ species specific antibodies. Such assay would only detect one specific species of aggregates. Since the identity of the most relevant Aβ aggregates for AD diagnosis or even prognosis is currently an active and controversal research topic, it would require additional evidence to support the use of such assays for diagnostic use. Additionally, care needs to be taken to characterize these antibodies regarding their cross-reactivity with other Aβ aggregate species and monomers.

Assays that Claim to Achieve Single Aggregate Sensitivity

Using fluorescence techniques being suitable for sensitive single molecule detection as fluorescence correlation spectroscopy (FCS), confocal laser scanning microscopy and flow cytometry, the detection of low amounts or even single aggregates is possible. This is substantially different to aggregate detection by the methods described above, where one integrated signal for all Aβ particles in the sample is obtained as a primary read-out. Single aggregate detection methods should be, in theory, more sensitive than the methods reviewed in the previous section. In comparison to methods based on species-specific antibodies, all different species of Aβ aggregates can theoretically be detected and differentiated.

In 1998, the first study describing single particle detection of aggregated Aβ species in CSF was published by Riesner and coworkers. In this study, the principle of "seeded polymerization" was used in combination with fluorescence correlation spectroscopy (FCS). In FCS, developed originally by Eigen & Rigler [37], a laser is focused into a sample volume with a diameter less than a micrometer, and the emitted fluorescence light is confocally detected, which enables to measure fluctuations of the fluorescence intensity within a femtoliter volume. Fluorescence labeled Aβ was added to human CSF samples of AD patients and non-demented controls. Aβ multimers in the sample acted as seeds for quick polymerization, leading to fluorescence bursts (high fluorescence intensities during time course of measurement) during FCS measurements. Each burst represented a single multimeric particle in the sample. Each of the 15 AD patient derived samples lead to numerous fluorescence bursts as observed with FCS, indicating rapid aggregation of the fluorescence labelled synthetic Aβ onto the "seeds". This was not observed for any of the 19 non-demented controls [28].

In 2007, Henkel *et al.* evaluated the diagnostic potential of the technique used by Pitschke *et al.*, again. The set up was slightly modified. Using an improved dynamic "flow through" set up and a self-made confocal spectroscopy system, the detection sensitivity was claimed to be improved 20-fold. Again, a CSF sample was mixed up with fluorescence-labelled synthetical Aβ and after an incubation time of 15 to 25 min, fluorescence from the flowing sample was detected. The authors also found large so called Aβ-peptide binding particles (LAPs), but those were not specific for AD. Instead, they were present in both AD patients and controls with large inter-individual variations. For further insights into LAPs, confocal microscopy was used to distinguish between four different classes of LAPs. Differences were made between brightness, area, shape and texture of the particles based on fully automated quantitative computer-assisted morphometry. Again, the different classes of LAPs were not suitable for diagnostic purposes. Interestingly, two kinds of LAPs seem to consist of Aβ-IgGs, one of them being present in some (41.1 %) non-AD humans only, not in AD patients. This strikes the hypothesis of a circulating IgG based Aβ(1-42) clearence system in CSF, being possibly absent in AD patients [29].

Why both of the two studies based on the seeded polymerization principle lead to contradicting results cannot be clarified at the moment. One has to keep in mind that different modifications of the method and different setups were used. As an example, in the study described by Henkel and co-workers, only bright LAPs of greater than 3000 kHz photon counts were included in the analysis which is a value three times the threshold used by Pitschke and co-workers. More importantly, both protocols utilize seeded polymerization with synthetic Aβ peptides. This approach is likely to be influenced by multiple factors such as CSF sample preparation procedure, amount of synthetic Aβ peptide added and the amount of incubation time before fluorescence was measured. The different observations from these two studies highlight the fact that this assay methodology might not be very robust.

In 2007, Santos and co-workers published a method for Aβ oligomer detection in CSF, based on the concurrent binding of two fluorescence labelled antibodies to oligomers and subsequent detection by flow cytometry. An elegant fluorescence resonance energy transfer (FRET) setup, in which energy from an excited donor (Aβ-antibody with AlexaFluor 488 fluorescence dye) is transferred to an acceptor molecule (Aβ-antibody with different epitope and AlexaFluor 594 fluorescence dye) was used. Therefore, specificity was assured as FRET effects can be only observed if both antibodies are in a distance of at least 10 nm. Only oligomeric Aβ species can bind sufficient amounts of labelled antibody molecules emitting fluorescence after FRET effects to be detected by flow cytometry. Sensitivity of the assay is very high (Aβ concentrations in the pM range) as determined with synthetically prepared Aβ oligomers. In the study 200 μl CSF samples of only non AD patients were diluted with buffer and applied to the procedure, which seems to be nicely reproducible. There seemed to be only a weak correlation between age and the amounts of oligomers detected by the FRET/flow cytometry method [30]. In 2012, the same group used the method described above to detect Aβ oligomers in CSF samples of 14 AD patients, 12 non-demented controls and other neurological disorders (n = 4). The levels of Aβ oligomers were (non significantly, p = 0.07) elevated in the AD patients compared to the pooled control group, the ratio of Aβ oligomers/Aβ(1-42) was significantly elevated in AD subjects compared to non AD subjects. As described in the previous study, a negative correlation between Aβ oligomer count and MMSE score in AD patients was found (r = -0.65; p = 0.013) [31].

A strong advantage of the FRET/flow cytometry method is that flow cytometry is available in all leading biomedical research institutions. A major drawback of this approach might be that washing steps cannot be applied at all, possibly leading to decreased specificity of the results.

In 2006, Birkmann *et al.* published a method which is able to detect single prion protein (PrP) aggregates prepared from brain samples based on FCS [38]. As already shown by the article of Pitschke *et al.* [28], fluctuations from fluorescent monomers or oligomers can be differentiated from larger aggregates if the particle number is low. As several antibodies bind to one aggregate, aggregates lead to fluorescence bursts in the FCS confocal detection volume and can thus be easily distinguished from monomers. To enhance the specificity of the detection, FCS was applied in a dual-colour mode so that only coincidental signals of two fluorescent markers (PrP-specific antibodies labelled with two different fluorescent dyes) within the confocal volume are counted as specific events by cross correlation evaluation. In a second study, the authors developed an even more sensitive assay based on the earlier results by immobilizing the aggregates on a glass surface by capture antibodies. The so called surface-FIDA (sFIDA) assay has major advantages in comparison to the FIDA assay in solution. After surface immobilisation of the aggregates, the surface is then scanned systematically by one or more laser foci. In addition, washing steps can reduce the background signals and enhance the signal/noise ratio, making the method theoretically also applicable to samples other than CSF. Applying this method, PrP-aggregates purified of brain extracts as well as in 20 μl of crude CSF could be detected and quantitated [39]. In 2007, Funke *et al.* adapted the method for the detection of Aβ aggregates and validated it using synthetically prepared aggregated Aβ. The assay was shown to be linear over a wide range of Aβ aggregate amounts down to the pg range. Monomeric Aβ was not detected, excluded not only by coincidal two colour detection and crosscorrelation setup but also by using two detection antibodies binding to the same epitope. One of the advantages of the assay is its high specificity for Aβ aggregates. In the detection process, three different Aβ specific antibodies were used, one for immobilization of the aggregates, two for decorating them with fluorescence dyes. As long as at least two antibodies of the three are specific for overlapping epitopes, cross correlation analysis is leading to aggregate specific signals. As a first trial to use the sFIDA assay for analysing real CSF samples for its diagnostic capabilities, 20 μl crude CSF samples of three AD patients and two non-demented control patients was subjected to the assay. The CSF of the AD patients could be clearly distinguished from the control patients in those very preliminary studies. The count of Aβ aggregates was higher in AD patients than in healthy controls [32]. In 2010, the assay could be adapted to laser scanning microscopy (sFIDA imaging), leading to further improvement of sensitivity [33]. Recently, the same group published an article on a novel, optimized version of sFIDA, with even higher sensitivity, achieved by a new protocol for covalent immobilization of the capture antibody. In comparison to the previous protocol, in which the capture antibody was immobilized to the glass surface by unspecific adsorption, unspecific fluorescent background was significantly reduced, and whereas synthetic Aβ monomers were not detected at all, size-exclusion chromatography prepared Aβ oligomers could be detected in a linear way even in low concentrations in the pM scale. The newly established assay was challenged by application of CSF samples from 14 AD patients and 12 non-demented controls. Although only 12.5 μl sample volume was used, both groups could be clearly distinguished by sFIDA. The mean value of the readout of the AD group was significantly higher than that of the control group, which showed homogenously low levels of Aβ oligomers. The AD group showed higher variations, but still, for the small number of samples tested, this yielded a sensitivity of 93 % and a specificity of 100 %. In addition, a negative correlation of the sFIDA readout with the MMSE score (r^2 = 0.35; p = 0.0016) was found, therefore, the sFIDA readout seems to reflect the severity of the disease [34].

OUTLOOK

A diagnostic tool is essential to follow the progression of AD at preclinical stages and to understand disease associated or causative mechanisms and to monitor potential therapeutical approaches. Techniques which are able to detect even single aggregates in body fluids will be the most sensitive methods by definition. A challenge for the analytic system is to reliably count only those aggregates or oligomers that consist of Aβ. Monomeric molecules need to be clearly distinguished because Aβ is a normal product of APP metabolism and hence a natural component of CSF and plasma [20]. So far it is unclear, which Aβ form is the most toxic one and which can aid early diagnosis of AD. Therefore, a method will be needed, which can not only quantify one type of aggregate, but rather distinguish between several Aβ aggregate species and determine aggregate form, size, number and composition. Then, a useful validation of the correlation between disease progression and aggregate content of body fluids can be performed.

As already shown by several studies [23-26,28,31-34], the count of Aβ aggregates was higher in body fluids of AD patients than in healthy controls. This somehow seems to contradict previous ELISA studies suggesting that the total Aβ amount decreases with disease progression. The "sink hypothesis" suggests that the count of measurable monomeric Aβ in CSF is decreased because aggregated Aβ is deposited in plaques [40,41]. However, one has to keep in mind that the employed ELISA measurements have not been suitable for the measurement of total Aβ. According to Stenh *et al.* and Englund and co-workers, [42,43], aggregated Aβ species are inefficiently measured by ELISA, leading to false low Aβ concentration measurements. Thus, the reported decrease of total Aβ, which in fact might just be a decrease of accessible monomeric Aβ, might well be in accordance with the observed increase of aggregated Aβ with disease progression.

Although CSF biomarkers are useful in demonstrating the relevance to the CNS compartment for neurological diseases such as AD, there will be some limitation due to the procedure required, even though lumbar puncture is moderately invasive and has low incidence of complications [44]. For wider use for diagnosis and to monitor therapy, a biomarker detectable in plasma would be of great value. It would be very useful to adapt the most robust and sensitive methodology developed based on CSF to plasma and serum samples.

In conclusion, we reviewed several recently developed methods attempting to detect diffusible Aβ aggregate species in CSF. Although some of the methods are innovative and hold promise for a much better biomarker for AD diagnosis and progression, parallel work is needed to elucidate the nature of the Aβ aggregates relavant to the disease as well as to improve the technical robustness of the methods employed.

ACKNOWLEDGEMENTS

The work was supported by EU Joint Programme Neurodegenerative Diseases (JPND) and the Kompetenznetz Degenerative Demenzen (KNDD) of the German Federal Ministry of Education and Research (BMBF).

CONFLICT OF INTEREST

Declared None.

DISCLOSURE

This chapter is an update of our previous publication in CAR "Detection and Quantitation of Amyloid-β Aggregates in Body Fluids may be Suitable for Early Diagnosis of Alzheimer's Disease" published in 'CAR', Volume 6, Number 3, June, pp. 285 to 289 [45].

REFERENCES

[1] Soto C. Plaque busters: strategies to inhibit amyloid formation in Alzheimer's disease. Mol. Med. Today 1999;5:343-350.

[2] Mattson MP. Pathways towards and away from Alzheimer's disease. Nature 2004;430:631-639.

[3] Golde, T. E., L. S. Schneider, Koo EH. Anti-abeta therapeutics in Alzheimer's disease: the need for a paradigm shift. Neuron 2011; 69(2):203-213.

[4] Haass C, Selkoe DJ. Cellular processing of beta-amyloid precursor protein and the genesis of amyloid beta-peptide. Cell 1993;75:1039-1042.

[5] Kang J, Lemaire HG, Unterbeck A, Salbaum JM, Masters CL, Grzeschik KH, Multhaup G, Beyreuther K, Muller-Hill B. The precursor of Alzheimer's disease amyloid A4 protein resembles a cell-surface receptor. Nature 1987;325:733-736.

[6] Weidemann A, Konig G, Bunke D, Fischer P, Salbaum JM, Masters CL, Beyreuther K. Identification, biogenesis, and localization of precursors of Alzheimer's disease A4 amyloid protein. Cell 1989;57:115-126.

[7] Hardy JA, and Higgins GA. Alzheimer's disease: the amyloid cascade hypothesis. Science 1992;256:184-185.

[8] Lue LF, Kuo YM, Roher E, Brachova L, Shen Y *et al.* Am. J. Pathol. 1999; 155: 853-862.

[9] Mc Lean CA, Cherny RA, Fraser FW, Fuller SJ, Smith MJ *et al.* Ann. Neurol. 1999;46:860-866.

[10] Wang J, Dickson DW, Trojanowski JQ, Lee VM. The levels of soluble *vs.* insoluble brain Abeta distinguish Alzheimer's disease from normal and pathologic aging. Exp. Neurol. 1999;158:328-337.

[11] Flirski M and Sobow T. Biochemical markers and risk factors of Alzheimer's disease. Curr. Alzheimer Res. 2225;2:47-64.

[12] Lewczuk P and Wiltfang J. Neurochemical dementia diagnostics: state of the art and research perspectives. Proteomics 2008;8:1292-1301

[13] Hansson O, Zetterberg H, Buchhave P, Andreasson U, Londos E, Blennow K, Minthon L. Association between CSF biomarkers and incipient Alzheimer's disease in patients with mild cognitive impairment: a follow-up study. Lancet Neurol. 2006;5:228-234.

[14] Andreasen N, Blennow K. CSF biomarkers for mild cognitive impairment and early Alzheimer's disease. Clin. Neurol. Neurosurg. 2005;107:165-173.

[15] Puzzo, D. and Arancio O. Amyloid-beta Peptide: Dr. Jekyll or Mr. Hyde? J. Alzheimers Dis. 2012; 33 Suppl 1:S111-20.

[16] Lesné S, Koh MT, Kotilinek L, Kayed R, Glabe CG, Yang A, Gallagher M, Ashe KH. A specific amyloid-beta protein assembly in the brain impairs memory. Nature. 2006;440:352-7.

[17] McLaurin J, Kierstead ME, Brown ME, Hawkes CA, Lambermon MH, Phinney AL, Darabie AA, Cousins JE, French JE, Lan MF, Chen F, Wong SS, Mount HT, Fraser PE, Westaway D, St George-Hyslop P. Cyclohexanehexol inhibitors of Abeta aggregation prevent and reverse Alzheimer phenotype in a mouse model. Nat Med. 2006;12:801-8.

[18] Klyubin I, Betts V, Welzel AT, Blennow K, Zetterberg H, Wallin A, Lemere CA, Cullen WK, Peng Y, Wisniewski T, Selkoe DJ, Anwyl R, Walsh DM, Rowan MJ. Amyloid beta protein dimer-containing human CSF disrupts synaptic plasticity: prevention by systemic passive immunization. J Neurosci. 2008;28:4231-7.

[19] Shankar GM, Li S, Mehta TH, Garcia-Munoz A, Shepardson NE, Smith I, Brett FM, Farrell MA, Rowan MJ, Lemere CA, Regan CM, Walsh DM, Sabatini BL, Selkoe DJ. Amyloid-beta protein dimers isolated directly from Alzheimer's brains impair synaptic plasticity and memory. Nat Med. 2008;8:837-42.

[20] Haass C, Koo EH, Mellon A, Selkoe DJ. Targeting of cell-surface beta-amyloid precursor protein to lysosomes: alternative processing into amyloid-bearing fragments. Nature 1992;359:322-325.

[21] Lambert MP, Barlow AK, Chromy BA, Edwards C, Freed R, Liosatos M, Morgan TE, Rozovsky I, Trommer B, Viola KL, Wals P, Zhang C, Finch CE, Krafft GA, Klein WL.

Diffusible, nonfibrillar ligands derived from Abeta1-42 are potent central nervous system neurotoxins. Proc Natl Acad Sci U S A. 1998 May 26;95(11):6448-53.

[22] Walsh DM, Hartley DM, Kusumoto Y, Fezoui Y, Condron MM, Lomakin A, Benedek GB, Selkoe DJ, Teplow DB.Amyloid beta-protein fibrillogenesis. Structure and biological activity of protofibrillar intermediates. J Biol Chem. 1999 ;274:25945-52.

[23] Georganopoulou DG, Chang L, Nam J-M, Thaxton S, Mufson EJ, Klein WL, and Mirkin CA. From the cover: Nanoparticle based detection in cerebral spinal fluid of a soluble pathogenic biomarker for Alzheimer's disease. Proc. Natl. Acad. Sci. USA 2005;102:2273-2276.

[24] A.J. Haes AJ, L. Chang L, W.L. Klein WL, and R. Van Dyne R. Detection of a biomarker for Alzheimer's disease from synthetic and clinical samples using a nanoscale optical biosensor. J. Am. Chem. Soc. 2005;127:2264-2271.

[25] Gao CM, Yam AY, Wang X, Magdangal E, Salisbury C, Peretz D, *et al.* Abeta40 oligomers identified as a potential biomarker for the diagnosis of Alzheimer's disease. PLoS One 5(12); e15725.

[26] Fukumoto H, Tokuda T, Kasai T, Ishigami N, Hidaka H, Kondo M, *et al.* High-molecular-weight {beta}-amyloid oligomers are elevated in cerebrospinal fluid of Alzheimer patients. FASEB J. 2010; 24(8):2716-26.

[27] Yang T, Hong S, O'Malley T, Sperling RA, Walsh DM, Selkoe DJ. New ELISAs with high specificity for soluble oligomers of amyloid β-protein detect natural Aβ oligomers in human brain but not CSF. Alzheimers Dement. 2013;9(2):99-112.

[28] Pitschke M, Prior R, Haupt M & Riesner D. Detection of single amyloid-β-protein aggregates in the cerebrospinal fluid of Alzheimer's patients by fluorescence correlation spectroscopy. Nat. Med. 1998;4:832-834.

[29] Henkel AW, Dittrich PS, Groemer TW, Lemke EA, Klingauf J, Klafki HW, Lewczuk P, Esselmann H, Schwille P, Kornhuber J, Wiltfang J. Immune complexes of auto-antibodies against A beta 1-42 peptides patrol cerebrospinal fluid of non-Alzheimer's patients. Mol. Psychiatry. 2007;12:601-610.

[30] Santos AN, Torkler S, Nowak D, Schlittig C, Goerdes M, Lauber T, Trischmann L, Schaupp M, Penz M, Tiller FW, Böhm G. Detection of amyloid-beta oligomers in human cerebrospinal fluid by flow cytometry and fluorescence resonance energy transfer. J. Alzheimers Dis. 2007;11:117-125.

[31] Santos AN, Ewers M, Minthon L, Simm A, Silber RE, Blennow K, Prvulovic D, Hansson O, Hampel H. Amyloid-β oligomers in cerebrospinal fluid are associated with cognitive decline in patients with Alzheimer's disease. J. Alzheimers Dis. 2012;29(1):171-6.

[32] Funke SA, Birkmann E, Henke F, Görtz P, Lange-Asschenfeldt, C Riesner D, Willbold D. Single particle detection of Aβ aggregates associated with Alzheimer's disease. Biochem. Biophys. Res. Commun. 2007;364:902-907.

[33] Funke SA, Wang L, Birkmann E, Willbold D. Single particle detection system for Aß: Adaptation of surface-FIDA to laser scanning microscopy. Rejuvenation Res. 2010;13:206-209.

[34] Wang-Dietrich L, Funke SA, Kühbach K, Wang K, Besmehn A, Willbold S, Cinar Y, Bannach O, Birkmann E, Willbold D. The Amyloid-β Oligomer Count in Cerebrospinal Fluid is a Biomarker for Alzheimer's Disease. J. Alzheimers Dis. 2013;34(4):985-94.

[35] Nam JM, Thaxton CS, Mirkin CA. Nanoparticle-based bio-bar codes for the ultrasensitive detection of proteins. Science 2003;301:1884-1886.

[36] Suzuki N, Cheung TT, Cai XD, Odaka A, Otvos L, Jr., Eckman C, *et al.* An increased percentage of long amyloid beta protein secreted by familial amyloid beta protein precursor (beta APP717) mutants. Science. 1994 May 27;264(5163):1336-40.

[37] Eigen M, and Riegler R. Sorting single molecules-application to diagnosis and evolutionary biotechnology. Proc. Natl. Acad. Sci. USA 1994;91:5740-5747.

[38] Birkmann E, Schäfer O, Weinmann N, Dumpitak C, Beekes M, Jackman R, Thorne L and Riesner D. Detection of prion particles in samples of BSE and scrapie by fluorescence correlation spectroscopy without proteinase K digestion. Biol. Chem. 2006;387:95-102.

[39] Birkmann E, Henke F, Weinmann N, Dumpitak C, Groschup M, Funke A, Willbold D, Riesner D. Counting of single prion particles bound to a capture-antibody surface (surface-FIDA). Vet. Microbiol. 2007;123:294-304.

[40] Kawarabayashi T, Younkin LH, Saido TC, Shoji M, Ashe KH, Younkin SG. Age-dependent changes in brain, CSF, and plasma amyloid (beta) protein in the Tg2576 transgenic mouse model of Alzheimer's disease. J. Neurosci. 2001;21 :372-381.

[41] DeMattos RB, Bales KR, Parsadanian M, O'Dell MA, Foss EM, Paul SM, Holtzman DM. Plaque-associated disruption of CSF and plasma amyloid-beta (Abeta) equilibrium in a mouse model of Alzheimer's disease. J Neurochem. 2002;81:229-236.

[42] Englund H, Seehlin D, Johansson AS, Nilsson LNG, Gellerfors P, Paulie S, Lannfelt L and Ekholm Pettersson F. Sensitive ELISA detection of amyloid-β protofibrils in biological samples. J. Neurochem. 2007;103:334-345.

[43] Stenh C, Englund H, Lord A, Johansson AS, Almeida CG, Gellerfors P, Greengard P, Gouras GK, Lannfelt L, Nilsson LN. Amyloid-beta oligomers are inefficiently measured by enzyme-linked immunosorbent assay. Ann Neurol. 2005;58:147-150.

[44] Andreasen N, Minthon L, Davidsson P, Vanmechelen E, Vanderstichele H, Winblad B, Blennow K. Evaluation of CSF-tau and CSF-Abeta42 as diagnostic markers for Alzheimer disease in clinical practice. Arch Neurol. 2001;58:373-379.

[45] Funke SA, Birkmann E, Willbold D. Detection of Amyloid-beta aggregates in body fluids: a suitable method for early diagnosis of Alzheimer's disease? Curr Alzheimer Res. 2009;6(3):285-9.

CHAPTER 12

Methods for Studying and Structure–Function Relationships of Non-Fibrillar Protein Assemblies in Alzheimer's Disease and Related Disorders

Farid Rahimi[1] and Gal Bitan[2,*]

[1]Research School of Biology, Division of Biomedical Science and Biochemistry, College of Medicine, Biology, and Environment, The Australian National University, Canberra, ACT, Australia, and [2]Department of Neurology, David Geffen School of Medicine, Brain Research Institute, and Molecular Biology Institute, University of California at Los Angeles, USA

Abstract: Several neurodegenerative diseases, including Alzheimer's, Parkinson's, Huntington's, and prion diseases, are characterized by intra- and/or extracellular deposition of fibrillar proteinaceous aggregates, and by extensive, neuron loss. Related non-neuropathic systemic diseases, *e.g.*, light-chain and senile systemic amyloidoses, and other organ-specific diseases, such as dialysis-related amyloidosis and type-2 diabetes, also are characterized by deposition of aggregated proteins. It is debated whether these hallmark lesions are causative. Substantial evidence suggests that the aggregates are the end state of protein misfolding whereas the actual culprits likely are transient, non-fibrillar assemblies preceding the aggregates. The non-fibrillar, oligomeric assemblies are believed to initiate pathogenesis, leading to synaptic dysfunction, neuron loss, and pathognomonic brain atrophy. It is hypothesized that non-fibrillar assemblies or fibril-derived fragments may promote anatomical progression of pathology, or even disease transmissibility, akin to misfolded prions.

Amyloid β-protein (Aβ), which is believed to cause Alzheimer's disease, is considered an archetypal amyloidogenic protein. Intense studies have led to nominal, functional, and structural descriptions of oligomeric Aβ assemblies. However, the dynamic and metastable nature of Aβ oligomers renders their study difficult. Different results generated using different methodologies under different experimental settings further complicate this complex area of research and identification of the exact pathogenic assemblies *in vivo* seems daunting.

In this chapter we review structural, functional, and biological experiments used to produce and study non-fibrillar Aβ assemblies, and highlight similar studies of proteins involved in related diseases. We discuss challenges that contemporary researchers are facing and future research prospects in this demanding, yet highly important, field.

***Corresponding author Gal Bitan:** David Geffen School of Medicine, University of California at Los Angeles, Neuroscience Research Building 1, Room 451, 635 Charles E. Young Drive South, Los Angeles, CA 90095-7334, USA; Tel: 310-2062082; Fax: 310-2061700; E-mail: gbitan@mednet.ucla.edu

D.K. Lahiri (Ed)

Keywords: Amyloid, neurodegeneration, Alzheimer's disease, amyloid β-protein, protein misfolding, non-fibrillar assemblies, oligomers, toxicity, prion

INTRODUCTION

The "amyloid cascade hypothesis" [1], suggesting that amyloid β-protein (Aβ) fibril formation and plaque deposition lead to neuronal dysfunction, dementia, and death in Alzheimer's disease (AD), had guided scientific research into discovery of etiologic and pathogenic mechanisms of AD. However, this hypothesis has been contentiously debated because: 1) fibrillar amyloid burden does not correlate well with neurological dysfunction [2], 2) cognitive impairment in transgenic murine models of AD is observed before and/or independently of amyloid plaque formation [3], 3) plaque-independent pathology can be explained by the neurotoxicity of soluble Aβ assembly intermediates, 4) oligomer-induced memory dysfunction occurs before neuronal death, and 5) brain, plasma, and cerebrospinal fluid (CSF) concentrations of soluble Aβ oligomers correlate with neurodegeneration better than those of fibrils [4]. These observations have led to a burgeoning yet encompassing alternative paradigm hypothesizing that soluble non-fibrillar protein assemblies, rather than mature fibrillar deposits, act as proximate neurotoxins that cause synaptic dysfunction, neuron loss, dementia, and death [4-11]. This new hypothesis has been supported by discovery of toxic non-fibrillar protein assemblies involved in other protein-misfolding diseases, such as, Parkinson's disease (PD), Huntington's disease (HD), transmissible spongiform encephalopathies (TSEs), amyotrophic lateral sclerosis, polyglutamine diseases, type-2 diabetes mellitus (T2D), and systemic amyloidoses [7, 12-15].

Diversity and sometimes inaccuracy in nominal definitions, and in structural/functional descriptions of soluble non-fibrillar Aβ assemblies, along with different methodologies to generate and study these assemblies, are confounding factors in this already vast and complex research area. Various forms of soluble non-fibrillar Aβ assemblies (reviewed in [10, 16-18]) including monomeric Aβ conformers [19], secreted cell- and brain-derived low-order oligomers [20-25], Aβ-derived diffusible ligands (ADDLs) [26, 27], protofibrils (PF) [28-30], Aβ*56 [31], paranuclei [32-34], amylospheroids [35], annular assemblies [36], amyloid pores [18, 36, 37], toxic fibrillar oligomers [38], and βamy balls [39] have been described Protein Asseblies. However, despite a global concerted scientific effort, the relationships amongst these Aβ-derived assemblies and their relevance to AD pathogenesis are unclear and the fundamental quest for a unanimous pathogenic "equivalent" active in AD-afflicted brain is ongoing [9].

We begin our discussion in the first step of studying non-fibrillar Aβ assemblies—protein preparation.

SOURCES AND METHODS OF Aβ PREPARATION

The low physiological concentration and the difficulty of procuring highly pure and homogeneous tissue-derived Aβ have precluded its routine use in experimental studies *in vitro*. Therefore, synthetic Aβ preparations have emerged as alternatives. Synthetic Aβ is produced either by standard solid-phase peptide synthesis (SPPS) [40, 41] or by recombinant DNA technology [42-45].

The Aβ sequence is recognized as a "difficult" target for SPPS owing to its high hydrophobicity and innate propensity to aggregate [46-48]. To overcome these issues, various deprotecting agents [46], novel solvent systems for coupling [47], solid-support modifications [49], or microwave-assisted SPPS [50] have been used to augment synthetic yield and improve purity of crude Aβ peptides. Application of an *O–N* acyl migration reaction, also called "*O*-acyl isopeptide" chemistry was proposed as an efficient alternative SPPS route for generating Aβ with increased solubility and purity [51, 52].

Similarly, tailored recombinant or semisynthetic expression systems have been used to produce Aβ in high yields. A strategy to increase solubility and facilitate purification is co-expression of Aβ with Aβ-specific affibodies [53] or as fusions with sequences affording high solubility, followed by cleavage of the fusion protein and purification by high-performance liquid chromatography (HPLC) [42-45, 54-56]. A semisynthetic procedure for generating full-length Aβ has been reported, producing 8–10 mg of pure Aβ(1–40) per liter of bacterial culture [57].

Because self-association of Aβ is believed to be central in the pathogenesis of AD, extensive research has been dedicated to developing methodologies to characterize Aβ assemblies structurally and biologically [58]. Multiple studies have shown that many of the neurotoxic effects of Aβ assemblies can be recapitulated by synthetic Aβ *in vitro* or *in vivo* [59]. However, differences in peptide quality, presence of trace contaminants in Aβ preparations from different sources, and compositional variation of Aβ preparations, even from the same source, have been serious problems leading to irreproducible or discrepant reports and study outcomes [60-62]. For example, under identical conditions, an Aβ oligomer-specific monoclonal antibody was shown to react only with oligomers derived from recombinant Aβ but not those derived from chemically synthesized Aβ [63]. In our hands, Photo-Induced Cross-linking of Unmodified Proteins (PICUP) using Aβ obtained from different sources, but prepared identically, yielded distinct results (Fig. **1**).

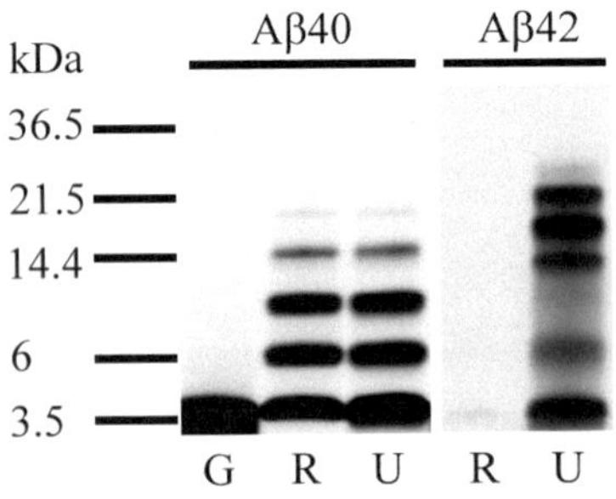

Figure 1: Comparison of photo-cross-linking using Aβ peptides from different sources. Synthetic Aβ from Global Peptide (G) and the UCLA Biopolymers Laboratory (U), and recombinant Aβ from rPeptide (R) were prepared in 10 mM sodium phosphate, pH 7.4, at 2 mg/mL nominal concentration and filtered through a 10-kDa molecular-weight cut-off filter [106]. Each filtered peptide was cross-linked using PICUP [98]. The resulting cross-linked oligomers were subjected to SDS-PAGE and silver-staining. The data suggest that Aβ40 from Global peptide contained contaminants that prevented cross-linking and that Aβ42 from rPeptide aggregated during the filtration step and was hardly detectable.

Neither SPPS nor recombinant methods can produce 100% pure Aβ. Failure sequences, oxidation of Met^{35}, and racemization may occur during various SPPS steps [58]. Similarly, Met^{35} oxidation may occur in bacterial inclusion bodies [57]. In recombinant preparations where a fusion protein is enzymatically cleaved to release Aβ, it is important to verify that the cleavage product is not contaminated with the uncleaved fusion protein, the cleaving enzyme, or adventitious proteolytic fragments [58]. Practically, it is important that the researcher verifies chemical purity of the preparation and ensures removal of residual components which could complicate solvation and stock preparation, potentially alter the biophysical and biological characteristics of the peptide, and render concentration measurements error-prone [58].

METHODS USED TO STUDY NON-FIBRILLAR Aβ ASSEMBLIES

Important biological functions of oligomeric Aβ assemblies have spurred extensive efforts to characterize them structurally. The non-crystalline nature of the oligomers and their slow tumbling time in aqueous solutions preclude high-resolution structural determination by X-ray crystallography and solution-state NMR [64], respectively. Moreover, the metastable nature of Aβ oligomers and their existence in rapidly changing mixtures have made their structural characterization particularly difficult [65, 66]. To address these issues, multiple low-resolution methods have been used to assess various structural features of non-fibrillar Aβ assemblies. Here, we outline some of the key methods used to provide structural and biophysical information on non-fibrillar Aβ assemblies.

Atomic-Resolution Techniques

NMR Spectroscopy

Solution-state NMR is a powerful high-resolution technique for determining peptide and protein structure in solution [67]. Typically, the structure is calculated based on distances and angles obtained through measurements of nuclear Overhauser effect and spin–spin scalar coupling interactions as constraints for computer-generated models. As mentioned above, peak broadening due to slow tumbling times [64] currently precludes solving structures of Aβ assemblies using solution-state NMR. However, multiple NMR studies have assessed structural properties of Aβ monomers. For instance, studies by Lee *et al.* introduced the concept of "plaque competence", which defines the propensity of near-physiological concentrations of soluble Aβ to deposit onto authentic amyloid plaques *in vitro* [68]. The plaque competence assay identified a central 26-residue fragment (Tyr^{10}–Met^{35}) which was deemed necessary to mimic plaque-deposition characteristics of the full-length Aβ [68]. Preliminary NMR conformational analyses showed that this 26-residue fragment had a different conformation from a plaque-incompetent fragment (Asp^{1}–Lys^{28}) [68]. Further NMR studies also confirmed that the central 26 residues of Aβ were sufficient to mimic amyloidogenic properties of Aβ40 and Aβ42 [69]. It was reported that the central hydrophobic cluster of full-length Aβ, and Aβ(10–35), both adopted well-defined, albeit irregular, conformations in solution, whereas the *C*- and *N*-terminal flanking regions of the full-length Aβ were partially disordered [69].

NMR studies also have highlighted differences between Aβ40 and Aβ42. Solution-phase NMR studies of non-oxidized [70] or Met-oxidized [71, 72] Aβ40 and Aβ42 showed that the *C*-terminus of Aβ42 is more rigid compared to that of Aβ40, likely due to the extended hydrophobic *C*-terminus of Aβ42. Similarly, a study combining molecular dynamics and NMR experiments, showed that the *C*-terminus of Aβ42 is more structured than that of Aβ40 [73]. NMR studies also revealed that common *C*-terminal peptide segments within Aβ40 and Aβ42 have distinct structures, which may be relevant to the strong disease association of elevated Aβ42 production [74]. Various types of NMR applications to studying of oligomeric assemblies of amyloid proteins have been reviewed recently by Bemporad *et al.* [75].

X-Ray Crystallography

X-ray crystallography examines atomic structures of crystals by X-ray diffraction techniques (reviewed in [76]). The signal is intensified by the coherent alignment and repetitive lattice of crystal structures. The wavelength of radiation used in X-ray crystallography is usually ~1.5 Å, about the length of a C–C bond. Use of X-rays with this wavelength theoretically allows resolution of individual atoms. Sawaya *et al.* reported that 33 peptide segments derived from 14 different amyloidogenic proteins formed amyloid-like fibrils, microcrystals, or both [77] and used X-ray crystallography to examine the atomic organization of molecules within microcrystals of these peptides. Microcrystals of three Aβ segments were resolved, Gly^{37}–Ala^{42}, Met^{35}–Val^{40}, and Val^{36}–Ala^{42}. The authors suggested that the structural organization of these peptides within the crystals is similar to those of Aβ fibrils and concluded that the fundamental unit of amyloid-like fibrils is a steric zipper arrangement formed by two tightly interdigitated β-sheets [77].

Hydrogen–Deuterium Exchange

Hydrogen–deuterium exchange is a powerful technique for probing protein structure and dynamics. The method involves studying of exchange rates of labile protons in proteins with deuterons from the solvent, typically D_2O. Labile protons are those bonded to nitrogen, sulfur, or oxygen. These protons can exchange with solvent hydrogen or deuterium cations. Labile protons that are solvent-exposed and are not involved in hydrogen bonding exchange rapidly, whereas buried or hydrogen-bonded protons exchange at substantially slower rates. This makes hydrogen–deuterium exchange sensitive to structural rearrangements occurring during protein aggregation. Thus, amide protons buried in the core of oligomeric and high-order assemblies or hydrogen-bonded in helices and sheets do not exchange readily with solvent deuterons. The exchange rate is detected using NMR and/or mass spectrometry [67]. For study of rapidly changing assemblies, mass spectrometric detection of exchange may be advantageous because NMR requires longer times (hours) to record the spectra, making the study of short-lived oligomers difficult. In addition, NMR requires prior assignment of protons and generally is limited to proteins smaller than 25 kDa. An additional advantage of mass spectrometric detection of exchange is requirement of substantially smaller amounts of proteins. However, assignment of specific exchanging protons using mass spectrometry requires tandem mass spectrometry and can be a daunting task, whereas for a previously assigned NMR spectrum, identification of exchanging protons is straightforward. Hydrogen–deuterium exchange coupled with mass spectrometry was used to map structural differences in Aβ PF and fibrils [78].

Determination of Oligomer Size Distribution

Sodium Dodecyl Sulfate–Polyacrylamide Gel Electrophoresis (SDS-PAGE)

SDS-PAGE is a routine and inexpensive method enabling separation of proteins based on their electrophoretic mobility, which is affected by a combination of primary, secondary, tertiary, and quaternary structures of proteins. In this method, protein mixtures are electrophoresed after treatment with SDS. SDS binds proteins *via* its hydrophobic dodecyl tail, leaving its sulfate group solvent-exposed, thus creating a negatively charged envelope that "coats" protein molecules [79]. SDS binds different polypeptides at an approximately constant mass ratio—1.4 g SDS per gram of polypeptide (reviewed in [67]). In most cases, SDS binding denatures secondary and non-disulfide-linked tertiary structures, negatively charging proteins approximately uniformly and proportionally to their mass. Under these conditions, electrophoretic migration of proteins through the gel matrix is governed directly by the molecular mass of the protein. Without SDS, different proteins of the same mass may electrophorese distinctly due to differences in overall charge (different isoelectric points) and folding.

It has been shown that at an appropriate protein–SDS molar ratio, SDS readily induces aggregation of diverse proteins at a pH two units below their respective isoelectric points (pI) with no aggregation at a pH two units above pI [80]. Electrostatic interactions were observed to play a leading role in the induction of amyloid under these conditions [80]. Importantly, the effect of SDS on all proteins is not equivalent [81]. Different proteins, different conformations of the same protein [82], or truncated versions of certain proteins [83] may not bind stoichiometric amounts of SDS. In many cases, SDS can induce or stabilize secondary and quaternary structures rather than denaturing them [82, 84, 85]. SDS may cause dissociation of some protein assemblies or conversely induce oligomerization and aggregation [85-88]. Aβ42-derived "globulomers", for example, are oligomeric assemblies produced by incubating Aβ42 with 0.2% SDS [89]. Therefore, resolution of apparently monomeric or low-molecular-weight (LMW) oligomeric components in a protein mixture does not necessarily indicate existence of such components under native conditions, *i.e.*, without SDS. Aβ is an amphipathic protein known to form SDS-stable oligomers [90]. Indeed, SDS-induced assembly of Aβ into insoluble aggregates has been capitalized on to purify Aβ from brain homogenates [91]. When treated with SDS, Aβ assembles rapidly into high-molecular-mass aggregates [63]. Furthermore, circular dichroism (CD) spectroscopy, thioflavin T fluorescence, nuclear magnetic resonance, and Fourier-transform infrared (FTIR) spectroscopy experiments have shown that Aβ40 undergoes structural transitions when treated with SDS or lithium dodecyl sulfate [92]. In this study, in solutions without SDS, Aβ40 yielded CD signals consistent with a random coil or a "statistical coil" structure [93], whereas at SDS concentration of ~4 mM (53-fold excess detergent to protein), this signal disappeared [92]. At 67-fold excess SDS, CD showed a typical β-sheet spectrum. At SDS concentrations of >10 mM (133-fold excess detergent), Aβ40 secondary structure was mainly α-helical [92]. Thus, the concept of "SDS stability" [94] in its essence is questionable in view of the fact that SDS has been used as amyloid [80, 92] or as α-helix inducer [92]. During electrophoresis of Aβ40, aggregates dissociate completely and only a monomer is observed following detection, whereas electrophoresis of Aβ42 yields apparent trimeric and tetrameric components [32]. Essentially identical monomer–trimer–tetramer distributions are observed when different preparations of Aβ42, including "monomeric", oligomeric, and fibrillar Aβ42 are analyzed by SDS-PAGE [95]. In a urea-containing SDS-PAGE system, Aβ and truncated versions thereof do not obey the law of mass–mobility relationship, likely because Aβ–SDS binding is proportional to the sum of the hydrophobicity indices, rather than the number, of constituent amino acids [83]. Thus, despite its wide use, SDS-PAGE is not a reliable method for characterization and size determination of non-covalently associated Aβ assemblies (see also [96] for a discussion of other analytical challenges in studying amyloid proteins).

Photo-Induced Cross-Linking of Unmodified Proteins (PICUP)

PICUP is a method originally developed to study stable protein homo- and hetero-oligomers [97]. PICUP was used by us and others to study oligomer size distribution of Aβ [66] and a variety of other proteins, including amyloidogenic proteins [98]. PICUP generates covalent bonds between closely interacting polypeptide chains within ≤1 *s* exposure to visible light without *pre facto* chemical modifications of the native sequence and without using spacers. The cross-linking is induced by rapid photolysis of a tris-bipyridyl Ru(II) complex in the presence of an electron acceptor. Illumination causes generation of a Ru(III) ion, which subsequently abstracts an electron from, and produces a carbon radical within, the polypeptide. The radical reacts rapidly with adjacent susceptible groups and forms covalent bonds. Therefore, PICUP stabilizes oligomer populations by covalent cross-linking, and "freezes" molecular interactions that exist before cross-linking. The mechanism, protocol, and limitations of PICUP were discussed in detail elsewhere [97-100]. Recently, a continuous-flow reactor, an "oligomerator", has been used to produce large-scale PICUP-stabilized amyloid oligomer mixtures [101]; however, purification of large quantities of single-order oligomers stabilized by PICUP still is a laborious and costly process.

Size-Exclusion Chromatography (SEC)

SEC (gel-permeation or gel-filtration chromatography) fractionates solutes based on their Stokes (hydrodynamic) radii, *i.e.*, hydrodynamic volumes (which can be correlated with molar mass) [102]. SEC is used to determine molar mass averages and molar mass distributions of solutes. SEC separation is achieved using a stationary phase comprising a porous matrix. When solutes of different sizes pass through a SEC column packed with porous material, larger molecules spend less time interacting with the solid phase and elute faster, whereas smaller molecules diffuse into the pores and therefore spend more time interacting with the solid phase and elute later. SEC affords an SDS-independent separation mechanism and covers a molecular mass range of ~10^3–10^6 Da. However, SEC provides lower resolution than SDS-PAGE and estimations of polypeptide molecular masses may be inaccurate because the elution profiles are sensitive to protein conformation. SEC analysis of Aβ assemblies does not resolve LMW assemblies but can distinguish between PF and small oligomers [90]. At this resolution, SEC may be useful for studying the kinetics involved in conversion of LMW Aβ to PF (or dissociation of PF into LMW Aβ). In addition to its use as an analytical method [39], SEC has been used extensively to purify fractions of particular Aβ assemblies [30, 32, 37, 103-105]. Description of the basic instrumentation and utilization of SEC for preparation of aggregate-free Aβ was published previously [106].

Analytical Ultracentrifugation

Analytical ultracentrifugation is a versatile technique used extensively to characterize the hydrodynamic and thermodynamic properties of proteins or macromolecules (reviewed in [67]). Conceptually, this method allows real-time quantitative analysis of spatial redistribution of soluble analytes under a high centrifugal force field. Unlabeled and unmodified proteins can be analyzed by this method in various excipients, obviating analyte–matrix interactions such as those occurring during SEC. Because molecular frictional forces oppose the centrifugal force, sedimentation depends, in addition to other parameters, on the hydrodynamic properties of the molecules, providing low-resolution information on the structure of protein complexes, thus enabling detection of conformational alterations.

This technique combines an ultracentrifuge, a multicompartmental rotor, and an optical detection system for measuring analyte concentration inside the centrifuge cell during sedimentation. The optical detection system is triggered by the revolution of the rotor, allowing data acquisition only during the extremely short intervals when a particular sample assembly aligns within the optical path. Coupled with data-analysis software, analytical ultracentrifugation can determine sample purity and molecular mass in the native state, measure sedimentation and diffusion coefficients, characterize assembly–disassembly mechanisms of complex analytes, determine subunit stoichiometry, detect and characterize macromolecular conformational changes, and measure equilibrium constants and thermodynamic parameters for homo- or hetero-associating assemblies. Two types of experiments are commonly performed using ultracentrifugation—sedimentation velocity [107, 108] and sedimentation equilibrium [109]. Typically, sedimentation-velocity experiments are conducted at relatively high rotor speeds. Under these conditions, each protein species in a mixture forms a unique boundary and sediments at a characteristic speed governed by its molecular mass, size, and shape. The velocity and shape of the moving concentration boundary is used to estimate the sedimentation coefficient, diffusion coefficient, molecular mass, and equilibrium constants of interacting species. In contrast, sedimentation-equilibrium experiments are performed at relatively low rotor speeds. The sedimentation of proteins under lower centrifugal forces than in sedimentation-velocity experiments is opposed by the diffusion, and eventually when equilibrium is reached, a time-invariant exponential concentration gradient is established throughout the centrifuge cell. The concentration gradient of proteins at equilibrium has been used widely to determine the molecular weight, stoichiometry, binding affinity, and virial coefficient of hetero-interacting or self-associating systems. Sedimentation-equilibrium experiments can analyze a mixture of moieties of different molecular masses. After each analyte reaches its equilibrium, high-molecular-mass species locate towards the cell bottom, whereas low-molecular-mass species dominate at the top. The equilibrium data can be fitted to calculated models for solute distribution. Using this type of analysis,

Huang *et al.* have reported that Aβ40 existed as an equilibrium mixture of monomers, dimers, and tetramers at neutral pH [110]. However, other equilibria, including monomer–dimer, monomer–trimer, or monomer–tetramer, produced equivalent residuals [110], hindering precise determination of the oligomerization state of the peptide. ADDLs, which are soluble, Aβ42-derived, non-fibrillar neurotoxic assemblies, have been shown to contain a high-molecular-mass component with an estimated mass of 175 kDa by sedimentation-velocity and 120–540 kDa by sedimentation-equilibrium experiments [95].

Dynamic Light Scattering (DLS) Spectroscopy

DLS, also known as quasielastic light scattering, intensity-fluctuation spectroscopy, or photon-correlation spectroscopy, is a non-invasive, nondestructive, quantitative, optical analytical method for determining diffusion coefficients of particles (0.1–3000-nm size range [111]) undergoing Brownian motion in solution (reviewed in [67]). DLS measures the temporal dependence of light scattering emanated from an analyte in solution over 10^{-7}–1 *s*. Temporal fluctuations in intensity of the scattered light relate to rate of the Brownian motion which is correlated to the diffusion coefficients, *D*, and radii of particles according to the Stokes–Einstein equation [112, 113]:

$$D = \frac{K_B T}{6\pi\eta R_h} = \frac{K_B T}{3\pi\eta D_h},$$

where K_B is Boltzmann's constant, T is the absolute temperature, η is the viscosity of the suspending liquid, and R_h and D_h are the hydrodynamic radius and diameter, respectively. Knowledge of diffusion coefficients of molecules allows determination of molecular features, including size and flexibility. Temporal changes in these parameters provide information about the kinetics and structural transitions occurring, *e.g.*, during protein assembly–disassembly processes. In a polydisperse mixture, a distribution of diffusion coefficients is obtained.

DLS is intrinsically biased for large aggregates because the intensity of the scattered light is proportional to the square of the particle mass [114]. Therefore, DLS is suited well to measure minute amounts of protein aggregates (<0.01% by weight) on the background of monomers and small oligomers. For large or extended proteins (rod-like/unfolded), scattering varies significantly with angle [115]. Determining scattering at additional angles by multi-angle laser-light scattering (MALLS) allows direct measurements of masses up to MDa ranges. Because the light-scattering signal is directly proportional to protein concentration and molecular mass, a combination of DLS signal and concentration measurements using refractive indexes or absorbance, allows calculation of the molecular mass of each component when proteins are fractionated chromatographically. DLS can resolve the monomeric and dimeric state of a protein if the shape of the protein is known, but it cannot distinguish among small oligomers when their hydrodynamic radii differ by less than a factor of 2 [116] or between, for example, a compact dimer and an extended monomer. Consequently, DLS is less useful for analyzing individual small oligomers than SEC-MALLS, PICUP coupled with SDS-PAGE, or sedimentation-velocity analytical ultracentrifugation. Because DLS allows monitoring protein assembly without analyte manipulation or consumption, it has been used widely to study Aβ aggregation and assembly processes [32, 104, 117-121]. Solution state and size distribution of ADDLs have been assessed by Hepler *et al.* using SEC coupled with MALLS [95]. Walsh *et al.* reported studies using DLS and other techniques examining early stages of Aβ oligomerization and characterization of Aβ intermediates during fibrillogenesis [90]. Detailed accounts of the theory and practice of DLS and its application to study of Aβ were given by Lomakin *et al.* [114, 122, 123].

Ion-Mobility Spectroscopy–Mass Spectrometry (IMS–MS)

IMS–MS is a mass-spectrometric method that can resolve molecules of identical mass-to-charge (*m/z*) values differing by collision cross-section, which in turn correlates with assembly state or conformation [124]. An IMS–MS instrument performs five basic processes: sample introduction, compound ionization, ion-mobility separation, mass separation, and ion detection [125]. Four types of IMS are used: drift-time, aspiration, differential, and traveling-wave IMS. Drift-time IMS is operated under either ambient pressure or reduced pressure. Aspiration and differential IMS are operated under ambient pressure, whereas traveling-wave IMS is performed under reduced-pressure conditions. Each of these IMS setups can be interfaced with a variety of mass spectrometers, including time-of-flight, quadrupole, ion-trap, ion-cyclotron, or magnetic-sector mass spectrometers.

In traditional drift-time IMS–MS, ions are carried by a weak, uniform electric field through a drift cell. In the drift cell, the anlytes collide at low velocity with a low-pressure inert gas (typically helium) such that the collision thermal energy due to the buffer gas is greater than the energy the ions obtain from the electric field. Under this principal condition, ions have energies similar to that of the buffer gas so that they undergo a directional diffusion process. Under these low-field conditions, the drift velocity of ions is directly proportional to the electric field but inversely proportional to their collision cross-section. This proportionality is defined by the ion-mobility constant, K, which is related to the ionic cross-section by

$$K = \left(\frac{3q}{16N}\right)\sqrt{\left(\frac{2\pi}{kT}\right)}\sqrt{\left(\frac{m+M}{mM}\right)}\left(\frac{1}{\Omega}\right),$$

where q is the ion charge, N is the number density of the buffer gas, k is Boltzmann's constant, T is the absolute temperature, m is the mass of the buffer gas, M is the mass of the ion, and Ω is the collision cross-section of the ion [124]. Under low-velocity, low-pressure conditions, the analyte ions quickly reach equilibrium resulting in a constant drift velocity. Because at equilibrium ion mobility is inversely proportional to collisional cross-section, in the case of a mixture of protein assemblies, conformers/ions with compact structures and smaller cross-section have higher mobility and drift faster through the cell than ions with larger cross-sections. The ions exit the drift cell, pass through a mass filter, and are detected as a function of time, producing a temporal arrival distribution. The traditional drift-time IMS is the only type allowing measurement of collision cross-section of ions.

Protein oligomers often have identical *m/z* ratio (*i.e.*, a singly charged monomer would have the same *m/z* as a doubly charged dimer, triply charged trimer, *etc.*). IMS–MS analysis can resolve these species yielding an assembly size distribution. IMS–MS studies of Aβ have shown that freshly prepared low-molecular-mass Aβ40 contained monomers, dimers, trimers, and tetramers, whereas similarly prepared solutions of Aβ42 comprised oligomers up to a dodecamer [126]. These results accord with earlier observations of distinct oligomer size distributions of Aβ40 and Aβ42 by PICUP [32] and may explain differences in neurotoxic effects of the two Aβ alloforms.

Utilization of gas-phase approaches such as IMS has led to accumulation of extensive evidence that ESI [and to some extent matrix-assisted laser desorption ionization (MALDI)] can produce ions that retain key structural aspects of proteins in solution [127]. In particular, the dependence of protein conformation on solution conditions, *e.g.*, pH and excipient composition, in IMS and field-asymmetric ion-mobility spectrometry (FAIMS) shows that gas-phase measurements can concord with protein conformations in solution [127]. Furthermore, 2D FAIMS–IMS separations coupled with MS can reveal many more protein conformations, including low-abundance conformations, than either FAIMS or IMS [127], suggesting that IMS–MS and IMS–IMS–MS offer great potential in the dissection of protein conformational dynamics, a feat currently unachievable by other biophysical techniques.

Analysis of Secondary Structure

Circular Dichroism (CD) Spectroscopy

CD is the change in the absorption of circularly polarized light as a function of wavelength exhibited by optically active molecules. Because secondary structural elements such as α-helices, β-strands, β-turns, and disordered regions display characteristic wavelength-dependent dichroism, CD is a useful method to determine secondary structure of proteins. Secondary structure analysis of peptides and proteins by CD spectroscopy uses "far-UV" spectra (180–250 nm), in which the chromophores are peptide bonds due to the effect of the dihedral angle of peptide bonds on the absorption of the chiral center at the α-carbon. In contrast, near-UV CD spectra (250–350 nm) reflect contributions of aromatic side-chains and disulfide bonds and provide information about polypeptide tertiary structure [128].

Samples for CD spectroscopy typically are dissolved in aqueous buffers with or without co-solvents. Because most of the structural information of proteins is obtained in the far-UV range, the buffer and co-solvent choices are critical. Several chemical bonds have strong absorption in this range. Hence, buffers with minimal absorption in the far-UV range should be chosen. A typical buffer used in CD experiments is 10 mM sodium phosphate [128].

The CD signal reflects an average of the entire ensemble of molecular structures. Quantitative assessment of secondary structures can be achieved by deconvolution of experimental spectra using libraries of existing known structures [129]. Therefore, CD can only determine the overall proportion of secondary structural elements, but not the amino acid residues involved or the fraction of molecules with a particular conformation. Thus, on the basis of CD data alone, it is impossible to distinguish, for example, between a situation in which part of a protein monomer is α-helical and another in β-sheet conformation, and a heterogeneous population in which a portion of the monomers are purely helical and another portion entirely in a β-sheet conformation.

CD has been used extensively to investigate secondary structures of Aβ peptides and to monitor structural transitions of Aβ during its oligomerization and aggregation [30, 130-133].

Fourier-Transform Infrared (FTIR) Spectroscopy

Complementary to CD, FTIR enables determination of the secondary structure of protein samples as thin films, as solids, or in solution. Characteristic bands in IR spectra of proteins and polypeptides include predominantly amide I and amide II. The amide-I band corresponds to the absorption in the vibrational spectrum of the C=O component of the amide bond (1600–1700 cm^{-1}), whereas C–N stretching and C–N–H bending vibrations give rise to absorption bands at 1550 cm^{-1} (amide II) and 1250 cm^{-1} (amide III), which are useful for assigning secondary structures. Because C=O and N–H bonds are involved in hydrogen bonding, the absorption wavelength of both amide-I and amide-II bands are sensitive to the secondary structure content of proteins. In many cases, instead of a series of well-resolved peaks for each type of secondary structure, one broad peak is observed. However, for proteins that cannot be studied by high-resolution methods, FTIR provides useful structural information. It is thought that FTIR is more sensitive to β-sheet content whereas CD measurements generally tend to underestimate β-sheet relative to α-helix content [134]. The main bands of interest in the amide-I region for detection of β-strand alignments are at 1626 and 1632 cm^{-1} for parallel β-sheet and at 1690 cm^{-1} for antiparallel β-sheet structures. The signature of statistical coil [93] (extended, irregular structure with distinct spectroscopic features) is a band at 1644 cm^{-1} and that of α-helix is a band at 1654 cm^{-1}. However, α-helical conformations also contribute to band intensities at 1644 and 1662 cm^{-1}, making distinction from statistical coil difficult. Non-α and non-β structures appear at <1660 cm^{-1}. Although strong signals corresponding to particular secondary structures exist in this region, information in IR spectra obtained in aqueous buffers is masked by a strong signal at 1630 cm^{-1} due to water bending vibrations. Hence, alternative strategies have been adopted to probe the secondary structure of proteins in general, and amyloidogenic proteins in particular, with IR spectroscopy. Isotopic substitution has far-reaching effects on IR absorption. The peak positions of $^{13}C{=}O$ and $C{=}^{18}O$ stretching bands shift to lower frequency relative to $^{12}C{=}^{16}O$ bands. Isotopic labeling thus allows assignment of secondary structures at a single-residue level. For example, for α-helix, the $^{13}C{=}O$ appears at 1600 cm^{-1}, whereas $^{13}C{=}O$ β-sheet bands are at 1586 cm^{-1} (parallel) and 1595 cm^{-1} (antiparallel). Another isotopic labeling strategy is changing the solvent from H_2O to D_2O. This shifts the water bending vibration peak from 1630 to 1290 cm^{-1} facilitating measurement in the amide-I region. FTIR has been used extensively to study the conformational changes of Aβ during assembly [135-139].

By two-dimensional IR and isotope labeling, Aβ40-derived amyloid fibrils were shown to contain significant amount of mobile water molecules trapped within the inter-sheet space in the fibril structures [140]. Woys *et al.* reported novel quantitative structural parameters for measuring parallel β-sheet vibrational couplings by two-dimensional IR [141]. Recently, isotope labeling and kinetic two-dimensional infrared spectroscopy were used to obtain residue-specific structural information in a complex of human islet amyloid polypeptide (IAPP, also called amylin) with rat IAPP, which inhibits the aggregation of human IAPP [142]. It was revealed that significant structural rearrangements continued to occur after the system had apparently reached equilibrium assessed by a thioflavin T (ThT) fluorescence assay. Rat IAPP was found to block *N*-terminal, rather than *C*-terminal, β-sheet formation at 8 h after mixing with human IAPP, whereas at 24 h, rat IAPP formed its own β-sheet fibrils without blocking human IAPP β-sheet formation [142]. These exemplary studies indicate that FTIR and 2D IR spectroscopic studies are important quantitative tools for elucidating amyloid structures or amyloid–inhibitor interactions.

Morphological Analysis

Transmission Electron Microscopy (TEM)

TEM uses a cathode-ray source that emits and accelerates a high-voltage electron beam focused by electrostatic and electromagnetic lenses. When the electron beam passes through a thin, electron-transparent specimen, it carries information about the inner structure of the sample as it reaches the TEM imaging system. There, the spatial variation in this information, which creates the image, is magnified by a series of electromagnetic lenses and detected by a fluorescent screen, photographic plate, or a light-sensitive sensor, *e.g.*, a charge-coupled device or a camera. Macromolecular specimens are applied typically onto a fine, metallic grid support coated by a thin, electron-transparent carbon film. Because biological macromolecules have nearly identical density to that of the carbon film, unstained macromolecules have intrinsically low contrast when viewed by TEM. To enhance contrast and reduce image noise, several strategies, including negative staining [143, 144], rotary shadowing [145], and cryo-EM [146], are used. In negative staining, the stain circumscribes the macromolecule, the shape of which is deduced from distribution of the stain, which scatters most of the electrons. In shadowing experiments, heavy metals are applied by evaporation to form a thin coating on specimens and enhance contrast. Metals may be evaporated unidirectionally either onto a static or a rotating specimen while shadowing takes place. In cryo-EM, the hydrated specimen is preserved in a thin vitreous film of ice maintained at −180°C preventing both its sublimation and crystallization. Cryo-EM also circumvents the need for staining. Examples for using TEM to characterize various assembly states of Aβ include LMW Aβ [32, 33], small Aβ oligomers [147-150], paranuclei [32, 33], PF [30, 104, 105, 121], and fibrils [90, 121, 151]. Cryo-EM was used to resolve the structure of Aβ42 fibrils, which comprised regularly spaced (~45 Å) protofilaments that twist regularly along the fibril axis [152].

Scanning Transmission Electron Microscopy (STEM)

In STEM, a high-energy (100 kV) electron beam scans the specimen and scattered electrons are collected by various types of detectors located behind the specimen. Commonly, the detectors include electron-energy-loss spectrometers, X-ray emission spectrometers, and cathodoluminiscence spectrometers (reviewed in [67]). The specimen image is generated as the focused beam moves step by step over the specimen. In a thin proteinaceous specimen, the image intensity is directly proportional to the mass of the irradiated region. Therefore, following background subtraction and calibration, the protein mass and mass-per-length unit (MPL) can be determined quantitatively [153]. Of note, other biophysical techniques, including DLS and analytical ultracentrifugation can monitor quaternary structural alterations during amyloid fibril formation and enable measuring average molecular masses reflecting the distribution of an ensemble of quaternary structures in solution. However, the size and morphological heterogeneity of the intermediate structures during fibrillogenesis preclude assignment of molecular mass averages to a particular quaternary structural element. In contrast, STEM captures images of isolated and unstained specimens, allowing for accurate, quantitative mass determination of individual molecules or macromolecular assemblies [154].

STEM is an excellent tool for characterizing the homogeneity and structural properties of transient quaternary structure intermediates in amyloid fibril-formation pathways. STEM has been used to characterize the MPL ratios of Aβ fibrils and PF [155-157]. A brief history of STEM, description of STEM mass mapping, and advantages and limitations of STEM have been reviewed by Wall *et al.* [158].

Atomic-Force Microscopy (AFM)

AFM captures high-resolution (≤1 nm) topography of a sample adsorbed on an atomically flat smooth surface, typically mica. A cantilever tip samples the surface contour of a specimen and when the tip contacts a spot on the adsorbed sample, an ionic repulsive force (pN–nN range) bends the cantilever upwards. The extent of bending, measured by a laser, is translated to force units by a photodetector. By keeping the force constant while scanning across the surface, the vertical movement of the tip generates the surface contour, which is recorded as a topographic map of the sample. AFM has been modified for specific applications and can be used in different modes. In "tapping mode" (also dubbed "intermittent-contact" or "dynamic-force mode"), a stiff cantilever oscillates close to the sample. Part of the oscillation extends into the repulsive regime so that the tip intermittently touches, or taps, the surface. This mode provides good resolution of soft samples and thus is useful for investigation of non-fibrillar Aβ species.

An advantage of AFM over TEM is that it allows continuous monitoring of the growth of Aβ oligomers [159]. Multiple studies on the structure of soluble oligomers have used conventional tapping-mode AFM [26, 30, 90, 160-163]. Individual Aβ42 oligomers have been studied by AFM following dilution of the sample to concentrations that practically arrest oligomer growth. The smallest size of individual oligomers that could be observed by AFM corresponded to a height of ~1–4 nm and were interpreted as folded monomers [139, 164].

Scanning Tunneling Microscopy (STM)

STM is a non-optical microscopic technique based on principles of quantum mechanics. The electron cloud of atoms in a sample extends a minute distance above the sample surface. An *x–y–z* piezoelectric translator controls the movement of the tip in three dimensions. When a probe, with a tip as sharp as a single atom, is brought sufficiently close to such a surface and a small voltage is applied, a strong interaction occurs between the electron cloud on the surface and the tip, leading to an electric tunneling current. The magnitude of the current depends exponentially on the distance between the probe and the surface. The tunneling current rapidly increases as the distance between the tip and the surface decreases. This rapid alteration in the current due to changes in distance results in construction of an atomically resolved image when the tip scans the structure. The feedback signal, applied to a piezoelectric element provides a measure of molecular surface contours. The principles and applications of STM in technology and biology have been reviewed by Hansma *et al.* [165]. Initial low-resolution STM studies of Aβ showed the ribbon-like filamentous nature of Aβ fibrils [166]. Later studies showed that Aβ fibrils contained laterally associated filaments that exhibited a right-handed twist [163]. STM was used to examine the structure of Aβ40 monomers, dimers, and oligomers on a surface of atomically flat gold [167]. At low concentrations (0.5 μM) small globular structures were observed. High-resolution STM measurements of Aβ samples, both immediately following preparation and after 24-h aging, found structures of ~3–4 nm in diameter corresponding to oligomeric Aβ. These results suggested that oligomer formation could potentially proceed through a mechanism involving linear association of monomers [167].

STRUCTURAL AND BIOLOGICAL STUDIES OF NON-FIBRILLAR Aβ ASSEMBLIES

The use of proper terminology to describe soluble non-fibrillar Aβ assemblies is crucial to forming consensus in the literature. However, achieving this goal is difficult because various *in vitro* oligomeric entities of Aβ have been described structurally, functionally, or both and the relationship or kinship amongst them are unclear [65]. Although all these structures are oligomeric, the use of the term "oligomer" to describe all the assemblies may be misleading for at least three reasons, as discussed before: 1) the structure of each assembly is unique; 2) the pathways leading to the formation of the assemblies or the ultimate path they may take towards fibrillization may differ; 3) the biological activities of each assembly may differ or similar activities may be mediated through different mechanisms [63]; and 4) methods used to study and determine the oligomeric state may differ. Adding to this complexity is the fact that no single oligomeric species remain structurally unique under test conditions because of the metastable nature of oligomers [65]. Furthermore, detection of oligomeric state has to be strictly defined and distinguished contextually—whether they have been studied or shown *in vitro* or *in vivo*. In the following section, we describe non-fibrillar Aβ species ranging from monomers to PF (Table **1**). In most cases, we begin with structural characterization of each species followed by discussion of its biological activity.

Table 1: Summary of structural and biological characteristics of non-fibrillar Aβ assemblies.

Assembly	**Structural Characteristics/Production**	**Biological Activity**
"Activated monomeric conformer" of Aβ	• Produced during aggregation of Aβ40 by constant rotary shaking. • Measured by turbidity assay and HPLC. • Postulated to be an oxidative or hydrolytic derivative of Aβ [19, 168]. • The monomeric nature of these conformers is not confirmed unambiguously.	• Forms 2–3-fold more complexes with apoE4 than apoE2 or apoE3 [168]. • Enhances toxicity and apoptotic activity in neurons [19]. • Inhibits action potential by blocking fast, inward tetrodotoxin-sensitive Na^+ channels [169]
Natural cell-derived Aβ oligomers	• Predominantly dimers, trimers, and tetramers, produced by CHO cells transfected with mutated or wild-type APP [23, 170]. • Resistant to SDS denaturation (see our discussions about "SDS stability" under "Determination of Oligomer Size Distribution") and to cleavage by insulin degrading enzyme [24].	• Inhibit LTP *in vivo* [24]. • Enhance LTD by mGluR or NMDAR activity [171]. • Impair short-term memory in rats [172]. • Cause dendritic spine loss [173]. • Affect synaptic structure and function. • Cognitive impairment in mice [94]. • It was suggested that apparent toxic effects mediated by dimers were attributable to relatively stable, dimer-derived PF [174].
Aβ-derived diffusible ligands (ADDLs)	• Synthetic species formed in the presence of apolipoprotein J [175], in F-12 media [176], or in PBS [177]. • Small globules 3–8 nm in diameter	• Highly neurotoxic [26, 179]. • Inhibit LTP [26]. • Bind to neuronal surfaces [59] co-localizing with neuronal proteins at

Assembly	Structural Characteristics/Production	Biological Activity
	measured by AFM [178]. • Polydisperse mixtures of 150–1,000 kDa determined by MALLS [95]. • A11-positive [65].	postsynaptic punctate sites [180, 181] and NR1 and NR2B subunits of NMDAR [180, 181]. • Promote oxidative stress and increased $[Ca^{2+}]_i$ [182]. • Induce τ phosphorylation [177] and misfolding [183]. • Induce IL-1β, iNOS, NO and TNF-α in astrocytes [184]. • Abnormal mitochondrial distribution in neurites caused by impaired τ-dependent axonal transport [183, 185]
Protofibrils (PF)	• Curvilinear fibril-like structures 6–8 nm in diameter and ≤200 nm long by TEM [90]; a periodicity of 20 nm and diameter of 4.3 nm were determined by AFM [161]. • Rich in β-sheet structure. • Bind Congo red and thioflavin T [10]. • Aβ40Ser26Cys dimers stabilized by disulfide bonding form stable PF (comprising ~100–450 monomers), which do not readily sediment unlike typical amyloid fibrils [174]. • These species were relatively stable because PF persisted even after a one-month-long incubation period in certain samples at 37°C [174].	• Increase EPSCs [29], and cause cell death [29, 30]. • May activate NMDAR in contrast to fibrils which activate non-NMDA glutamate receptors [186]. • Patch-clamping using Aβ42 PF induces reversible, Ca^{2+}-dependent increase in spontaneous action potentials and membrane depolarizations. • Can inhibit the A- and D-type K^+ currents, but not other outward/inward rectifying K^+ channels. • PF-induced membrane activity increases $[Ca^{2+}]_i$ spikes [187]. • Aβ40 containing the E22G substitution forms PF faster and in larger quantities than wild-type Aβ *in vitro*, suggesting that PF may be the main disease-causing agents in carriers of the Arctic mutation [188]. • Stable, dimer-derived PF inhibit LTP [174].
Aβ*56	• Extracted from brains of *Tg2576* mice and isolated by immunoaffinity and SEC [31].	• Concentration correlates with degree of cognitive deficits. • Cause defects in long-term spatial memory in rats (micromolar concentrations) [31, 94]. • NMDAR-dependent synaptotoxicity, but no cytotoxicity (reviewed in [65]). • Concentration-dependent cognitive deficits in rats by an Alternating Lever Cyclic Ratio (ALCR) cognitive assay [94]

Assembly	Structural Characteristics/Production	Biological Activity
Amyloid pores	• Channel-like structures of synthetic Aβ, having outer diameter of 8–12 nm and inner diameter of 2–2.5 nm, associated with artificial membrane bilayers [18, 36] .	• Pore- and channel-forming capacity that may lead to membrane leakage and increased $[Ca^{2+}]_i$ [18, 36].
Toxic fibrillar oligomers of Aβ (TABFOs)	• Aβ42-derived fibrillar conformation or lattice reactive with OC, but not A11, antibody [38, 189, 190]. • Can seed formation of additional fibrillar oligomers, but not fibrils [191]. • $M_r = 80{,}000 \pm 20{,}000$; β-sheet-rich; α-helix-poor [190].	• Cytotoxicity likely mediated by pore-forming capacity predicted by modeling studies [190]
Double-cysteine mutant Aβ42 PF	• Stabilized by intramolecular disulfide bonds, which forms a β-sheet-rich structure that does not form fibrils [192]. • Weak reactivity with A11 [192].	• Synaptotoxicity [65]. • Caspase activation in human neuroblastoma cells [192]
"SDS-stable" brain-derived dimers and synthetic dimers (Aβ40Ser26Cys)	• 8–12 kDa assemblies. • 3–4 nm height. • No detectable secondary structure. • For a discussion on the concept of "SDS-stability" refer to "Determination of Oligomer Size Distribution".	• LTP impairment [193]. • τ phosphorylation in primary neurons [194]. • Not cytotoxic to primary neurons (micromolar concentration), but toxic to neurons co-cultured with microglia [149]. • It was suggested that the Aβ40Ser26Cys dimers were not cytotoxic and the initial toxicity described for these dimers [193, 195] was attributed to PF, which may have formed during frozen storage of the Aβ40Ser26Cys samples [174].
Annular Aβ42-derived protofibrils (APF)	• Off-path Aβ42 assemblies arranged as hexamers [196]. • Weakly reactive with A11 [197]. • Form pores with outer diameter of 11–14 nm and inner diameter of 2.5–4 nm [196]. • Highly reactive with an anti-serum raised against APF (αAPF), which was shown to react also with fibrils and oligomeric assemblies of Aβ42 [197].	• Postulated to cause Ca^{2+} overload and cytotoxicity [196]. • Immunoreactivity of αAPF was observed in tissues from AD brains leading to the conclusion that annular amyloid pores are present in AD brain tissues [196]; however, the same antibody was shown to react with oligomeric and fibrillar assemblies of Aβ42 [197].
Amylospheroids	• 10–15-nm spherical Aβ40- or Aβ42-derived assemblies [35] which are A11-negative (reviewed in [65])	• τ protein kinase 1/GSK-3β activation [35]. • NMDAR-independent cytotoxicity in neurons at high picomolar to low nanomolar concentrations [198, 199].

"Activated Monomeric Conformer" of Aβ

Structural Characterization

Monomer activation denotes a conformational change preceding Aβ self-assembly that may render monomers toxic, or cause their nucleation and further aggregation, or both. Based on concepts taken from actin polymerization [200] and a kinetic model of Aβ aggregation induced by constant rotary shaking, Taylor *et al.* introduced the idea of "activated monomeric conformers" of Aβ40 [19], also called "intermediate aggregated species" [168]. It was postulated that this moiety was an oxidative or hydrolytic derivative or a slowly folding conformer of intact Aβ40 [19, 168]. It was proposed that the "inactive" monomer slowly converted into the "activated" monomeric conformer, several of which may cooperate to form growing nidi for oligomerization and progression of aggregation [19]. In these studies, the presence of the active monomeric Aβ conformer was tested by HPLC using acetonitrile and trifluoroacetic acid, which might have caused structural alterations in Aβ sequence by increasing its β-sheet content [201]. Lee *et al.* have provided evidence that Aβ aggregation intermediates and final structures formed under slowly agitated or quiescent conditions at 37°C differed in their toxicity, stability to denaturants, and apparent morphologies [202], emphasizing that parametrical consideration of methods used to prepare Aβ for structural or biological studies and proper methods to assess the assembly state of the resulting preparations are paramount [58]. Similarly, NMR studies emphasize the importance of performing structural studies under physiological conditions [71] rather than "structure-inducing" milieus as reported by Taylor *et al.* [19].

Other studies also have shown presence of Aβ intermediates; however, the assembly states of these were not determined unambiguously. A study by Chimon *et al.* described Aβ40 intermediates that contained a β-sheet-rich character and were thought to originate from a monomeric state, preceding PF and fibril formation [203]. Filtration experiments showed that these intermediates were not monomeric but were likely larger than decamers, indicating that unambiguous determination of the assembly intermediates is difficult. By electron microscopy, these intermediates had a spherical morphology similar to ADDLs [178], amylospheroids [35], and βamy balls [39]. NMR studies showed that the intermediate species were well-ordered in the hydrophobic core and the *C*-

terminal region [203]. Aβ40 was used in this study at higher concentrations than those found in biological specimens and the possibility that the intermediates could have undergone fibril formation during preparation for NMR studies was not excluded. Similarly, Lim *et al.* provided evidence for presence of monomeric intermediates using CD and NMR studies of Aβ40 and Aβ42 under both non-amyloidogenic (<5°C) and amyloid-promoting conditions (>5°C) at physiological pH [132]. CD studies suggested that the initially unfolded Aβ peptides at low temperature gradually transformed to β-sheet-containing monomeric intermediates at stronger amyloidogenic conditions (higher temperatures) [132]. However, exclusive presence of monomers after dialysis of 1,1,1,3,3,3-hexafluoro-2-isopropanol (HFIP)-treated Aβ species against phosphate buffer was not confirmed [132]. Providing formal proof for the presence of Aβ monomers exclusively is difficult and has not been achieved unambiguously in the studies mentioned above. Therefore, whether a critical conformational change in the monomer occurs before self-assembly, or the conformational change and the assembly occur concurrently and co-dependently remains an open question.

Biological Activity

In cell biological studies, toxicity and apoptotic activity were enhanced when the concentration of the "activated monomeric conformer" described by Taylor *et al.* was maximal during the aggregation continuum [19]. Similarly, in electrophysiologic experiments, Aβ species described as monomeric conformers obtained between ~60–120 min during rotary-shaken aggregation inhibited neuronal action potentials [169]. This neurotoxicity was attributed only to the "active" monomeric conformers detected at 60 min after the initiation of aggregation but not to inactive monomers or fully formed aggregates [19, 168, 169]. In these studies, the kinetics of aggregation was monitored by turbidity and the loss of the starting low-molecular-mass material was monitored by HPLC [19]. The sensitivity of turbidity measurements for detection of small particles is substantially lower than that of DLS and it is thus unlikely that the method can distinguish monomers from small oligomers. Also of note is that biological activities similar to those obtained by Taylor *et al.* [19] have been described for Aβ oligomers [59], thus it is unclear that these toxicity data can be ascribed to monomeric Aβ.

Brain- and Cell-Derived Low-Order Aβ Oligomers

Structural Characterization

Dimeric and trimeric assemblies of Aβ have been isolated from amyloid plaque cores [20], CSF [22], and human cortical homogenates [21], and produced by cells transfected with amyloid β-protein precursor (APP) [23]. Dimeric and trimeric Aβ (apparent SDS-PAGE mobility corresponding to ~9 and ~13.5 kDa) purified from neuritic plaques and leptomeningeal mural amyloid, were characterized by SEC, AFM, and electron microscopy [149]. MALDI mass spectrometry was used to determine the mass of the "dimeric" components [149]. However, to extract Aβ from tissue sources, SDS was included in extraction buffers and the possibility that these Aβ species could form during the extraction process, *ex vivo*, was not excluded. In fact, SDS has been shown to be a useful amyloid inducer under certain pH and protein–SDS stoichiometric conditions [80]. Immunoaffinity purification, HPLC, and MALDI analyses of CSF from patients suffering from meningitides and other neurological conditions, including dementia, revealed Aβ species of various length, including two truncated trimer species—$(Asp^{1}–Met^{35})_3$ and $(His^{6}–Ala^{42})_3$— and an Aβ40 dimer, $(Asp^{1}–Val^{40})_2$ [22]. Aβ in CSF was shown to be associated with high-density-lipoprotein particles in an apparently monomeric form detected by SDS-PAGE [204, 205]. Similarly, 24% and 27% of brain Aβ40 and Aβ42, respectively, were shown to be concentrated in lipid-raft extracts as dimers determined by SDS-PAGE in the *Tg2576* murine model of AD [206]. However, as discussed previously, SDS-PAGE is not a reliable method for Aβ size determination [63] and presence of SDS in buffers used to extract Aβ species makes assessment of these *ex vivo* findings questionable [63, 65] in relation to what is actually present *in vivo*.

Walsh *et al.* have reported "natural" Aβ oligomers that are "SDS-stable", low-order oligomers (dimers, trimers, and tetramers) detected in the conditioned media and/or lysates of cells [23, 25, 170, 207, 208]. These oligomers are produced by Chinese hamster ovarian cells that express human mutant (V717F, V717I, or E693Q, cells referred to as 7PA2), or wild-type APP [23, 209]. Low-abundance species of masses ~10, 14, and sometimes 16 kDa, which were reactive with antibodies against Aβ also were detected in the culture media of these cells [23]. The nature of these low-order oligomers is not fully understood but the observation that they are not disassembled by several types of denaturants suggests that they may be covalently linked [25].

Biological Activity

Initially, biological effects of oligomeric Aβ fractions purified from neuritic plaques and leptomeningeal mural deposits were investigated in an *ex vivo* astroglial–neuronal co-culture system believed to approximate *in vivo* conditions [149]. Neuronal viability was compromised by AD-derived Aβ only when microglial cells were co-cultured, indicating that toxicity was mediated through a microglia-dependent mechanism [149].

Ease of maintenance and fast growth-rate of 7PA2 cells facilitated investigations of the biological activities of "natural", cell-derived Aβ oligomers. Intracerebroventricular microinjection of small volumes (~1.5 μL containing ~3 ng/mL Aβ) of SEC-fractionated cell-culture media to anesthetized wild-type rats was shown to inhibit hippocampal long-term potentiation (LTP) [24, 210]. This inhibition was predominantly mediated by Aβ trimers in wild-type murine hippocampal brain slices, whereas dimers and tetramers had intermediate potencies, and monomers were apparently ineffective [208]. Cell-derived oligomers were shown to interfere primarily with LTP induction, but not its expression, once the signaling cascades responsible for LTP were initiated [208]. These results suggested that cell-derived oligomeric Aβ assemblies altered certain aspects of hippocampal synaptic plasticity both *in vivo* and *in vitro* (reviewed in [211]).

The validity of LTP as an electrophysiological paradigm for learning and memory composition has been debated [212]. To test the effect of the "natural Aβ oligomers" in a non-LTP paradigm, Cleary *et al.* used an *in vivo* behavioral model in rats that were injected with cell-conditioned media containing Aβ assemblies into the dorsal lateral cerebral ventricles. This treatment was found to transiently interrupt pre-learned behaviors [172]. This was attributed to Aβ oligomers because SEC fractions containing oligomers caused the deficits, whereas monomer-containing fractions were ineffective [172].

Actin-based cytoskeletal network dynamics is critical for regulation of neuronal spine morphology and function [213]. Alterations in spine morphology and actin-regulatory mechanisms recently have emerged as sensitive measures of early neuronal functional deficits and neurotoxicity [180, 214, 215]. Because loss of synaptic termini strongly correlates with the severity of dementia, Shankar *et al.* assessed the effect of cell-derived soluble oligomers on synapses [173]. They showed that the density of dendritic spines decreased substantially in neurons treated with sub-nanomolar levels of cell-derived Aβ oligomers [173]. This effect was shown to be specific to Aβ oligomers, *i.e.*, SEC monomer fractions alone were ineffective. The decrease in spine density was reversed by monoclonal immunodepletion of Aβ, by transfer of cells back into the control media, and by *scyllo*-inositol [173], a molecule thought to stabilize synthetic Aβ as nontoxic species, possibly preventing Aβ interaction with neuronal target proteins [216, 217].

In cultures of dissociated cortical neurons, synthetic Aβ was shown to activate nicotinic acetylcholine receptors (nAchRs) and trigger internalization of *N*-methyl-D-aspartate (NMDA) receptors (NMDARs) [218]. However, Shankar *et al.* found that an irreversible nAchR antagonist did not affect Aβ-oligomer-mediated spine loss, indicating that nAchR activity was unnecessary for this effect [173]. Signaling cascades involving NMDARs, cofilin, and calcineurin were found to be involved in Aβ-induced spine loss as determined by inhibition studies [173]. Together, these data demonstrated that cell-derived low-order Aβ oligomers could cause reduction of synapse density and loss of electrophysiologically active synapses in hippocampal pyramidal neurons, suggesting that their deleterious effects may be important mechanistic contributors to synaptic dysfunction in AD *in vivo* [211].

Aβ-Derived Diffusible Ligands (ADDLs)

Structural Characterization

ADDLs are exclusively Aβ42-derived soluble non-fibrillar assemblies that morphologically appear as 3–8-nm globules by AFM [26, 178] and have estimated masses between 17–42 kDa [26] (reviewed in [176]). It was first observed that apolipoprotein J (also called clusterin, a ubiquitous multifunctional glycoprotein co-localizing with fibrillar deposits in systemic/localized amyloid disorders [219]) partially inhibited Aβ aggregation and caused formation of "slowly precipitating" Aβ42 complexes of >200 kDa [175]. Follow-up studies showed that ADDLs with the same biochemical and neurotoxic characteristics could be produced in clusterin-free solutions by incubating aggregate-free Aβ42 in phenol-red-free F-12 medium at

4–8°C for 24 h, in clusterin-free brain-slice culture media at 37°C for 24 h [26, 176], or even in phosphate-buffered saline [177].

By SEC, ADDL preparations contained two distinct peaks—an early-eluting high-mass component, which exhibited punctate binding to primary neurons, and a late-eluting low-mass component (13 kDa), which lacked this property [178]. These peaks are similar to those reported by Walsh *et al.* for protofibrillar and LMW preparations of Aβ, respectively (see below) [90]. However, Walsh *et al.* showed by TEM that the early-eluting peak contained abundant PF whereas the late-eluting peak was reported later to contain a mixture of monomer and small oligomers detected using PICUP [103]. When SEC coupled with MALLS and analytical ultracentrifugation was used to determine the size distribution of ADDLs, the SEC peaks corresponding to 75 and 13 kDa showed oligomer masses ranging from 150–1,000 kDa, and a monomeric component of 4.5 kDa by MALLS [95]. This study suggested that previous reports identifying low-molecular-mass components as a composite of low-number oligomers were misrepresentations of what might actually be a monomeric Aβ42 fraction [95]. ADDLs found in the early-eluting peak were shown to be in a dynamic equilibrium comprising a polydisperse population of oligomers [95]. Multiple parameters such as peptide concentration, temperature, pH, storage duration, and excipient addition were shown to affect this equilibrium dramatically [220].

Importantly, Aβ40 does not form ADDLs [95]. NMR studies have shown that the *C*-terminus of Aβ42 is more rigid compared to that of Aβ40 [70-72] potentially due to the extended hydrophobic *C*-terminus of Aβ42. This *C*-terminal difference and potentially the different monomeric Aβ42 conformers generated due to this structural difference may account for the increased toxicity and plaque competence of Aβ42 compared to Aβ40 [70, 71]. Indeed, some oligomeric moieties (ADDLs, paranuclei, and globulomers, see below) were shown to form by Aβ42 only. In fact, the exclusive Aβ42 derivation of ADDLs and paranuclei, and the fact that ADDLs and paranuclei are indistinguishable morphologically (compare [26, 178] with [32]), suggests that ADDLs and paranuclei may be related to each other or even be the same species obtained under different conditions [26, 32].

ADDLs have been shown to resist dissociation by low SDS concentrations (0.01%) [175]. However, when supramicellar SDS concentrations were used, ADDLs and fibrils migrated with the same electrophoretic profile yielding monomeric, trimeric, and tetrameric moieties [95]. A similar profile was observed for LMW Aβ42 [32] produced by SEC or filtration [106]. At submicellar concentrations of SDS, oligomers were detected both by denaturing electrophoresis and SEC [95]. When Aβ42 was electrophoresed in the presence of submicellar or supramicellar concentrations of SDS, high-molecular-mass aggregates and intermediate-sized assemblies formed, respectively [63]. During SDS-PAGE, these aggregates may partially dissociate as diffuse Aβ42 trimer/tetramer components [63] as observed for ADDLs [95]. These observations re-emphasize that visualization of SDS-stable oligomeric Aβ likely misrepresent the actual assembly state.

Biological Activity

Initial clusterin-induced ADDL preparations (0.34 mg/mL) were neurotoxic [175]. Later studies showed that ADDLs selectively targeted the principal neurons in the hippocampal *strata pyramidale* and *granulosum* in organotypic murine brain slices [26] and inhibited LTP in rat hippocampal brain slices [221, 222]. ADDLs also were shown to augment the negative synaptic plasticity of long-term depression (LTD) [223]. Prolonged maintenance of LTD along with LTP inhibition leads to an overall synapse-inhibitory effect (reviewed in [59]).

When cultured hippocampal neurons were incubated with synthetic ADDLs, F-12-prepared soluble brain extracts, or crude human CSF, and probed with ADDL-specific antibodies a punctate binding pattern reminiscent of synaptic termini was observed [181] (Fig. **2**). The antibodies used were shown to be 100-fold more sensitive to ADDLs (femtomole levels) than to monomeric Aβ [27, 180, 181, 224, 225]. The ADDL-binding sites were demonstrated to coincide with dendritic spines at postsynaptic termini of excitatory synapses [181]. ADDL binding also overlapped with NMDAR subunit NR1 on highly arborized neurons positive for α calcium-calmodulin kinase II [181] which accumulates in postsynaptic termini of neurons involved in memory function [181]. In addition, ADDLs specifically bound to excitatory pyramidal, but not GABAergic, neurons [180], and to neurons positive for NMDAR subunits NR1 and NR2B [180]. Similarly, ADDLs did not bind astrocytes or inhibitory neurons expressing glutamic acid decarboxylase [180]. Preferential binding of ADDLs to excitatory synapses at postsynaptic sites was consistent with the inhibitory impact of ADDLs on NMDAR-dependent LTP [26, 223] and NMDAR-mediated phosphorylation of cAMP-response-element-binding protein [226], demonstrating that ADDLs could impact crucial receptors involved in synaptic plasticity.

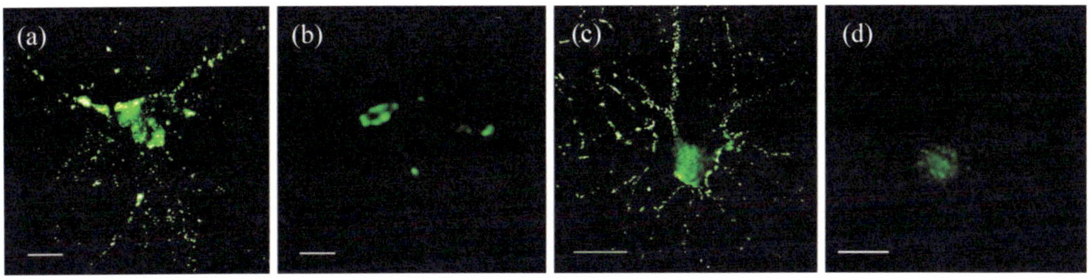

Figure 2: Punctate ADDL-binding to neurons. ADDLs isolated from AD brain or prepared *in vitro* show identical punctate binding to neuronal cell-surface proteins. Cultured hippocampal neurons were incubated with soluble extracts of human brain or synthetic ADDLs. Immunoreactivity against ADDLs was visualized by microscopy using M93 antibody. Soluble AD-brain proteins (a), soluble control-brain proteins (b), synthetic ADDLs (c), and synthetic ADDLs pre-treated (1 h) with oligomer-specific antibody M71 (d) are shown. Small puncta distributed along neurites, are evident for AD extracts and synthetic ADDLs, but not for control extracts or antibody-preadsorbed ADDLs (Scale bar = 10 μm). Adopted with permission from [27].

Defective neuronal actin-regulatory machinery is an underlying factor in dendritic and synaptic dysfunctions in many neurological disorders accompanied by cognitive deficits, including AD and Down syndrome (reviewed in [213]). ADDLs were shown to affect spine shape, which, like receptor expression is a facet of spine cell biology with ramifications for signaling and plasticity [227, 228]. ADDL-induced alterations of spine morphology which resembled the morphology of immature and diseased spines associated with mental retardation and prionoses [229].

ADDL binding to neuritic spines was reported to induce expression of the activity-regulated cytoskeleton-associated protein (Arc), a synaptic immediate-early gene [181, 230]. Proper expression of Arc is essential for LTP, but its ectopic and aberrant expression causes failure of long-term memory formation [231]. ADDLs generated a rapid and sustained increase in synaptic Arc protein expression [181], which interfered with long-term memory formation [231] and was hypothesized to lead to synapse failure and memory loss. De Felice *et al.* showed that ADDL treatment of mature primary hippocampal neurons led to reproducible and dose-dependent generation of reactive oxygen species (ROS) in the vicinity of synaptic ADDL-binding sites [182]. It was shown that ADDL binding to the NR1 subunit of NMDAR and NMDA-mediated Ca^{2+} influx led to ROS generation, further delineating the mechanisms of ADDL neurotoxicity [182]. Interestingly, ADDL treatment was shown to induce τ hyperphosphorylation in neuroblastoma cells and rat hippocampal primary neurons before neuronal death occurred [177]. Intrahippocampal injection of an oligomer-specific antibody was sufficient to reverse the effect of amyloid and τ pathologies, providing an additional insight into ADDL-mediated neurotoxicity [232].

Although *in vitro* experiments demonstrated that ADDLs interfered specifically with memory-associated experimental phenomena, a crucial question is whether ADDLs exist, and cause the same toxic effects, *in vivo*. Conformation-specific polyclonal [233] and monoclonal antibodies [179] shown to discriminate between ADDLs and Aβ monomers have been used to address this question. Dot-blot assays have detected ADDL immunoreactivity in transgenic mice and in AD brains which were extracted without detergents or harsh chemicals precluding extraction-induced alterations of the assembly structures [27, 225]. ADDL concentrations were 70-fold higher in AD brains compared to controls [27]. In the nontransgenic mouse brain, no ADDLs (detection limit <10 fmol/μg) were detected by dot-blotting brain extracts using an ADDL-specific antibody [225]. However, in brains of transgenic mice, ADDL concentrations varied from ~20–250 fmol/μg depending on the brain region tested [225]. Soluble brain proteins extracted in F-12 culture medium by ultracentrifugation contained ADDL immunoreactivity that correlated with presence of AD [27, 181] (reviewed in [59]). These findings support the hypothesis that ADDLs may be an important component in the amyloid cascade, as opposed to the poor correlation between insoluble amyloid deposits and cognitive impairment [59].

Protofibrils

Structural Characterization

PF are Aβ40- and Aβ42-derived curvilinear, soluble assemblies, which were described originally by Walsh *et al.* [90] and Harper *et al.* [28]. Walsh *et al.* reported studies using SEC, DLS, and TEM examining initial stages of Aβ oligomerization and characterizing Aβ intermediates during fibrillogenesis. By SEC, PF had apparent mass >100 kDa. They predominantly comprised curved, fibril-like structures of 6–8 nm in diameter and ≤200 nm long as observed by TEM [90]. Harper *et al.* detected the same protofibrillar assemblies of Aβ during polymerization by AFM [28]. They noted that Aβ40 PF, which appeared during the first week of incubation, had diameters of 3.1 nm and were 20–70 nm long [28]. The PF showed a periodic diametrical variation every 20 nm. In contrast, Aβ42 PF formed within the first day of incubation and had larger diameters (4.2 nm) than those of Aβ40. Aβ42 PF elongated overtime with diametrical periodicity similar to Aβ40 [28].

TEM examination of Aβ PF with rotary shadowing [30] demonstrated flexible rods up to ~200 nm long, with larger diameters than those observed by regular TEM or AFM. PF appeared more beaded with a periodicity of 3–6 nm, and the proportion of small PF (<10 nm) was higher, suggesting that these smaller structures might have been overlooked using TEM with routine negative staining or that the preparations were simply different [30]. The beaded structures were shown to be typical of early PF, whereas at later time points, PF appeared smoother [234]. High-resolution AFM studies have demonstrated that Aβ40 PF had a diameter of ~4.3 nm, with periodicity of ~20 nm, and coexisted with spherical species of the same diameter [161]. Spheres similar to those have been hypothesized by us and others to be precursors which join together to form PF [32, 159].

PF have a high β-sheet content, a characteristic similar to that of mature amyloid fibrils [30] and are recognized by antibody WO1, which reacts with the fibrillar form of various amyloid proteins [235]. Thus, PF are the latest precursors on the pathway of fibril formation described to date. Nevertheless, apparently a substantial conformational rearrangement occurs upon maturation of PF into fibrils as evidenced by the observations that PF can be readily disassembled into LMW Aβ, whereas mature fibrils do not typically disaggregate back into PF [30]. Proline substitution experiments showed that Aβ40 PF were "less structured" in the region Glu^{22}–Gly^{29} compared to mature fibrils [235]. Hydrogen–deuterium exchange data demonstrated that the *C*-terminal Met^{35}–Val^{40} and the *N*-terminal Asp^{1}–Phe^{19} regions of Aβ40 were highly exposed to solvent both in fibrils and PF. In contrast, the Phe^{20}–Leu^{34} segment was highly protected from hydrogen–

deuterium exchange in fibrils but much less so in PF [78]. The β-structure (β-sheet and β-turn) content of PF was similar to that of fibrils as assessed by CD studies [90]. Collectively, these data suggested that the β-sheet elements comprising the amyloid fibrils were already present in PF. These elements could be expanded into adjacent residues and other elements, such as lateral association of filaments, may contribute to the maturation of amyloid fibrils.

Biological Activity

Initial studies to assess the biological activity of PF were performed in cultured primary rat cortical neurons over a time scale of minutes to hours, presumably before PF convert to fibrils [30]. In these experiments, compromise of cell viability by SEC-isolated PF was evaluated using the 3-(4,5-dimethylthiazol-2-yl)-2,5-diphenyltetrazolium bromide (MTT) assay [236]. It was found that PF and fibrils altered the normal physiology of cultured neurons, whereas LMW Aβ did not [30]. To explore and compare the toxic effects of LMW Aβ, PF, and fibrils further, Hartley *et al.* used rat cerebral primary mixed cultures (containing neurons, astrocytes, and microglia) and showed that PF caused neuronal injury and altered electrophysiological activities, ultimately causing cell death [30]. Although LMW Aβ caused a rapid but transient increase in excitatory post-synaptic currents (EPSCs), PF or fibrils (~3 μM) invariably produced rapid and sustained increases in electrical activity, six-fold greater than that induced by LMW Aβ [30]. Similarly, PF and fibrils significantly increased the frequency of action potentials and augmented the frequency and size of membrane depolarization compared to LMW Aβ preparation [29]. Substantial neuron loss (80% as opposed to 10% non-treated cells) was observed consistently using the lactate dehydrogenase assay [237] and immunostaining against neuron-specific, microtubule-associated protein-2, after 5 days exposure to LMW and protofibrillar Aβ [29]. It was hypothesized that LMW Aβ could either convert to PF that cause the neurotoxicity or it could induce neurotoxicity by a mechanism independent of PF [29]. Relevant to this hypothesis, it was initially shown that human brain-derived Aβ dimers inhibited LTP, enhanced LTD, and reduced dendritic spine density in rodent hippocampal neurons [193]. However, it was found later that covalently stabilized Aβ dimers readily formed relatively stable PFs, which mediated the above-mentioned toxic activities (see Table **1**) [174].

Important insight into the clinical relevance of PF came from investigation of a family in Northern Sweden, members of which carry a mutation in the *app* gene that leads to a single amino acid substitution in the Aβ region, E22G (dubbed the Arctic mutation) [188]. Surprisingly, even though carriers of this mutation have decreased plasma levels of Aβ40 and Aβ42 compared to non-carriers, they develop early-onset AD [188]. *In vitro* fibrillization studies showed that Aβ containing the E22G substitution formed PF faster and in larger quantities than wild-type Aβ, suggesting that PF may be the main disease-causing agents in carriers of the Arctic mutation [188]. These findings, along with the observations of PF formation by most other amyloidogenic proteins, have positioned PF as a likely primary pathogenic assembly state and an important target for drug development efforts for amyloidosis [238].

Concentrations of 4-hydroxy-2-nonenal (HNE), a metabolite of oxidative stress resulting from fatty-acid peroxidation, and of HNE-derived lipid peroxidation products, have been shown to increase in AD [239]. HNE has been shown to modify Aβ by 1,4 conjugation to primary amino groups and Schiff base formation, which could result in putative covalent intermolecular cross-linking of Aβ monomers [240]. Aβ40 prepared after a 285-h incubation with HNE predominantly had a PF-like, curved morphology when examined by AFM, whereas preparations formed in the absence of HNE comprised straight fibrils predominantly [240]. Both the long, straight fibrils formed in the absence of HNE and the curved fibrillar aggregates formed in the presence of HNE were rich in β-sheet structure, based on their CD spectra. In the presence of HNE, accelerated formation of protofibrillar Aβ40 species was observed, whereas generation of mature straight fibrils even upon extended incubations was inhibited [240]. These data suggested that HNE could cause accumulation of toxic Aβ PF by preventing their maturation to the less toxic fibrils [239]. Similarly, docosahexaenoic acid was shown to stabilize soluble Aβ42 PF and hinder their conversion to insoluble fibrils, thus leading to a sustained Aβ-induced neurotoxicity measured using cultured PC12 cells [241]. These observations suggest that toxic effects of PF could be promoted by molecular interactions that prevented downstream fibril formation.

Aβ*56

Lesné and colleagues have identified an oligomeric Aβ species, termed Aβ*56, that caused cognitive deficits in middle-aged transgenic *Tg(APPSWE)2576Kahs (Tg2576)* mice [31]. The *Tg2576* mice express high levels of a human APP variant, which carries a familial AD-linked double mutation originating in a Swedish lineage (K670N, M671L) [242, 243]. Aβ concentrations in these mice increase rapidly at 6 months of age, and abundant amyloid plaques are apparent between 9–12 months [242]. *Tg2576* mice recapitulate many other neurological features of AD, including neuroinflammation and oxidative stresses, dystrophic neurites, and significant cognitive deficits (reviewed in [242]). However, other important features, such as neurofibrillary tangles and significant neuron loss are not found in this model [244].

Because in these and other APP transgenic mice administration of Aβ-specific antibodies has been shown to rapidly ameliorate memory decline, and because memory deficits were thought to precede plaques, Lesné *et al.* reasoned that a particular Aβ species could promote cognitive decline preceding plaque maturation [31]. They found that insoluble Aβ accumulated over 7 months without noticeable spatial memory decline. In contrast, certain soluble and extracellular Aβ species, which migrated as LMW bands in SDS-PAGE/Western blots, correlated strongly with memory deficits at 6 months of age, suggesting that these oligomers, particularly those with apparent gel mobility of Aβ dodecamers, were important neurotoxins in this model. Based on these data, it was proposed that similar species could be causing AD [31]. In support of this hypothesis, when pathophysiologically relevant concentrations of Aβ*56 (8.5 pmol) were administered into the lateral cerebral ventricles of healthy young rats pre-trained in the Morris water maze, the rats developed defective long-term spatial memory. These are important findings supporting the central role of oligomeric Aβ in the disease mechanism of AD.

The structural characterization of Aβ*56 as a putative dodecamer should be interpreted cautiously because the apparent electrophoretic migration of this oligomer, corresponding to 56 kDa, may not represent accurately its *in vivo* mass given the artifactual effects of SDS [63], which was included in the initial steps of the extraction protocol. Of note, Jacobsen *et al.* have found that cognitive deficits in *Tg2756* mice occurred before the reported time of appearance of Aβ*56 [245].

Longitudinal water-maze spatial training was reported to reduce Aβ and τ neuropathology transiently but significantly, and improve later learning performance in a triple transgenic (3×Tg) murine model of AD [246]. The 3×Tg-AD mice harbor human APP containing the Swedish mutations (KM670/671NL), human τ containing the frontotemporal dementia-associated mutation, P301L, and a human presenilin 1 gene (*PSEN1*) containing the AD-linked mutation, PS1M146V [246]. The improvement in performance in 3×Tg-AD mice occurred at 6–12 months and depended strongly on spatial training [246]. To achieve this effect, pre-training was required before development of overt neuropathology, presumably because it delayed Aβ redistribution to extracellular plaques and reduced the concentration of Aβ oligomers, including one with an apparent SDS-PAGE mobility similar to Aβ*56 [246]. These findings suggest that Aβ*56 is a neurotoxic form of Aβ that may be important in the etiology of AD. Currently, the structural relationships of this species to PF and ADDLs are unknown, although under certain conditions, ADDLs also display electrophoretic migration corresponding to a dodecamer [27].

Aβ Pores

Aβ pores are channel-like structures believed to disrupt cell membranes and cellular ionic homeostasis [247]. In lipid bilayers *in vitro*, Aβ was shown to form uniform pore-like structures with 8–12 nm outer and 2 nm inner diameters [247, 248]. These are thought to serve as Ca^{2+} channels and thus have been hypothesized to cause excitotoxicity and mediate Aβ-induced neurotoxicity in AD [249, 250]. Reports of various models including artificial phospholipid membrane bilayers, excised neuronal membrane patches, whole-cell patch-clamp experiments, and phospholipid vesicles support a channel-forming property of Aβ [247, 250-262]. In these studies, imaging techniques [247, 254, 256, 257], electrophysiological experiments [250, 251, 253-255, 257, 258, 261, 262], or cation-sensitive dyes [257] were used to assess channel-like properties of Aβ. However, other studies have reported general disruption of the plasma membrane homeostasis without channel formation [263-265]. In a study by Kayed *et al.* the effect of spherical Aβ42 oligomers on membrane conductivity was assessed using planar lipid bilayers [265]. It was found that these Aβ42 oligomers specifically increased the conductance of the bilayer in a concentration-dependent manner whereas no increase in conductance was observed for LMW Aβ species (monomer or dimer) or for Aβ fibrils [265]. The increase in membrane conductance in response to spherical oligomers occurred in the absence of evidence for discrete ion-channel or pore formation [265]. It was postulated that soluble oligomers enhanced movement of ions through the lipid bilayer by a channel-independent mechanism [265]. High sensitivity recording has indicated that there was little change in the noise level of the current trace as the current increased from 0 to ~100 pA after oligomer addition.

Aβ42 was reported to be more prone to forming channels than Aβ40 [18]. High-resolution examination of individual Aβ42 channel-like structures revealed two subunit arrangements: rectangular and hexagonal structures, putatively comprising tetramers and hexamers, respectively [247]. The disease-associated mutant E22G form of Aβ40 was shown to form pore-like structures akin to those formed by Aβ42 [36, 266]. Treatment of the hypothalamic neuronal cells GT1-7 with Aβ40 has led to simultaneous formation of Ca^{2+} channels and increased intracellular Ca^{2+} concentration ($[Ca^{2+}]_i$) as determined by fluorometric measurements, suggesting that Aβ40 also could disrupt biological and artificial membranes, possibly *via* formation of pores [252, 267].

Paranuclei

Using PICUP followed by SDS-PAGE analysis, Aβ40 and Aβ42 were shown to form distinct oligomer size distributions, suggesting that the two Aβ alloforms oligomerized through distinct pathways [32]. In those experiments, Aβ42 preferentially formed pentamer/hexamer units termed paranuclei, which self-associated into larger assemblies, including dodecamers and octadecamers [32]. In contrast, Aβ40 formed a roughly equimolar, quasi-equilibrium mixture of monomers, dimers, trimers, and tetramers [103].

A systematic study using PICUP assessed oligomerization of 34 Aβ alloforms [34], including those containing familial AD-linked amino acid substitutions, *N*-terminal truncations found in AD plaques, and modifications that altered the charge, hydrophobicity, or conformation of Aβ [34]. *C*-terminal length was found to be the most important structural determinant in early oligomerization, and the side-chain of Ile^{41} in Aβ42 was found to be important both for effective formation of paranuclei and for their self-association [34]. Thus, Aβ41 and longer alloforms formed abundant paranuclei whereas Aβ40 and shorter alloforms did not [32]. The side-chain of Ala^{42}, and the *C*-terminal carboxyl group, affected paranucleus self-association [34]. In a related study, oxidation of Met^{35} in Aβ42 was found to preclude paranucleus formation and led to generation of oligomers indistinguishable from those produced by Aβ40 [33]. These data demonstrated that modification of even a single atom could induce dramatic effects on Aβ paranucleus formation and downstream assembly, providing important insights into mechanisms of Aβ assembly into neurotoxic oligomers potentially relevant to AD pathogenesis. As discussed above, the difference in toxicity between Aβ40 and Aβ42 [268] correlates with observations that certain oligomeric Aβ forms, such as paranuclei and ADDLs, are produced by Aβ42 only, emphasizing strong correlation of the latter to the pathogenic process of AD.

βamy Balls

βamy balls are Aβ40-derived structures that form spontaneously when high concentrations of Aβ40 (60–600 μM) are incubated in phosphate-buffered saline at 30°C for 8–13 days [39]. βamy balls, have diameters of 20–200 μm and were shown to be composed of birefringent 6–10-nm diameter Aβ fibrils with random orientation [39]. Although such high Aβ concentrations used to generate βamy balls are unlikely to occur *in vivo* [22, 269], it was argued that these concentrations could possibly occur locally at microfoci circumscribing the amyloid plaques in AD brain [39]. Interestingly, *in vivo* extracellular retinal deposits called drusen have an apparent similarity to βamy balls. Drusen are Aβ-containing macromolecular assemblies and are a pathologic sign in age-related macular degeneration [270]. However, these structures have larger diameters and unlike βamy balls, which are produced from synthetic Aβ40 *in vitro* in the absence of other proteins, the retinal deposits contain other Aβ-binding proteins [270].

Amylospheroids

Amylospheroids, were described as Aβ40- and Aβ42-derived assemblies with 10–15-nm diameters [35]. Aβ40 amylospheroids formed by incubating 350 μM of the peptide in phosphate-buffered saline under slow rotation for 5–7 days at 37°C [35]. Aβ42 amylospheroids were produced by incubating 0.01–1 μM peptide in the same buffer for 8–10 h at 4°C [35]. Indeed, it was observed that Aβ42 amylospheroids, which formed faster and at substantially lower concentration than those of Aβ40, were also more toxic than Aβ40 amylospheroids [35], correlating with the higher toxicity and pathogenicity of Aβ42 in AD compared to Aβ40. Although these Aβ42 assemblies are spherical [35], they are morphologically distinct from ADDLs in their diameter (2.5 nm by AFM [95] *vs.* 10 nm by TEM, respectively).

Using antibodies reactive to amylospheroids, Noguchi *et al.* reported immunoisolation of neurotoxic, 10–15-nm, spherical Aβ assemblies, from brains affected by AD or dementia with Lewy bodies, which they termed native amylospheroids [198]. The amount of native amylospheroids correlated with disease severity. These native amylospheroids were non-reactive with antibody A11, had a high mass (>100 kDa), and induced degeneration of human neurons *in vitro*. Amylospheroid-induced neuronal degeneration was reverted only by anti-amylospheroid antibodies. Immunospecificity of the antibodies for amylospheroids was suggested to be indicative of their tertiary surface topology distinct from those of other reported assemblies, including dimers, ADDLs, or A11-reactive assemblies [198]. Amylospheroid-specific polyclonal antibodies were generated in immunized rabbits (rpASD1; K_d = 5 pM) and monoclonal antibodies in hamsters (haASD1; K_d = 0.5 pM). These antibodies reacted with epitopes distinct from those on dimers, A11-reactive 12-mers, or fibrils [198]. Amylospheroids bound neuronal presynaptic target(s) and demonstrated a mode of toxicity independent of NMDAR-mediated synaptic transmission [198].

Globulomers

Globulomers are Aβ42 oligomers produced by incubating 400 μM Aβ42 in phosphate-buffered saline in the presence of 0.2% SDS at 37°C for 6 h [89]. These species also have been produced by incubation of Aβ42 with lauric, oleic, or arachidonic acids [89], suggesting that they are generated by interaction of Aβ42 with micelles of SDS or fatty acids. Aβ42 globulomers were neurotoxic to rat brain slices and antibodies generated against globulomers detected immunoreactive epitopes in tissue sections [89]. Similar globular structures of Aβ40 were reported to form after 18 h incubation in 25 mM 2-morpholinoethanesulfonic acid buffer (pH 4.5) in a "hanging-drop" environment [271]. Hanging-drop environment is used extensively for protein crystallization and provides a static, low-convection environment with a markedly increased hydrophobic air–buffer interfacial area compared to that of the microfuge-tube environment [271].

Toxic Fibrillar Oligomers of Aβ

Based on reactivity of antibodies specific for epitopes generically associated with distinct aggregation states of different amyloid assemblies, at least two types of oligomeric amyloid assemblies were proposed: fibrillar and non-fibrillar oligomers [38]. Accordingly, monomers of amyloidogenic proteins aggregate to form non-fibrillar oligomers reactive with polyclonal antibody A11, but not OC. Non-fibrillar oligomers are transient intermediates that may undergo further aggregation and form fibrils ultimately. On the other hand, amyloidogenic proteins also can self-associate into fibrillar oligomers that are reactive with OC, but not A11. These fibrillar oligomers likely represent fibril nuclei or seeds which can elongate by recruiting additional monomers [38]. Interestingly, in the presence of Zn^{2+}, Aβ40 was found to form toxic, fibrillar oligomers that upon incubation self-associated into large, non-fibrillar structures and lost their toxicity [164]. The OC antibody has been generated in rabbits immunized with Aβ fibrils [189], suggesting that Aβ-derived fibrillar oligomers share surface structural features with Aβ fibrils. Furthermore, fibrillar oligomers are similar to fibrils in terms of their ability to seed formation of additional fibrillar oligomers, but not Aβ fibrils [191], suggesting that they likely have a lattice distinct from the fibrils.

James *et al.* recently characterized a particular preparation of toxic Aβ42-derived fibrillar oligomers (TABFOs) [190]. This TABFO preparation had similar morphology and OC reactivity to fibrillar oligomers reported previously [191]. To prepare TABFOs, recombinant wild-type Aβ42 was dissolved in HFIP initially. After removing HFIP by evaporation, Aβ42 was resuspended in dilute ammonium hydroxide, which prevents fibrillation and allows formation of TABFOs. TABFOs were stable in SEC, which was the final purification step. TABFOs converted into fibrils in phosphate-buffered saline. TABFO-derived fibrils had typical amyloid features by TEM and ThT fluorescence and contained significant β-structure and negligible α-helical content by CD spectroscopy [190]. Structural studies showing the fibril-like cross-β structure of TABFOs may explain the reactivity of the antibody OC with fibrillar oligomers and mature amyloid fibrils [38].

Functionally, TABFOs were found to be toxic to neurons and HeLa cells by MTT assays at ≥2.25 μg/mL (0.5 μM of Aβ42 monomer equivalent). It was proposed that TABFO toxicity may be related to their potential to form membrane pores. Pore formation has been implicated in the toxicity of Aβ oligomers [36, 272].

OLIGOMERS OF DISEASE-RELATED AMYLOIDOGENIC PROTEINS OTHER THAN Aβ

Over twenty human amyloidoses are caused by aberrant protein folding and aggregation [273-275]. As Aβ often is considered an archetypal protein in studies of these diseases, the discoveries of toxic non-fibrillar Aβ assemblies and their centrality in AD have led to a search for similar assemblies of other amyloidosis-related proteins. To date, at least 24 different proteins have been identified as causative agents of amyloidoses [276]. In essentially all cases, such assemblies have been found and had adverse biological effects similar to those of Aβ oligomers [5, 7, 11, 277]. Because this review focuses on non-fibrillar assemblies of Aβ, we do not intend to cover assemblies of other amyloidogenic proteins in detail, but rather to highlight a few examples and discuss current features that are common to all or most of these assemblies.

The structures reported for amyloidogenic protein oligomers, in general, have been similar to those described for Aβ, namely PF, annular (pore-like) PF, and spherical oligomers. In several cases, annular PF have been the predominant structures found. However, as discussed elsewhere [63], it is important to note that in many cases the term PF has been used even though the morphologies of the assemblies under study were distinct from those originally defined as PF.

One of the most studied amyloidogenic proteins is α-synuclein, the function of which is not clear although it is believed to be part of the ubiquitin system that marks proteins for proteasomal degradation [278, 279]. α-Synuclein is the predominant component in Lewy bodies, the pathological hallmarks in PD brain, and has been implicated in other degenerative disorders (synucleinopathies), including dementia with Lewy bodies and multiple system atrophy [280]. Similar to Aβ, α-synuclein belongs to a growing family of "intrinsically unstructured" proteins [281, 282], a characteristic that perhaps renders these proteins more prone to undergoing amyloidogenic assembly. Mutant α-synuclein alloforms linked to familial PD were found to oligomerize faster than the wild-type protein, whereas the rate of fibril formation did not correlate with the presence of disease-causing mutations [283]. Non-fibrillar assemblies of both wild-type and mutant α-synuclein included spherical oligomers, protofibrillar structures, and most abundantly, annular PF [266, 284]. The latter morphology suggested that the mechanism whereby α-synuclein induces toxicity is pore formation in cell membranes. In agreement with this idea, protofibrillar α-synuclein was found to permeabilize synthetic vesicles [285]. Interestingly, this effect was increased by the familial PD-linked mutants A30P and A53T [286], but not by the mutant E46K [287]. Thus, although pore formation may be involved in α-synuclein-induced toxicity, other mechanisms also have been implicated, but these are not well-understood [288].

Two amyloidogenic proteins involved in sugar metabolism are insulin and IAPP. Insulin aggregation is not associated with disease but has been studied by multiple groups as a convenient *in vitro* model [289-292]. Biophysical investigation of insulin fibrillogenesis has identified oligomeric populations with conformations distinct from those of natively folded insulin dimer and hexamer [293]. Taking advantage of the relative stability of insulin oligomers and using special instrumentation, Robinson and co-workers have provided one of the first examples of mass spectrometric investigation of amyloidogenic protein oligomers, and demonstrated the power of this experimental approach for studying the effects of pH and metal ion binding on oligomerization [294]. In a study combining structural characterization and cytotoxicity experiments, Grudzielanek *et al.* found no toxicity for low-order insulin oligomers, whereas substantial toxicity was measured for high-order, β-sheet-rich aggregates that displayed either fibrillar or amorphous morphology [295].

In contrast to insulin, IAPP aggregation is believed to be causative in T2D. IAPP is a 37-residue peptide hormone produced in pancreatic β-cells and co-secreted with insulin. Early stages of T2D are characterized by insulin resistance followed by increased insulin and IAPP secretion. Elevated IAPP concentrations lead to its assembly into toxic oligomers and insoluble aggregates [14]. Oligomeric and protofibrillar IAPP were shown to interact with synthetic membranes [296], a characteristic that decreases with further aggregation, providing a clue for the mechanism of IAPP toxicity [297]. The interaction with biological membranes may induce a transient α-helical conformation in IAPP, presumably facilitating penetration of the oligomers into the membrane resulting in solute leakage across the membrane [298, 299]. Strong evidence for the neurotoxic role of IAPP oligomers in T2D was given in a study in which rifampicin, an inhibitor of IAPP fibril, but not oligomer formation, did not protect pancreatic β-cells against apoptosis induced by either endogenously expressed or externally applied IAPP [300]. More recent data have suggested that *in vivo*, toxic IAPP oligomers are formed intracellularly and therefore, oligomer-specific antibodies do not prevent cell death *in vitro* and *in vivo* [301].

Numerous other examples have demonstrated the important roles of oligomers of amyloidogenic proteins as disease-causing agents. Before the focus in the amyloid field shifted from fibrils to oligomers, it had been known that although no sequence similarity was found among amyloidogenic proteins, the fibril structures of all were highly similar, characterized by fibrillar morphology with periodic helical twist and cross-β structures [302, 303]. The realization that the precursor oligomers may be the proximate disease-causing agents in the amyloidoses related to these proteins raised the question whether oligomer structures also were similar. High-resolution microscopic studies of oligomeric structures, mostly by TEM and AFM, have demonstrated that in most cases the morphologies observed were spherical, annular, or protofibrillar (worm-like). Conformational studies of oligomers have been difficult because the oligomers typically are metastable and exist in mixtures. Structural insight has been offered by Glabe and co-workers who developed antibodies that showed specificity for oligomers of proteins with unrelated sequences but did not bind the monomeric or fibrillar forms of these proteins [304]. The first polyclonal antibody, A11, and similar antibodies developed in follow-up studies showed remarkable ability to bind to oligomers formed by proteins as diverse as Aβ, α-synulein, IAPP, lysozyme, insulin, poly Q, and prion fragments [304]. These observations strongly suggested that a predominant mechanism whereby these oligomers injure cells is through permeabilization of the plasma membrane because toxic oligomers sharing a common structure formed by both intracellular and extracellular proteins [264, 265]. As discussed above, oligomers may interact with membranes by several mechanisms, including pore-formation and shallow penetration under the surface resulting in thinning of the membrane and a net increase in its permeability. Further delineation of the specific mechanisms governing these interactions requires additional studies and will be highly important for designing reagents that block them.

NON-FIBRILLAR ASSEMBLIES OF DISEASE-UNRELATED PROTEINS

In his 1972 Nobel-Prize acceptance speech, Anfinsen stated that "the native conformation [of proteins] is determined by the totality of inter-atomic interactions and hence by the amino acid sequence, in a given environment" which does not always favor the normally functional and folded state of proteins. Consistent with Anfinsen's theory, the conformational-change hypothesis postulates that one of 17 normally soluble and functional human proteins could undergo structural alterations under partially denaturing conditions leading to self-assembly and amyloid fibril formation [305]. Besides disease-associated amyloid-forming proteins, and proteins that naturally form non-pathological, functional amyloid-like fibrils (reviewed in [306]), disease-unrelated proteins [307] and artificially designed peptides [308-310] have been found to form amyloid under particular non-native conditions. To the best of our knowledge, the ability of disease-unrelated peptides and proteins to form amyloid fibrils was first reported by Guijarro *et al.* [311] and Litvinovich *et al.* [312]. The src-homology 3 (SH3) domain of bovine phosphatidyl inositol 3-kinase (PI3K), an 85-residue, β-structured protein, was shown to aggregate slowly and form amyloid fibrils under acidic pH [311]. Thenceforth, the disease-unrelated SH3 domain has served as an excellent model for systematic studies examining structural properties of amyloid fibrils and molecular mechanisms of amyloid formation [313-316]. The PI3K-SH3 was shown to adopt a compact denatured state under acidic conditions before formation of amyloid fibrils [317]. Limited proteolysis studies showed that PI3K-SH3 at low pH had a partially folded conformation [318] and progressively displayed enhanced susceptibility to proteolysis, suggesting that the protein became more unfolded in the early stages of aggregation [318]. In contrast, the amyloid fibrils that formed over longer periods of time were resistant to proteolysis [318]. It was suggested that the protein aggregates formed initially were relatively dynamic and this flexibility allowed for the particular interactions leading to formation of the highly ordered fibrils [318].

After Litvinovich *et al.* demonstrated formation of amyloid-like fibrils by self-association of murine fibronectin type III module [312], others reported that similar conversions in a number of disease-unrelated proteins could be induced *in vitro* by a deliberate, rational choice of excipient conditions [317, 319]. Examples (reviewed in [307]) include human apolipoprotein CII, ADA2H, amphoterin, stefin B and endostatin, murine V1 domain, equine acylphosphatase (AcP) and apomyoglobin, monellin (*Dioscoreophyllum camminsii*), and yeast phosphoglycerate kinase. Fezoui *et al.* reported *de novo* design of a monomeric α-helix-turn-α-helix peptide (αtα) which converted to β-sheet-rich amyloid-type, protease-resistant, 6–10 -nm fibrils at 37°C in a neutral aqueous buffer [308]. Formation of fibrils from full-length proteins requires solution conditions that partially or completely disrupt the native structure of the protein, but not completely disturb hydrogen bonds [317]. It was observed that proteins with as few as four residues, and amino-acid homopolymers that are unable to fold into stable globular structures, form fibrils readily [307, 320, 321]. Therefore, it has been suggested that the ability to form amyloid fibrils could be a generic property of polypeptide chains [307].

In one study of non-fibrillar assemblies of disease-unrelated proteins, tapping-mode AFM was used to follow the process of HypF-N aggregation which was induced by incubating the protein in the presence of trifluoroethanol (TFE) [322]. HypF-N was shown to aggregate hierarchically through a number of distinct steps with morphologically different intermediates [322]. Initially, globular assemblies appeared, which subsequently self-assembled into beaded chains, similar to those found for amyloidogenic proteins [323-325]. Subsequently, these organized into crescents, large annular and ribbon-like structures (Fig. **3**), and eventually assembled into mature fibrils of different sizes [322]. The globule height was measured to be 2.8–3.0 nm [322]. Although HypF-N and AcP are similarly prone to conversion from a predominantly α-helical conformation to one rich in β-sheet, HypF-N aggregation rate was found to be dramatically higher (~1,000-fold) than AcP, possibly due to the higher hydrophobicity and lower net charge of HypF-N compared to AcP [326].

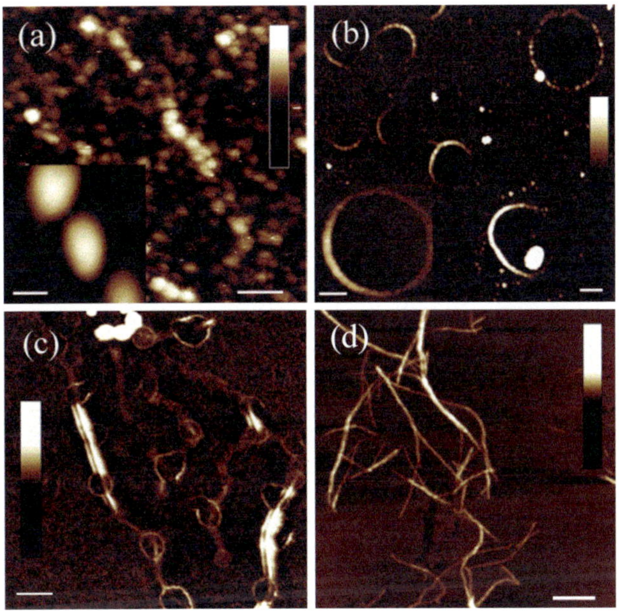

Figure 3: Hierarchical aggregation process of HypF-N. (a) Tapping AFM images taken under liquid (height data, scan size 670 nm, Z range 20 nm) of HypF-N globular aggregates observed a few hours after the onset of the aggregation process in the presence of 30% TFE. Scale bar = 100 nm. Inset, STM image (height data, scan size 42 nm, Z range 15 nm) of globular aggregates obtained under the same conditions, but diluted 1:50 prior to deposition onto the substrate; the globules are apparently asymmetric and tend to form a defined mutual orientation. Scale bar = 10 nm. (b) HypF-N crescents and a ring observed after 3 days of incubation in 30% TFE (scan size 5.3 μm, Z range 45 nm). Inset, high resolution image of a ring (scan size 1.9 μm, Z range 120 nm), revealing its globular components, taken after 5 days of incubation in 30% TFE. Scale bars = 400 nm. (c) Tapping-mode AFM image taken in air (height data) after three days of incubation in 30% TFE showing the co-existence of annular structures with thin and wide ribbon-like fibrils. Scan size 4.8 μm, Z range 40 nm. Scale = 500 nm. (d) Tapping-mode AFM images taken in air (height data) of mature fibrils obtained in 30% TFE showing supercoiled fibrils obtained after eight days (scan size 3.6 μm, Z range 80 nm). Adopted with permission from [322].

In contrast to fibrils of disease-causing amyloidogenic proteins, those formed by disease-unrelated proteins did not cause cytotoxicity in cell-culture experiments.

For example, fibrils formed by the aforementioned αtα peptide displayed no neurotoxicity, even though they were morphologically indistinguishable from Aβ and IAPP fibrils, which were toxic [308]. It was therefore unexpected that the non-fibrillar assemblies of PI3K-SH3 and HypF-N were shown to be highly toxic to PC12 cells and murine fibroblasts *in vitro* [327]. The extent of cellular injury caused by the cytotoxic oligomers was comparable to that of Aβ42 oligomers, whereas the corresponding fibrils of both PI3K-SH3 and HypF-N were benign.

Early non-fibrillar HypF-N assemblies were shown to permeabilize artificial phospholipid membranes more efficiently than mature fibrils, indicating that this disease-unrelated protein displayed the same toxic properties as non-fibrillar assemblies of pathological peptides and proteins [322]. Further investigation of the cellular effects of HypF-N oligomers revealed that they entered the cytoplasm and caused an acute rise in ROS levels and $[Ca^{2+}]_i$, leading to cell death [328]. In a study where murine fibroblasts and endothelial cells were treated with non-fibrillar HypF-N assemblies, the two cell types underwent two different death mechanisms—fibroblasts exposed for 24 h to 10 μM HypF-N oligomers underwent necrosis, whereas endothelial cells treated similarly sustained apoptosis [329]. A similar study comparing cytotoxic effects of non-fibrillar and fibrillar HypF-N assemblies using a panel of normal and pathological cell-lines showed that cells were variably affected by the same amount of non-fibrillar aggregates, whereas mature fibrils showed little or no toxicity [330]. This difference in the extent of compromise of cell viability was significantly related to the cell-membrane cholesterol content and to different cellular Ca^{2+}-buffering and antioxidant capacities of the various cell types [330]. Recently, it has been shown that microinjection into rat brain nucleus basalis magnocellularis of PI3K-SH3 or HypF-N assemblies, but not the corresponding mature fibrils, compromised neuronal viability dose-dependently [8]. Taken together, these data clearly demonstrate that the non-fibrillar assemblies of disease-unrelated proteins are highly toxic whereas the corresponding mature fibrils are not [8]. The toxic effect of the oligomers may arise when these assemblies assume a "misfolded" conformation which may expose hydrophobic residues that are natively entombed within the core structure. Such aggregation-prone regions may interact with membranes and other cellular components modifying their structural/functional homeostasis.

Dobson and co-workers have proposed that evolutionary mechanisms may have been in force to ensure propagation of proteins that resist aggregation for efficient function [331]. However, genetic, environmental, and metabolic factors that decrease the solubility or increase the concentration of susceptible proteins *in vivo* may act against those forces and induce protein misfolding disorders including neurodegenerative diseases [331].

The fact that aggregates of some disease-unrelated proteins could function similarly to those formed by amyloidogenic, disease-related peptides and proteins, has profound implications for understanding the mechanistic fundamentals of abnormal protein deposition in amyloidoses. These observations facilitate investigation and discovery of the general mechanistic features underlying protein misfolding and aggregation [307] and help defining likely targets for drug design.

CRYSTALLOGRAPHIC STUDIES OF AMYLOID OLIGOMER MODELS

The dynamic, polymorphic, transient, and non-crystalline behaviors of oligomeric amyloid species have precluded determination of their structures at atomic resolution. However, recent X-ray crystallographic studies have provided structural details of oligomers of peptides derived from amyloidogenic protein sequences, shedding light on oligomer structures [332-335]. In one study, nanobodies were used to trap and characterize intermediates of β_2-microglobulin (β_2m) fibrillation for X-ray crystallographic studies [335]. A single-domain antibody that blocks fibrillogenesis of a proteolytic amyloidogenic β_2m fragment ($\Delta N6\beta_2m$) was used to trap and crystalize $\Delta N6\beta_2m$ for crystallography. This approach identified two extended hinge loops, which folded into a two-stranded antiparallel β-sheet. The β-strands of this sheet self-associated and stacked perpendicularly to the strand direction to form intermolecular β-sheets running parallel to the axis of oligomer growth, providing an elongation mechanism by a self-template growth mechanism [335].

Another study used microcrystals of a cyclic, 42-membered peptide ring consisting of two densely packed β-sheets. The individual β-strands, joined by two δ-linked, β-turn-mimicking ornithine residues, were antiparallel to each other [333]. Key amyloidogenic segments of Aβ and τ were selected and incorporated into these macrocyclic structures to model their respective oligomeric arrangements [333]. These macrocycles assembled into dimers through backbone hydrogen bonds in parallel or antiparallel β-strand arrangements. Tetramer formation occurred through complementary side-chain interactions, forming a variety of β-sheet–β-sheet packing geometries, deviating by 0° to 45° from the typical fibrillar cross-β arrangements [333]. Despite architectural and interfacial similarities between macrocyclic oligomers and fibrillar structures, the macrocyclic oligomers differed from fibrillar structures by an additional degree of freedom in the sheet–sheet packing. In the cross-β structure of fibrils, the strands in opposing sheets are constrained to either parallel or antiparallel orientations. In contrast, in the oligomeric macrocyles the opposing β-sheet orientations ranged from orthogonal to parallel arrangements, likely accommodating additional (non-cross-β) sheet–sheet packing geometries, which potentially limit extension of β-structures into macrocyclic oligomers [333]. Further work will be needed to test whether this is a general structural phenomenon in all oligomers.

Laganowski *et al.* [336] used a Rosetta-Profile algorithm to identify amyloid-forming fragments in αB-crystallin, a chaperone protein found in the ocular lens [337]. The algorithm identified polypeptide sequence fragments, which formed the steric-zipper spines of amyloid fibrils [338, 339]. The authors chose αB-crystallin because it formed amyloid fibrils more slowly than Aβ or IAPP, facilitating trapping of αB-crystallin and studying them before fibrillation onset. After characterizing αB-crystallin fragments as amyloid oligomers, they studied them by X-ray crystallography [336]. One of these fragments produced a stable cytotoxic oligomer, which was termed cylindrin. This oligomer had six antiparallel strands woven into a single sheet rolled into a nonporous barrel (Fig. **4**). Each strand was composed of a sequence of 11 amino acid residues, Lys-Val-Lys-Val-Leu-Gly-Asp-Val-Ile-Glu-Val. The axial interior of the cylinder was closed by the Val triplet, forming hydrophobic interactions and excluding water molecules. The cylindrin structure was similar to a steric zipper, but it was cylindrical rather than nearly flat as in amyloid fibrils [336]. Each antiparallel pair of β-strands in the cylindrin sheet is out of register with neighboring pairs in contrast to β-strands in amyloid fibrils [340-342] or short steric zippers [77]. This indicates that an "unrolled cylindrin sheet would not be an in-register structure, ready to bond with an identical sheet to form the steric zipper spine of an amyloid fiber" [336]. This study suggests that the transition from cylindrin to an antiparallel fibril-like structure would require crossing a high free-energy barrier.

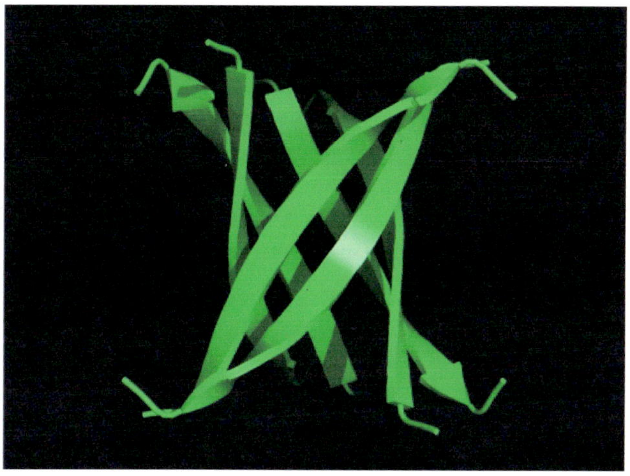

Figure 4: Ribbon representation of the crystal structure of cylindrin—the first model structure for amyloid oligomers. Pairs of β-strands form antiparallel dimers, assembled around an axis through the barrel of the cylindrin. Figure is courtesy of Dr. David Eisenberg, UCLA.

Liu *et al.* designed β-sheet amyloid mimics derived from β_2m, IAPP, τ, and Aβ, based on β-sheet mimics described by Cheng *et al.* [343]. These mimics, studied by crystallography and molecular dynamics simulations, were found to form out-of-register, antiparallel, cylindrin-like, oligomeric structures. The oligomeric structures were found to form out-of-register fibrils upon longer incubation duration [344]. Interestingly, the oligomeric structures were reactive with antibody A11 [344]. This study raises the hypothesis that oligomeric assemblies containing antiparallel, out-of-register β-sheets may promote distinct amyloid aggregation pathways in which the resultant fibrillar aggregates, besides being toxic themselves, may function as a source for toxic, out-of-register, cylindrin-like oligomers [344].

PRION-LIKE PROPAGATION AND TRANSMISSION OF MISFOLDED PROTEIN STRUCTURES

In 1967, a heretical hypothesis was proposed to explain the transmission and infectivity mechanisms of scrapie, an ovine/caprine TSE [345, 346]. Based on this hypothesis and other studies [347], the causal infectious agents of TSEs were identified to be misfolded forms of the prion protein (PrP^{Sc}), which replicate in affected individuals by converting the normal, cellular prion protein (PrP^{C}), into more of the misfolded, β-sheet-rich isoform, PrP^{Sc} [348]. After being debated and researched for decades, this hypothesis was confirmed finally by demonstrating that the infectious prions can be generated *in vitro*, without any genetic material, by self-template misfolding and resultant replication [349-352]. Thus, prion replication requires minute quantities of PrP^{Sc}, which convert the host PrP^{C} into PrP^{Sc} autocatalytically. Thus, PrP^{Sc} particles form a nucleus to recruit additional monomeric PrP^{C} that undergoes a conformational transition and polymerizes as fibrillar PrP^{Sc} [353]. Seeding of additional polymerization can occur also by fragmentation of large PrP^{Sc} aggregates into several smaller particles that serve as seeds and cause exponential accumulation of PrP^{Sc} [354].

This mechanism was thought to be exclusive to prion diseases, yet recent literature suggests that protein culprits in other protein-misfolding diseases, including AD and PD, also undergo a similar seeding–nucleation process. The similarity between the mechanisms of protein misfolding in TSEs and other protein-misfolding diseases has raised the hypothesis that the latter diseases may also be transmissible and the implicated proteins may behave as infectious agents [355-363]. Experiments testing this hypothesis have generated accumulating evidence showing prion-like transmission and/or propagation mechanisms in common neurodegenerative diseases though actual infectivity remains highly debated (Table **2**) [364, 365]. For example, it was found that a single intrastriatal inoculation of α-synuclein fibrils caused cell–cell transmission of pathologic α-synuclein and formation of Lewy-body pathology in anatomically interconnected regions in transgenic [366] and wild-type non-transgenic mice [367]. Lewy-body-like pathology resulted in progressive loss of dopaminergic neurons in the *substantia nigra pars compacta*, but not in the adjacent ventral tegmental area, and was accompanied by reduced dopamine levels culminating in motor deficits [367]. The possibility that AD pathology may be transmitted akin to prions was studied in transgenic mice expressing the human amyloid protein injected intracerebrally with dilute brain homogenates from AD patients [368-372]. In these experiments, pre-formed Aβ aggregates were necessary to seed Aβ accumulation as plaques in the brains of inoculated animals. In a separate study, Aβ seeds that accelerated cerebral Aβ amyloidosis were characterized and shown to consist of a range of aggregated Aβ species of varying sizes and sensitivities to proteinase K digestion [373]. The Aβ in the brain extracts was more resistant to proteinase K than synthetic fibrillar Aβ, and this proteinase-K-resistant fraction in the brain extracts was capable of inducing amyloid deposition by intracerebral injection in young transgenic mice [373]. However, induction of Aβ deposition in the above studies is only an accelerated version of pathology, which otherwise would develop spontaneously due to the genetic manipulations in these animal models. This is unlike prion diseases, which onset *de novo* in humans and animals that mostly do not have a predisposition to develop the disease. On the other hand, studies in transgenic animals expressing low levels of wild-type human APP show that pathologic changes, which would not have developed otherwise during the animals' lifespans, are inducible by human brain extracts containing Aβ aggregates [374, 375]. Another piece of evidence supporting the similarity between Aβ and prion transmission has been the observation that pathology was induced by a peripheral route—intraperitoneal injection of transgenic mice with AD brain extracts [371]. However, because the source of the misfolded Aβ used in these experiments was diseased brain homogenates, the relevance of these findings for AD transmissibility in otherwise normal individuals remains uncertain.

Table 2: Prion-like properties of proteins involved in protein-misfolding diseases.

Protein	Seed-Mediated Propagation of Misfolding	Intercellular Transmission	Tissue Migration	Transmissibility	Only Protein Sufficient for Infection	Protease Resistance of Aggregates	Cross-Seeding with Other Proteins
Prion protein [376]	Yes	Yes	Yes	Yes	Yes	Yes	Yes: between recombinant murine and Syrian hamster prion protein [377]
Serum amyloid A in captive cheetahs [378, 379] (reviewed in [365])	Seeded aggregates cause polymerization of native protein *in vitro*.	No, amyloid formation occurs interstitially.	No, diffuse simultaneous deposition in many tissues	Yes, but only in cheetahs [378, 379].	Amyloid fibrils can cause infection on the background of an inflammatory predisposition in host [380, 381].	Yes.	Yes: fibrils of medin (AMed amyloidosis) [382] *in vitro*; apolipoprotein A-II amyloid (AApoAII) and protein A amyloid (AA) both cross-seed and cross-compete

Protein	Seed-Mediated Propagation of Misfolding	Intercellular Transmission	Tissue Migration	Transmissibility	Only Protein Sufficient for Infection	Protease Resistance of Aggregates	Cross-Seeding with Other Proteins
							in amyloid formation in a murine model [383].
Amyloid β-protein (Aβ)	Seeded polymerization of native protein by aggregates *in vitro* [384, 385] and *in vivo* [368, 369, 371-374].	Aggregation takes place extracellularly; however, oligomeric assemblies of Aβ are transmitted amongst neurons with distinct connections, leading to transfer of cytotoxicity *in vitro* [386].	Defined spatiotemporal pattern of lesion propagation and progression during pathogenesis may be explained by cell–cell transmission of oligomers through axonal transport between different brain regions [387-389].	Transmission in murine models by intracerebral or intraperitoneal inoculation of preformed aggregates [368, 369, 371, 372, 375].	Natural transmission of AD is undocumented. Experimental evidence indicates transmission in mice or rats with a genetic predisposition to pathogenesis [368, 369, 371-374].	Yes [373, 390].	Yes: with tau and α-synuclein [391, 392].
Microtubule-associated protein tau	Seeded polymerization of native protein by aggregates has been documented *in vitro* [393].	Extracellular aggregates are taken up by cells *in vitro* and *in vivo* in transgenic mice by intracerebral inoculation [393-398].	Outward pattern of lesion propagation from transentorhinal cortex in AD may explain transmission of misfolding through axonal transport between different brain regions [389, 399].	Transmission in mice with a genetic predisposition by intracerebral inoculation of preformed aggregates [393-398].	Natural transmission of tauopathies is undocumented.	No evidence to date	Yes. Cross-seeding occurs with α-synuclein, Aβ, and IAPP [392, 395, 400].
Superoxide dismutase 1 (SOD-1) [360]	Native and mutant SOD-1 variants co-associate, forming aggregates and fibrils under non-denaturing conditions [401, 402] in familial ALS [403], in transgenic models [404], and in	Mutant SOD-1 aggregates enter neurons efficiently by macropinocytosis and seed aggregation of the normally soluble SOD-1 [362, 407].	Motor neuron degeneration initiates focally and spreads to contiguous regions with disease progression, providing indirect evidence for tissue spreading of pathology [408, 409].	Undocumented	Possible because intercellular misfolding progression was blocked by antibodies against misfolded SOD-1 (reviewed in [365])	Misfolded protein is highly susceptible to proteases [406].	Seeds of S100A6, an EF-hand Ca^{2+}-binding protein, promote SOD-1 aggregation [410].

Protein	**Seed-Mediated Propagation of Misfolding**	**Intercellular Transmission**	**Tissue Migration**	**Transmissibility**	**Only Protein Sufficient for Infection**	**Protease Resistance of Aggregates**	**Cross-Seeding with Other Proteins**
	cell-culture systems [362, 405, 406].						
α-Synuclein [358]	Seeded polymerization of aggregation *in vitro* [411], in cell cultures [412] and *in vivo* [413].	α-Synuclein misfolding is transferred to transplanted stem cell grafts in patients with PD [414, 415], murine [413, 416], and rat models [417]. Endocytosis likely mediates uptake of α-synuclein *in vivo*, and transferred α-synuclein causes seeded aggregation of endogenous α-synuclein in recipient neurons [417]. Lipid peroxidation product, HNE, induces α-synuclein oligomerization and promotes cell–cell transfer of seeding-capable assemblies [418].	Contiguous, progressive spread of PD lesions from brainstem to cortex [419-423] provides indirect evidence for tissue migration of misfolding.	Undocumented	Undocumented	Cell-transmitted α-synuclein aggregates were shown to be sensitive to protease treatment [417].	Cross-seeding occurs with, γ-synuclein [424], tau [392], and Aβ [391].
Huntingtin	Polyglutamine peptides exceeding a critical length aggregate *in vitro* and *in vivo* [425, 426]. Brain extracts of patients and transgenic mice accelerate seeded polyglutamine amyloid formation [427].	Aggregates are internalized by cells in culture [428].	Systematic, contiguous dissemination of pathology in HD [429] has been documented.	Unlikely because genetic susceptibility in host is necessary.	No, because etiology constitutes underlying genetic mutations.	Yes.	Fibrillar aggregates of huntingtin function as a structural template to induce, *in vitro* and *in vivo*, fibrillation of TIA-1, an RNA-binding protein containing a Q/N-rich sequence [430].

Whether infectious or not, propagation of protein misfolding may be one of the mechanisms responsible for the findings that pathological changes in various neurodegenerative diseases, including AD, PD, and HD, progress temporally in a characteristic, step-wise, anatomical pattern. Neuropathological studies by Braak *et al.* and others have shown that Lewy bodies in PD and neurofibrillary tangles in AD initiate early in the course of these diseases in circumscribed brain regions while progressing in predictable topographies through anatomical connections [387, 389, 399, 422]. Similarly, in an AD mouse model, the pathology progresses from the entorhinal cortex to all of the hippocampal subregions and cortical areas through anatomical connections, such as the perforant pathway [388]. Neurodegenerative changes in HD progress simultaneously in two defined anatomical directions in the striatum [431]. Among the first affected in HD are the striatal projection neurons, particularly those expressing encephalin [432]. Brain-imaging studies show that cortical regions processing motor, sensory, and visual functions undergo thinning in asymptomatic huntingtin gene carriers, and cortical areas that subserve more advanced functions are affected later in the course of HD [429]. This defined spatiotemporal pattern of lesion propagation and progression in neurodegenerative diseases may be explained by cell–cell transmission of misfolded proteins through axonal transport between different brain regions. Indeed, oligomeric, fluorescently tagged Aβ microinjected into electrophysiologically defined primary hippocampal rat neurons were shown to transfer between differentiated neurons through direct connections [386]. With progressive accumulation of such oligomers, the acceptor cells gradually showed signs of neurite damage and cytotoxicity [386]. In this study, time-lapse imaging showed that diffuse, intracellular Aβ oligomers gradually accumulated into vesicular structures corresponding to lysosomes and Aβ-containing vesicles travelled in neurites at a speed of 61 nm/s, the velocity of late endosomes or lysosomes [386]. Collectively, it was postulated that macroautophagic formation of endosomes/lysosomes might have mediated intraneuritic transfer of Aβ oligomers, which were then exocytosed from the donor cells and rapidly endocytosed by the acceptor cells [386]. Other mechanisms of transmission such as exosomes [433] and tunneling nanotubes [434] also have been discussed as potential means of cell–cell transmission of Aβ or other amyloidogenic proteins.

The studies described above demonstrate that regional spreading of protein misfolding may play an important role in the pathogenesis and progression of many protein-misfolding diseases. Furthermore, these studies strongly indicate that at least some prion characteristics, including the molecule–molecule transmission of misfolding and cell–cell spreading of misfolded protein moieties occur in other protein-misfolding diseases. Contextually, another noteworthy phenomenon is the cross-seeding mechanism whereby misfolded aggregates of one protein may interact and promote aggregation of a different protein [391, 435].

CONCLUSIONS

Since the amyloid-cascade hypothesis was formulated [1], intensive research has led to an exponential accumulation of data elucidating the pathogenic mechanisms of AD. In mid-December, 2012, PubMed database searches, using the queries "Alzheimer's disease", "amyloid", and "protein misfolding disease" returned 87,702, 53,493, and 32,184 hits, respectively. Importantly, as our understanding of the devastating *morbus* Alzheimer, and other neurodegenerative and protein-misfolding diseases has been growing, an alternative, encompassing paradigm has been emerging. This paradigm postulates that non-fibrillar protein assemblies rather than mature amyloidogenic fibrils likely are the key neurotoxins responsible for most of the pathogenic mechanisms in protein-misfolding and neurodegenerative diseases, including AD. Accordingly, oligomeric species with different degrees of structural order are thought to mediate various pathogenic mechanisms that may lead to cytotoxicity and cell loss eventuating in organic and systemic morbidity. It is thought that histopathological progression of neurodegenerative lesions and symptom development likely occur by dissemination of protein-misfolding through connected brain regions. With the progressive use of classical techniques, and the advent of novel, sophisticated methodologies, several different forms of non-fibrillar assemblies of Aβ and those of other amyloidogenic proteins have been described. This has led to considerable progress in the elucidation of structural and functional features and fundamentals of the assembly of these proteins at the molecular level. Overall, it is postulated that some of the non-fibrillar amyloidogenic assemblies are on path to fibrillogenesis. The resulting protein fibrils are thought to be the end-stage sinks for the toxic non-fibrillar species. Fibrillar assemblies accumulate progressively into intra- and/or extracellular proteinaceous amyloid aggregates generating the disease-specific lesions *in vivo*. However, recent crystallographic studies of disease-related model peptides, having shed light on the structures of oligomeric amyloid assemblies, may have reignited the counter-argument that out-of-register, antiparallel amyloid fibrils may be cytotoxic in their own right [344].

In AD research, various forms of non-fibrillar Aβ assemblies, including activated monomeric conformers, ADDLs, PF, cell-derived dimers and trimers, and annular assemblies have been described (Table **1**). In many cases, the structural and functional interrelationships amongst these assemblies are still elusive and their atomically resolved structural relationships with out-of-register, antiparallel "cylindrins" are yet to be examined. Nevertheless, some have been shown to be pathogenic through one or several common pathways, suggesting that they may share structural features and possibly mechanisms of action. Understanding these intricate structure–function correlations will decipher a complex and interconnected array of pathogenic mechanisms.

Global research efforts have established a framework for understanding the fundamentals of Aβ assembly [7, 10, 11]. A remaining challenge is to assess how these fundamental structural principles are linked to cellular and tissular microenvironments during progression of AD. Many experimental conditions have been used to study the structure and function of non-fibrillar assemblies, but it is difficult to regenerate and scrutinize the actual *in vivo* milieus and conditions in which protein assembly, oligomerization, fibrillization, and deposition occur. Similarly, it is extremely difficult to assess all the possible interactions these assemblies may have with various cellular components and organelles. A multitude of detrimental mechanisms, including disruption of cellular metabolism, synapse structure and function deregulation, membrane damage, ionic imbalance, oxidative/inflammatory stress, apoptotic, and other cytotoxic effects, have been shown to be mediated by non-fibrillar Aβ assemblies, emphasizing that a single therapeutic approach likely will be insufficient to prevent or treat AD progression. By inference, this likely is true also for other amyloidoses. The intricacy of the pathogenic mechanisms in these diseases calls for rational diagnostic and therapeutic approaches that would target not only a single assembly or a single mechanism, but a multitude of assemblies and mechanisms. It is important to design and discover therapeutic agents that could target various assemblies that potentially become active early or are continuously active throughout the course of disease. Successful targeting of non-fibrillar assemblies *in vitro* and in animal models could have crucial diagnostic and prognostic implications for amyloid-related diseases.

ACKNOWLEDGEMENTS

We acknowledge Mr. Sean M. Spring for conducting the experiment described in Fig. **1**. The work was supported by funding from the Jim Easton Consortium for Alzheimer's Drug Discovery and Biomarker Development at UCLA, Team Parkinson/Parkinson Alliance, grant 20095024 from the RJG Foundation, a grant from the Cure Alzheimer's Fund, and a UCLA Alzheimer's Disease Research Center Pilot Award (from NIH/NIA P50AG016570).

CONFLICT OF INTEREST

The authors confirm that this chapter content has no conflict of interest.

DISCLOSURE

This chapter is an update of our previous publication in CAR "Structure–Function Relationships of Pre-Fibrillar Protein Assemblies in Alzheimer's Disease and Related Disorders" published in 'CAR', Volume 5, Number 3, June, pp. 319 to 341.

ABBREVIATIONS

αtα	=	α-helix-turn-α-helix
β_2m	=	β_2-microglobulin
AcP	=	Acylphosphatase
AD	=	Alzheimer's disease
ADDLs	=	Aβ-derived diffusible ligands

AFM = Atomic-force microscopy

APF = Annular Aβ42-derived protofibrils

APP = Amyloid β-protein precursor

Arc = Activity-regulated cytoskeleton-associated protein

Aβ = Amyloid β-protein

$[Ca^{2+}]_i$ = Intracellular Ca^{2+} concentration

CD = Circular dichroism

CSF = Cerebrospinal fluid

DLS = Dynamic light scattering

EPSC = Excitatory post-synaptic current

FAIMS = Field-asymmetric ion-mobility spectrometry

FTIR = Fourier-transform infrared spectroscopy

HD = Huntington's disease

HFIP = 1,1,1,3,3,3-hexafluoro-2-isopropanol

HNE = 4-hydroxy-2-nonenal

HPLC = High-performance liquid chromatography

HypF-N = Hydrogenase maturation-factor

IAPP = Islet amyloid polypeptide

IMS–MS = Ion-mobility spectrometry–mass spectrometry

LMW = Low molecular weight

LTD	=	Long-term depression
LTP	=	Long-term potentiation
MALDI	=	Matrix-assisted laser-desorption ionization
MALLS	=	Multi-angle laser light scattering
MPL	=	Mass-per-length
MTT	=	3-(4,5-Dimethylthiazol-2-yl)-2,5-diphenyltetrazolium bromide
nAchR	=	Nicotinic acetylcholine receptor
NMDA	=	*N*-methyl-D-aspartate
NMDAR(s)	=	NMDA receptor(s)
PD	=	Parkinson's disease
PF	=	Protofibrils
PI3K	=	Phosphatidyl inositol 3-kinase
PICUP	=	Photo-induced cross-linking of unmodified proteins
PrP^{C}	=	Cellular prion protein
PrP^{Sc}	=	Misfolded prion protein
ROS	=	Reactive oxygen species
SDS	=	Sodium dodecyl sulfate
SEC	=	Size-exclusion chromatography
SH3	=	Src-homology 3
SPPS	=	Solid-phase peptide synthesis

STEM = Scanning transmission electron microscopy

STM = Scanning tunneling microscopy

SOD1 = Superoxide dismutase 1

T2D = Type-2 diabetes mellitus

TABFOs = Toxic Aβ42-derived fibrillar oligomers

TEM = Transmission electron microscopy

TFE = Trifluoroethanol

ThT = Thioflavin T

TSE = Transmissible spongiform encephalopathies

REFERENCES

[1] Hardy JA, Higgins GA. Alzheimer's disease: the amyloid cascade hypothesis. Science 1992; 256: 184-5.

[2] Terry RD, Masliah E, Salmon DP, *et al.* Physical basis of cognitive alterations in Alzheimer's disease: synapse loss is the major correlate of cognitive impairment. Ann Neurol 1991; 30: 572-80.

[3] Mucke L, Masliah E, Yu GQ, *et al.* High-level neuronal expression of $A\beta_{1-42}$ in wild-type human amyloid protein precursor transgenic mice: synaptotoxicity without plaque formation. J Neurosci 2000; 20: 4050-8.

[4] Klein WL, Krafft GA, Finch CE. Targeting small Aβ oligomers: the solution to an Alzheimer's disease conundrum? Trends Neurosci 2001; 24: 219-24.

[5] Kirkitadze MD, Bitan G, Teplow DB. Paradigm shifts in Alzheimer's disease and other neurodegenerative disorders: the emerging role of oligomeric assemblies. J Neurosci Res 2002; 69: 567-77.

[6] Hardy J, Selkoe DJ. The amyloid hypothesis of Alzheimer's disease: progress and problems on the road to therapeutics. Science 2002; 297: 353-6.

[7] Caughey B, Lansbury PT. Protofibrils, pores, fibrils, and neurodegeneration: separating the responsible protein aggregates from the innocent bystanders. Annu Rev Neurosci 2003; 26: 267-98.

[8] Baglioni S, Casamenti F, Bucciantini M, *et al.* Prefibrillar amyloid aggregates could be generic toxins in higher organisms. J Neurosci 2006; 26: 8160-7.

[9] Lansbury PT, Lashuel HA. A century-old debate on protein aggregation and neurodegeneration enters the clinic. Nature 2006; 443: 774-9.

[10] Haass C, Selkoe DJ. Soluble protein oligomers in neurodegeneration: lessons from the Alzheimer's amyloid β-peptide. Nat Rev Mol Cell Biol 2007; 8: 101-12.

[11] Ferreira ST, Vieira MN, De Felice FG. Soluble protein oligomers as emerging toxins in Alzheimer's and other amyloid diseases. IUBMB life 2007; 59: 332-45.

[12] Fleming Outeiro T, Tetzlaff J. Mechanisms of disease II: cellular protein quality control. Semin Pediatr Neurol 2007; 14: 15-25.

[13] Agorogiannis EI, Agorogiannis GI, Papadimitriou A, Hadjigeorgiou GM. Protein misfolding in neurodegenerative diseases. Neuropathol Appl Neurobiol 2004; 30: 215-24.

[14] Marzban L, Park K, Verchere CB. Islet amyloid polypeptide and type 2 diabetes. Exp Gerontol 2003; 38: 347-51.

[15] Lachmann HJ, Hawkins PN. Systemic amyloidosis. Curr Opin Pharmacol 2006; 6: 214-20.

[16] Finder VH, Glockshuber R. Amyloid-β aggregation. Neurodegener Dis 2007; 4: 13-27.

[17] Teplow DB. Structural and kinetic features of amyloid β-protein fibrillogenesis. Amyloid 1998; 5: 121-42.

[18] Lashuel HA, Lansbury PT, Jr. Are amyloid diseases caused by protein aggregates that mimic bacterial pore-forming toxins? Q Rev Biophys 2006; 39: 167-201.

[19] Taylor BM, Sarver RW, Fici G, *et al.* Spontaneous aggregation and cytotoxicity of the β-amyloid Aβ1–40: a kinetic model. J Protein Chem 2003; 22: 31-40.

[20] Roher AE, Palmer KC, Yurewicz EC, Ball MJ, Greenberg BD. Morphological and biochemical analyses of amyloid plaque core proteins purified from Alzheimer disease brain tissue. J Neurochem 1993; 61: 1916-26.

[21] Enya M, Morishima-Kawashima M, Yoshimura M, *et al.* Appearance of sodium dodecyl sulfate-stable amyloid β-protein (Aβ) dimer in the cortex during aging. Am J Pathol 1999; 154: 271-9.

[22] Vigo-Pelfrey C, Lee D, Keim P, Lieberburg I, Schenk DB. Characterization of β-amyloid peptide from human cerebrospinal fluid. J Neurochem 1993; 61: 1965-8.

[23] Podlisny MB, Ostaszewski BL, Squazzo SL, *et al.* Aggregation of secreted amyloid β-protein into sodium dodecyl sulfate-stable oligomers in cell culture. J Biol Chem 1995; 270: 9564-70.

[24] Walsh DM, Klyubin I, Fadeeva JV, *et al.* Naturally secreted oligomers of amyloid β protein potently inhibit hippocampal long-term potentiation *in vivo*. Nature 2002; 416: 535-9.

[25] Walsh DM, Tseng BP, Rydel RE, Podlisny MB, Selkoe DJ. The oligomerization of amyloid β-protein begins intracellularly in cells derived from human brain. Biochemistry 2000; 39: 10831-9.

[26] Lambert MP, Barlow AK, Chromy BA, *et al.* Diffusible, nonfibrillar ligands derived from $A\beta_{1-42}$ are potent central nervous system neurotoxins. Proc Natl Acad Sci USA 1998; 95: 6448-53.

[27] Gong Y, Chang L, Viola KL, *et al.* Alzheimer's disease-affected brain: presence of oligomeric Aβ ligands (ADDLs) suggests a molecular basis for reversible memory loss. Proc Natl Acad Sci USA 2003; 100: 10417-22.

[28] Harper JD, Wong SS, Lieber CM, Lansbury PT. Observation of metastable Aβ amyloid protofibrils by atomic force microscopy. Chem Biol 1997; 4: 119-25.

[29] Hartley DM, Walsh DM, Ye CP, *et al.* Protofibrillar intermediates of amyloid β-protein induce acute electrophysiological changes and progressive neurotoxicity in cortical neurons. J Neurosci 1999; 19: 8876-84.

[30] Walsh DM, Hartley DM, Kusumoto Y, *et al.* Amyloid β-protein fibrillogenesis. Structure and biological activity of protofibrillar intermediates. J Biol Chem 1999; 274: 25945-52.

[31] Lesné S, Koh MT, Kotilinek L, *et al.* A specific amyloid-β protein assembly in the brain impairs memory. Nature 2006; 440: 352-7.
[32] Bitan G, Kirkitadze MD, Lomakin A, *et al.* Amyloid β-protein (Aβ) assembly: Aβ40 and Aβ42 oligomerize through distinct pathways. Proc Natl Acad Sci USA 2003; 100: 330-5.
[33] Bitan G, Tarus B, Vollers SS, *et al.* A molecular switch in amyloid assembly: Met35 and amyloid β-protein oligomerization. J Am Chem Soc 2003; 125: 15359-65.
[34] Bitan G, Vollers SS, Teplow DB. Elucidation of primary structure elements controlling early amyloid β-protein oligomerization. J Biol Chem 2003; 278: 34882-9.
[35] Hoshi M, Sato M, Matsumoto S, *et al.* Spherical aggregates of β-amyloid (amylospheroid) show high neurotoxicity and activate tau protein kinase I/glycogen synthase kinase-3β. Proc Natl Acad Sci USA 2003; 100: 6370-5.
[36] Lashuel HA, Hartley D, Petre BM, Walz T, Lansbury PT, Jr. Neurodegenerative disease: amyloid pores from pathogenic mutations. Nature 2002; 418: 291.
[37] Lashuel HA, Hartley DM, Petre BM, *et al.* Mixtures of wild-type and a pathogenic (E22G) form of Aβ40 *in vitro* accumulate protofibrils, including amyloid pores. J Mol Biol 2003; 332: 795-808.
[38] Glabe CG. Structural classification of toxic amyloid oligomers. J Biol Chem 2008; 283: 29639-43.
[39] Westlind-Danielsson A, Arnerup G. Spontaneous *in vitro* formation of supramolecular β-amyloid structures, "betaamy balls", by β-amyloid 1–40 peptide. Biochemistry 2001; 40: 14736-43.
[40] Merrifield B. Concept and early development of solid-phase peptide synthesis. Methods Enzymol 1997; 289: 3-13.
[41] Kim YS, Moss JA, Janda KD. Biological tuning of synthetic tactics in solid-phase synthesis: application to Aβ(1–42). J Org Chem 2004; 69: 7776-8.
[42] Sharpe S, Yau WM, Tycko R. Expression and purification of a recombinant peptide from the Alzheimer's β-amyloid protein for solid-state NMR. Protein Expr Purif 2005; 42: 200-10.
[43] Lee EK, Hwang JH, Shin DY, Kim DI, Yoo YJ. Production of recombinant amyloid-β peptide 42 as an ubiquitin extension. Protein Expr Purif 2005; 40: 183-9.
[44] Dobeli H, Draeger N, Huber G, *et al.* A biotechnological method provides access to aggregation competent monomeric Alzheimer's 1–42 residue amyloid peptide. Biotechnology (NY) 1995; 13: 988-93.
[45] Carrotta R, Di Carlo M, Manno M, *et al.* Toxicity of recombinant β-amyloid prefibrillar oligomers on the morphogenesis of the sea urchin *Paracentrotus lividus*. FASEB J 2006; 20: 1916-7.
[46] Tickler AK, Barrow CJ, Wade JD. Improved preparation of amyloid-β peptides using DBU as N^{α}-Fmoc deprotection reagent. J Pept Sci 2001; 7: 488-94.
[47] Zarándi M, Soós K, Fülöp L, *et al.* Synthesis of Aβ[1–42] and its derivatives with improved efficiency. J Pept Sci 2007; 13: 94-9.
[48] Tickler AK, Clippingdale AB, Wade JD. Amyloid-β as a "difficult sequence" in solid phase peptide synthesis. Protein Pept Lett 2004; 11: 377-84.
[49] García-Martín F, Quintanar-Audelo M, García-Ramos Y, *et al.* ChemMatrix, a poly(ethylene glycol)-based support for the solid-phase synthesis of complex peptides. J Comb Chem 2006; 8: 213-20.

[50] Bacsa B, Bosze S, Kappe CO. Direct solid-phase synthesis of the β-amyloid (1–42) peptide using controlled microwave heating. J Org Chem 2010; 75: 2103-6.
[51] Sohma Y, Sasaki M, Hayashi Y, Kimura T, Kiso Y. Design and synthesis of a novel water-soluble Aβ1–42 isopeptide: an efficient strategy for the preparation of Alzheimer's disease-related peptide, Aβ1–42, *via O-N* intramolecular acyl migration reaction. Tetrahedron Lett 2004; 45: 5965-68.
[52] Sohma Y, Taniguchi A, Yoshiya T, *et al.* 'Click peptide': a novel '*O*-acyl isopeptide method' for peptide synthesis and chemical biology-oriented synthesis of amyloid β peptide analogues. J Pept Sci 2006; 12: 823-8.
[53] Macao B, Hoyer W, Sandberg A, *et al.* Recombinant amyloid β-peptide production by coexpression with an affibody ligand. BMC Biotechnol 2008; 8: 82.
[54] Cornista JC, Koga Y, Takano K, Kanaya S. Amyloidogenecity and pitrilysin sensitivity of a lysine-free derivative of amyloid β-peptide cleaved from a recombinant fusion protein. J Biotechnol 2006; 122: 186-97.
[55] Yonemoto IT, Wood MR, Balch WE, Kelly JW. A general strategy for the bacterial expression of amyloidogenic peptides using BCL-XL-1/2 fusions. Protein Sci 2009; 18: 1978-86.
[56] Garai K, Crick SL, Mustafi SM, Frieden C. Expression and purification of amyloid-β peptides from *Escherichia coli*. Protein Expr Purif 2009; 66: 107-12.
[57] Bockhorn JJ, Lazar KL, Gasser AJ, *et al.* Novel semisynthetic method for generating full length β-amyloid peptides. Biopolymers 2010; 94: 511-20.
[58] Teplow DB. Preparation of amyloid β-protein for structural and functional studies. Methods Enzymol 2006; 413: 20-33.
[59] Klein WL, Stine WB, Jr., Teplow DB. Small assemblies of unmodified amyloid β-protein are the proximate neurotoxin in Alzheimer's disease. Neurobiol Aging 2004; 25: 569-80.
[60] Howlett DR, Jennings KH, Lee DC, *et al.* Aggregation state and neurotoxic properties of Alzheimer β-amyloid peptide. Neurodegeneration 1995; 4: 23-32.
[61] Simmons LK, May PC, Tomaselli KJ, *et al.* Secondary structure of amyloid β peptide correlates with neurotoxic activity *in vitro*. Mol Pharmacol 1994; 45: 373-9.
[62] Soto C, Castaño EM, Kumar RA, Beavis RC, Frangione B. Fibrillogenesis of synthetic amyloid-β peptides is dependent on their initial secondary structure. Neurosci Lett 1995; 200: 105-8.
[63] Bitan G, Fradinger EA, Spring SM, Teplow DB. Neurotoxic protein oligomers—what you see is not always what you get. Amyloid 2005; 12: 88-95.
[64] Zeeb M, Balbach J. Protein folding studied by real-time NMR spectroscopy. Methods 2004; 34: 65-74.
[65] Benilova I, Karran E, De Strooper B. The toxic Aβ oligomer and Alzheimer's disease: an emperor in need of clothes. Nat Neurosci 2012; 15: 349-57.
[66] Bitan G, Teplow DB. Rapid photochemical cross-linking—a new tool for studies of metastable, amyloidogenic protein assemblies. Acc Chem Res 2004; 37: 357-64.
[67] Li H, Rahimi F, Sinha S, *et al.* Amyloids and Protein Aggregation—Analytical Methods. Encyclopedia of Analytical Chemistry: John Wiley & Sons, Ltd; 2009.
[68] Lee JP, Stimson ER, Ghilardi JR, *et al.* 1H NMR of Aβ amyloid peptide congeners in water solution. Conformational changes correlate with plaque competence. Biochemistry 1995; 34: 5191-200.

[69] Zhang S, Iwata K, Lachenmann MJ, *et al.* The Alzheimer's peptide Aβ adopts a collapsed coil structure in water. J Struct Biol 2000; 130: 130-41.

[70] Yan Y, Wang C. Aβ42 is more rigid than Aβ40 at the C terminus: implications for Aβ aggregation and toxicity. J Mol Biol 2006; 364: 853-62.

[71] Riek R, Güntert P, Döbeli H, Wipf B, Wüthrich K. NMR studies in aqueous solution fail to identify significant conformational differences between the monomeric forms of two Alzheimer peptides with widely different plaque-competence, Aβ(1–40)^{ox} and Aβ(1–42)^{ox}. Eur J Biochem 2001; 268: 5930-6.

[72] Hou L, Shao H, Zhang Y, *et al.* Solution NMR studies of the Aβ(1–40) and Aβ(1–42) peptides establish that the Met35 oxidation state affects the mechanism of amyloid formation. J Am Chem Soc 2004; 126: 1992-2005.

[73] Sgourakis NG, Yan Y, McCallum SA, Wang C, Garcia AE. The Alzheimer's peptides Aβ40 and 42 adopt distinct conformations in water: a combined MD/NMR study. J Mol Biol 2007; 368: 1448-57.

[74] Lazo ND, Grant MA, Condron MC, Rigby AC, Teplow DB. On the nucleation of amyloid β-protein monomer folding. Protein Sci 2005; 14: 1581-96.

[75] Bemporad F, Chiti F. Protein misfolded oligomers: experimental approaches, mechanism of formation, and structure-toxicity relationships. Chem Biol 2012; 19: 315-27.

[76] MacArthur MW, Driscoll PC, Thornton JM. NMR and crystallography—complementary approaches to structure determination. Trends Biotechnol 1994; 12: 149-53.

[77] Sawaya MR, Sambashivan S, Nelson R, *et al.* Atomic structures of amyloid cross-β spines reveal varied steric zippers. Nature 2007; 447: 453-7.

[78] Kheterpal I, Chen M, Cook KD, Wetzel R. Structural differences in Aβ amyloid protofibrils and fibrils mapped by hydrogen exchange–mass spectrometry with on-line proteolytic fragmentation. J Mol Biol 2006; 361: 785-95.

[79] Laemmli UK. Cleavage of structural proteins during the assembly of the head of bacteriophage T4. Nature 1970; 227: 680-5.

[80] Khan JM, Qadeer A, Chaturvedi SK, *et al.* SDS can be utilized as an amyloid inducer: a case study on diverse proteins. PLoS One 2012; 7: e29694.

[81] Gudiksen KL, Gitlin I, Whitesides GM. Differentiation of proteins based on characteristic patterns of association and denaturation in solutions of SDS. Proc Natl Acad Sci USA 2006; 103: 7968-72.

[82] Leffers KW, Schell J, Jansen K, *et al.* The structural transition of the prion protein into its pathogenic conformation is induced by unmasking hydrophobic sites. J Mol Biol 2004; 344: 839-53.

[83] Kawooya JK, Emmons TL, Gonzalez-DeWhitt PA, Camp MC, D'Andrea SC. Electrophoretic mobility of Alzheimer's amyloid-β peptides in urea–sodium dodecyl sulfate–polyacrylamide gel electrophoresis. Anal Biochem 2003; 323: 103-13.

[84] Montserret R, McLeish MJ, Böckmann A, Geourjon C, Penin F. Involvement of electrostatic interactions in the mechanism of peptide folding induced by sodium dodecyl sulfate binding. Biochemistry 2000; 39: 8362-73.

[85] Yamamoto S, Hasegawa K, Yamaguchi I, *et al.* Low concentrations of sodium dodecyl sulfate induce the extension of β_2-microglobulin-related amyloid fibrils at a neutral pH. Biochemistry 2004; 43: 11075-82.

[86] Rangachari V, Moore BD, Reed DK, *et al.* Amyloid-β(1–42) rapidly forms protofibrils and oligomers by distinct pathways in low concentrations of sodium dodecylsulfate. Biochemistry 2007; 46: 12451-62.
[87] Rangachari V, Reed DK, Moore BD, Rosenberry TL. Secondary structure and interfacial aggregation of amyloid-β(1–40) on sodium dodecyl sulfate micelles. Biochemistry 2006; 45: 8639-48.
[88] Piening N, Weber P, Hogen T, *et al.* Photo-induced crosslinking of prion protein oligomers and prions. Amyloid 2006; 13: 67-77.
[89] Barghorn S, Nimmrich V, Striebinger A, *et al.* Globular amyloid β-peptide$_{1-42}$ oligomer—a homogenous and stable neuropathological protein in Alzheimer's disease. J Neurochem 2005; 95: 834-47.
[90] Walsh DM, Lomakin A, Benedek GB, Condron MM, Teplow DB. Amyloid β-protein fibrillogenesis. Detection of a protofibrillar intermediate. J Biol Chem 1997; 272: 22364-72.
[91] Mori H, Takio K, Ogawara M, Selkoe DJ. Mass spectrometry of purified amyloid β protein in Alzheimer's disease. J Biol Chem 1992; 267: 17082-6.
[92] Wahlström A, Hugonin L, Perálvarez-Marín A, Jarvet J, Gräslund A. Secondary structure conversions of Alzheimer's Aβ(1–40) peptide induced by membrane-mimicking detergents. FEBS J 2008; 275: 5117-28.
[93] Yang M, Teplow DB. Amyloid β-protein monomer folding: free-energy surfaces reveal alloform-specific differences. J Mol Biol 2008; 384: 450-64.
[94] Reed MN, Hofmeister JJ, Jungbauer L, *et al.* Cognitive effects of cell-derived and synthetically derived Aβ oligomers. Neurobiol Aging 2011; 32: 1784-94.
[95] Hepler RW, Grimm KM, Nahas DD, *et al.* Solution state characterization of amyloid β-derived diffusible ligands. Biochemistry 2006; 45: 15157-67.
[96] Rahimi F, Bitan G. Overview of Fibrillar and Oligomeric Assemblies of Amyloidogenic Proteins In: Rahimi F, Bitan G, editors. Non-fibrillar Amyloidogenic Protein Assemblies—Common Cytotoxins Underlying Degenerative Diseases. Netherlands: Springer Netherlands; 2012. p. 1–36.
[97] Fancy DA, Kodadek T. Chemistry for the analysis of protein-protein interactions: rapid and efficient cross-linking triggered by long wavelength light. Proc Natl Acad Sci USA 1999; 96: 6020-4.
[98] Bitan G. Structural study of metastable amyloidogenic protein oligomers by photo-induced cross-linking of unmodified proteins. Methods Enzymol 2006; 413: 217-36.
[99] Lopes DH, Sinha S, Rosensweig C, Bitan G. Application of photochemical cross-linking to the study of oligomerization of amyloidogenic proteins. Methods Mol Biol 2012; 849: 11-21.
[100] Rahimi F, Maiti P, Bitan G. Photo-induced cross-linking of unmodified proteins (PICUP) applied to amyloidogenic peptides. Journal of visualized experiments: JoVE 2009.
[101] Hayden EY, Teplow DB. Continuous flow reactor for the production of stable amyloid protein oligomers. Biochemistry 2012.
[102] Squires TM, Brady JF. A simple paradigm for active and nonlinear microrheology. Physics of Fluids 2005; 17: 073101.
[103] Bitan G, Lomakin A, Teplow DB. Amyloid β-protein oligomerization: prenucleation interactions revealed by photo-induced cross-linking of unmodified proteins. J Biol Chem 2001; 276: 35176-84.

[104] Nichols MR, Moss MA, Reed DK, *et al.* Growth of β-amyloid(1–40) protofibrils by monomer elongation and lateral association. Characterization of distinct products by light scattering and atomic force microscopy. Biochemistry 2002; 41: 6115-27.

[105] Kheterpal I, Lashuel HA, Hartley DM, *et al.* Aβ protofibrils possess a stable core structure resistant to hydrogen exchange. Biochemistry 2003; 42: 14092-8.

[106] Bitan G, Teplow DB. Preparation of aggregate-free, low molecular weight amyloid-β for assembly and toxicity assays. Methods Mol Biol 2005; 299: 3-9.

[107] Urbanke C, Witte G, Curth U. Sedimentation velocity method in the analytical ultracentrifuge for the study of protein-protein interactions. Methods Mol Biol 2005; 305: 101-14.

[108] Mok YF, Howlett GJ. Sedimentation velocity analysis of amyloid oligomers and fibrils. Methods Enzymol 2006; 413: 199-217.

[109] Lebowitz J, Lewis MS, Schuck P. Modern analytical ultracentrifugation in protein science: a tutorial review. Protein Sci 2002; 11: 2067-79.

[110] Huang TH, Yang DS, Plaskos NP, *et al.* Structural studies of soluble oligomers of the Alzheimer β-amyloid peptide. J Mol Biol 2000; 297: 73-87.

[111] Philo JS. Is any measurement method optimal for all aggregate sizes and types? AAPS J 2006; 8: E564-71.

[112] Einstein A. On the motion of small particles suspended in liquids at rest required by the molecular-kinetic theory of heat. Annalen der Physik 1905; 17: 549-60.

[113] Sutherland W. A dynamical theory of diffusion for non-electrolytes and the molecular mass of albumin. Philos Mag 1905; 9: 781-85.

[114] Lomakin A, Benedek GB, Teplow DB. Monitoring protein assembly using quasielastic light scattering spectroscopy. Methods Enzymol 1999; 309: 429-59.

[115] Wyatt P. Light scattering and the absolute characterization of macromolecules. Anal Chim Acta 1993; 272: 1-40.

[116] Oliva A, Llabrés M, Fariña JB. Applications of multi-angle laser light-scattering detection in the analysis of peptides and proteins. Curr Drug Discov Technol 2004; 1: 229-42.

[117] Tomski SJ, Murphy RM. Kinetics of aggregation of synthetic β-amyloid peptide. Arch Biochem Biophys 1992; 294: 630-8.

[118] Shen CL, Scott GL, Merchant F, Murphy RM. Light scattering analysis of fibril growth from the amino-terminal fragment β(1–28) of β-amyloid peptide. Biophys J 1993; 65: 2383-95.

[119] Lomakin A, Chung DS, Benedek GB, Kirschner DA, Teplow DB. On the nucleation and growth of amyloid β-protein fibrils: detection of nuclei and quantitation of rate constants. Proc Natl Acad Sci USA 1996; 93: 1125-9.

[120] Murphy RM, Pallitto MM. Probing the kinetics of β-amyloid self-association. J Struct Biol 2000; 130: 109-22.

[121] Ward RV, Jennings KH, Jepras R, *et al.* Fractionation and characterization of oligomeric, protofibrillar and fibrillar forms of β-amyloid peptide. Biochem J 2000; 348 Pt 1: 137-44.

[122] Lomakin A, Teplow DB. Quasielastic light scattering study of amyloid β-protein fibril formation. Protein Pept Lett 2006; 13: 247-54.

[123] Lomakin A, Teplow DB, Benedek GB. Quasielastic light scattering for protein assembly studies. Methods Mol Biol 2005; 299: 153-74.

[124] Kanu AB, Dwivedi P, Tam M, Matz L, Hill HH, Jr. Ion mobility-mass spectrometry. J Mass Spectrom 2008; 43: 1-22.

[125] Tang K, Li F, Shvartsburg AA, Strittmatter EF, Smith RD. Two-dimensional gas-phase separations coupled to mass spectrometry for analysis of complex mixtures. Anal Chem 2005; 77: 6381-8.

[126] Bernstein SL, Wyttenbach T, Baumketner A, *et al.* Amyloid β-protein: monomer structure and early aggregation states of Aβ42 and its Pro^{19} alloform. J Am Chem Soc 2005; 127: 2075-84.

[127] Shvartsburg AA, Li F, Tang K, Smith RD. Characterizing the structures and folding of free proteins using 2-D gas-phase separations: observation of multiple unfolded conformers. Anal Chem 2006; 78: 3304-15.

[128] Greenfield NJ. Using circular dichroism spectra to estimate protein secondary structure. Nat Protoc 2006; 1: 2876-90.

[129] Whitmore L, Wallace BA. Protein secondary structure analyses from circular dichroism spectroscopy: methods and reference databases. Biopolymers 2008; 89: 392-400.

[130] Kirkitadze MD, Condron MM, Teplow DB. Identification and characterization of key kinetic intermediates in amyloid β-protein fibrillogenesis. J Mol Biol 2001; 312: 1103-19.

[131] Gursky O, Aleshkov S. Temperature-dependent β-sheet formation in β-amyloid $A\beta_{1-40}$ peptide in water: uncoupling β-structure folding from aggregation. Biochim Biophys Acta 2000; 1476: 93-102.

[132] Lim KH, Collver HH, Le YT, Nagchowdhuri P, Kenney JM. Characterizations of distinct amyloidogenic conformations of the Aβ(1–40) and (1–42) peptides. Biochem Biophys Res Commun 2007; 353: 443-9.

[133] Hou L, Kang I, Marchant RE, Zagorski MG. Methionine 35 oxidation reduces fibril assembly of the amyloid Aβ-(1–42) peptide of Alzheimer's disease. J Biol Chem 2002; 277: 40173-6.

[134] Ahting U, Thieffry M, Engelhardt H, *et al.* Tom40, the pore-forming component of the protein-conducting TOM channel in the outer membrane of mitochondria. J Cell Biol 2001; 153: 1151-60.

[135] Hetényi C, Szabó Z, Klement E, *et al.* Pentapeptide amides interfere with the aggregation of β-amyloid peptide of Alzheimer's disease. Biochem Biophys Res Commun 2002; 292: 931-6.

[136] Lin SY, Chu HL. Fourier transform infrared spectroscopy used to evidence the prevention of β-sheet formation of amyloid β(1–40) peptide by a short amyloid fragment. Int J Biol Macromol 2003; 32: 173-7.

[137] Kakio A, Yano Y, Takai D, *et al.* Interaction between amyloid β-protein aggregates and membranes. J Pept Sci 2004; 10: 612-21.

[138] Brzyska M, Trzesniewska K, Gers T, Elbaum D. Discrete conformational changes as regulators of the hydrolytic properties of beta-amyloid (1–40). FEBS J 2006; 273: 5598-611.

[139] Mastrangelo IA, Ahmed M, Sato T, *et al.* High-resolution atomic force microscopy of soluble Aβ42 oligomers. J Mol Biol 2006; 358: 106-19.

[140] Kim YS, Liu L, Axelsen PH, Hochstrasser RM. 2D IR provides evidence for mobile water molecules in β-amyloid fibrils. Proc Natl Acad Sci USA 2009; 106: 17751-6.

[141] Woys AM, Almeida AM, Wang L, *et al.* Parallel β-sheet vibrational couplings revealed by 2D IR spectroscopy of an isotopically labeled macrocycle: quantitative benchmark for the interpretation of amyloid and protein infrared spectra. J Am Chem Soc 2012; 134: 19118-28.

[142] Middleton CT, Marek P, Cao P, *et al.* Two-dimensional infrared spectroscopy reveals the complex behaviour of an amyloid fibril inhibitor. Nat Chem 2012; 4: 355-60.
[143] De Carlo S, Harris JR. Negative staining and cryo-negative staining of macromolecules and viruses for TEM. Micron 2011; 42: 117-31.
[144] Harris JR. Negative staining of thinly spread biological particulates. Methods Mol Biol 1999; 117: 13-30.
[145] Sherratt MJ, Meadows RS, Graham HK, Kielty CM, Holmes DF. ECM macromolecules: rotary shadowing and transmission electron microscopy. Methods Mol Biol 2009; 522: 175-81.
[146] Jonic S, Vénien-Bryan C. Protein structure determination by electron cryo-microscopy. Curr Opin Pharmacol 2009; 9: 636-42.
[147] Nybo M, Svehag SE, Holm Nielsen E. An ultrastructural study of amyloid intermediates in $A\beta_{1-42}$ fibrillogenesis. Scand J Immunol 1999; 49: 219-23.
[148] Modler AJ, Gast K, Lutsch G, Damaschun G. Assembly of amyloid protofibrils *via* critical oligomers—a novel pathway of amyloid formation. J Mol Biol 2003; 325: 135-48.
[149] Roher AE, Chaney MO, Kuo YM, *et al.* Morphology and toxicity of Aβ-(1–42) dimer derived from neuritic and vascular amyloid deposits of Alzheimer's disease. J Biol Chem 1996; 271: 20631-5.
[150] Selenica ML, Wang X, Ostergaard-Pedersen L, Westlind-Danielsson A, Grubb A. Cystatin C reduces the *in vitro* formation of soluble Aβ1–42 oligomers and protofibrils. Scand J Clin Lab Invest 2007; 67: 179-90.
[151] Wood SJ, Maleeff B, Hart T, Wetzel R. Physical, morphological and functional differences between pH 5.8 and 7.4 aggregates of the Alzheimer's amyloid peptide Aβ. J Mol Biol 1996; 256: 870-7.
[152] Lührs T, Ritter C, Adrian M, *et al.* 3D structure of Alzheimer's amyloid-β(1–42) fibrils. Proc Natl Acad Sci USA 2005; 102: 17342-7.
[153] Engel A, Colliex C. Application of scanning transmission electron microscopy to the study of biological structure. Curr Opin Biotechnol 1993; 4: 403-11.
[154] Lashuel HA, Wall JS. Molecular electron microscopy approaches to elucidating the mechanisms of protein fibrillogenesis. Methods Mol Biol 2005; 299: 81-101.
[155] Goldsbury C, Frey P, Olivieri V, Aebi U, Müller SA. Multiple assembly pathways underlie amyloid-β fibril polymorphisms. J Mol Biol 2005; 352: 282-98.
[156] Goldsbury CS, Wirtz S, Müller SA, *et al.* Studies on the *in vitro* assembly of Aβ1–40: implications for the search for Aβ fibril formation inhibitors. J Struct Biol 2000; 130: 217-31.
[157] Petkova AT, Leapman RD, Guo Z, *et al.* Self-propagating, molecular-level polymorphism in Alzheimer's β-amyloid fibrils. Science 2005; 307: 262-5.
[158] Wall JS, Simon MN, Lin BY, Vinogradov SN. Mass mapping of large globin complexes by scanning transmission electron microscopy. Methods Enzymol 2008; 436: 487-501.
[159] Blackley HK, Sanders GH, Davies MC, *et al.* *In-situ* atomic force microscopy study of β-amyloid fibrillization. J Mol Biol 2000; 298: 833-40.
[160] Kowalewski T, Holtzman DM. *In situ* atomic force microscopy study of Alzheimer's β-amyloid peptide on different substrates: new insights into mechanism of β-sheet formation. Proc Natl Acad Sci USA 1999; 96: 3688-93.

[161] Harper JD, Wong SS, Lieber CM, Lansbury PT, Jr. Assembly of Aβ amyloid protofibrils: an *in vitro* model for a possible early event in Alzheimer's disease. Biochemistry 1999; 38: 8972-80.
[162] Arimon M, Díez-Pérez I, Kogan MJ, *et al.* Fine structure study of Aβ1–42 fibrillogenesis with atomic force microscopy. FASEB J 2005; 19: 1344-6.
[163] Wang Z, Zhou C, Wang C, *et al.* AFM and STM study of β-amyloid aggregation on graphite. Ultramicroscopy 2003; 97: 73-9.
[164] Solomonov I, Korkotian E, Born B, *et al.* Zn^{2+}–Aβ40 complexes form metastable quasi-spherical oligomers that are cytotoxic to cultured hippocampal neurons. J Biol Chem 2012.
[165] Hansma PK, Elings VB, Marti O, Bracker CE. Scanning tunneling microscopy and atomic force microscopy: application to biology and technology. Science 1988; 242: 209-16.
[166] Shivji AP, Brown F, Davies MC, *et al.* Scanning tunnelling microscopy studies of β-amyloid fibril structure and assembly. FEBS Lett 1995; 371: 25-8.
[167] Losic D, Martin LL, Mechler A, Aguilar MI, Small DH. High resolution scanning tunnelling microscopy of the β-amyloid protein (Aβ1–40) of Alzheimer's disease suggests a novel mechanism of oligomer assembly. J Struct Biol 2006; 155: 104-10.
[168] Stratman NC, Castle CK, Taylor BM, *et al.* Isoform-specific interactions of human apolipoprotein E to an intermediate conformation of human Alzheimer amyloid-beta peptide. Chem Phys Lipids 2005; 137: 52-61.
[169] Sun XD, Mo ZL, Taylor BM, Epps DE. A slowly formed transient conformer of $A\beta^{1-40}$ is toxic to inward channels of dissociated hippocampal and cortical neurons of rats. Neurobiol Dis 2003; 14: 567-78.
[170] Xia W, Zhang J, Kholodenko D, *et al.* Enhanced production and oligomerization of the 42-residue amyloid β-protein by Chinese hamster ovary cells stably expressing mutant presenilins. J Biol Chem 1997; 272: 7977-82.
[171] Li S, Hong S, Shepardson NE, *et al.* Soluble oligomers of amyloid β protein facilitate hippocampal long-term depression by disrupting neuronal glutamate uptake. Neuron 2009; 62: 788-801.
[172] Cleary JP, Walsh DM, Hofmeister JJ, *et al.* Natural oligomers of the amyloid-β protein specifically disrupt cognitive function. Nat Neurosci 2005; 8: 79-84.
[173] Shankar GM, Bloodgood BL, Townsend M, *et al.* Natural oligomers of the Alzheimer amyloid-β protein induce reversible synapse loss by modulating an NMDA-type glutamate receptor-dependent signaling pathway. J Neurosci 2007; 27: 2866-75.
[174] O'Nuallain B, Freir DB, Nicoll AJ, *et al.* Amyloid β-protein dimers rapidly form stable synaptotoxic protofibrils. J Neurosci 2010; 30: 14411-9.
[175] Oda T, Wals P, Osterburg HH, *et al.* Clusterin (apoJ) alters the aggregation of amyloid β-peptide ($A\beta_{1-42}$) and forms slowly sedimenting Aβ complexes that cause oxidative stress. Exp Neurol 1995; 136: 22-31.
[176] Klein WL. Aβ toxicity in Alzheimer's disease: globular oligomers (ADDLs) as new vaccine and drug targets. Neurochem Int 2002; 41: 345-52.
[177] De Felice FG, Wu D, Lambert MP, *et al.* Alzheimer's disease-type neuronal tau hyperphosphorylation induced by Aβ oligomers. Neurobiol Aging 2007.
[178] Chromy BA, Nowak RJ, Lambert MP, *et al.* Self-assembly of Aβ(1–42) into globular neurotoxins. Biochemistry 2003; 42: 12749-60.
[179] Lambert MP, Velasco PT, Chang L, *et al.* Monoclonal antibodies that target pathological assemblies of Aβ. J Neurochem 2007; 100: 23-35.
[180] Lacor PN, Buniel MC, Furlow PW, *et al.* Aβ oligomer-induced aberrations in synapse composition, shape, and density provide a molecular basis for loss of connectivity in Alzheimer's disease. J Neurosci 2007; 27: 796-807.

[181] Lacor PN, Buniel MC, Chang L, *et al.* Synaptic targeting by Alzheimer's-related amyloid β oligomers. J Neurosci 2004; 24: 10191-200.
[182] De Felice FG, Velasco PT, Lambert MP, *et al.* Aβ oligomers induce neuronal oxidative stress through an *N*-methyl-D-aspartate receptor-dependent mechanism that is blocked by the Alzheimer drug memantine. J Biol Chem 2007; 282: 11590-601.
[183] Zempel H, Thies E, Mandelkow E, Mandelkow EM. Aβ oligomers cause localized Ca^{2+} elevation, missorting of endogenous Tau into dendrites, Tau phosphorylation, and destruction of microtubules and spines. J Neurosci 2010; 30: 11938-50.
[184] White JA, Manelli AM, Holmberg KH, Van Eldik LJ, Ladu MJ. Differential effects of oligomeric and fibrillar amyloid-β 1–42 on astrocyte-mediated inflammation. Neurobiol Dis 2005; 18: 459-65.
[185] Wang X, Perry G, Smith MA, Zhu X. Amyloid-β-derived diffusible ligands cause impaired axonal transport of mitochondria in neurons. Neurodegener Dis 2010; 7: 56-9.
[186] Ye C, Walsh DM, Selkoe DJ, Hartley DM. Amyloid β-protein induced electrophysiological changes are dependent on aggregation state: *N*-methyl-D-aspartate (NMDA) *versus* non-NMDA receptor/channel activation. Neurosci Lett 2004; 366: 320-5.
[187] Ye CP, Selkoe DJ, Hartley DM. Protofibrils of amyloid β-protein inhibit specific K^+ currents in neocortical cultures. Neurobiol Dis 2003; 13: 177-90.
[188] Nilsberth C, Westlind-Danielsson A, Eckman CB, *et al.* The 'Arctic' APP mutation (E693G) causes Alzheimer's disease by enhanced Aβ protofibril formation. Nat Neurosci 2001; 4: 887-93.
[189] Kayed R, Canto I, Breydo L, *et al.* Conformation dependent monoclonal antibodies distinguish different replicating strains or conformers of prefibrillar Aβ oligomers. Mol Neurodegener 2010; 5: 57.
[190] Stroud JC, Liu C, Teng PK, Eisenberg D. Toxic fibrillar oligomers of amyloid-β have cross-β structure. Proc Natl Acad Sci USA 2012; 109: 7717-22.
[191] Wu JW, Breydo L, Isas JM, *et al.* Fibrillar oligomers nucleate the oligomerization of monomeric amyloid β but do not seed fibril formation. J Biol Chem 2010; 285: 6071-9.
[192] Sandberg A, Luheshi LM, Söllvander S, *et al.* Stabilization of neurotoxic Alzheimer amyloid-β oligomers by protein engineering. Proc Natl Acad Sci USA 2010; 107: 15595-600.
[193] Shankar GM, Li S, Mehta TH, *et al.* Amyloid-β protein dimers isolated directly from Alzheimer's brains impair synaptic plasticity and memory. Nat Med 2008; 14: 837-42.
[194] Jin M, Shepardson N, Yang T, *et al.* Soluble amyloid β-protein dimers isolated from Alzheimer cortex directly induce Tau hyperphosphorylation and neuritic degeneration. Proc Natl Acad Sci USA 2011; 108: 5819-24.
[195] Hu NW, Smith IM, Walsh DM, Rowan MJ. Soluble amyloid-β peptides potently disrupt hippocampal synaptic plasticity in the absence of cerebrovascular dysfunction *in vivo*. Brain 2008; 131: 2414-24.
[196] Lasagna-Reeves CA, Glabe CG, Kayed R. Amyloid-β annular protofibrils evade fibrillar fate in Alzheimer disease brain. J Biol Chem 2011; 286: 22122-30.
[197] Kayed R, Pensalfini A, Margol L, *et al.* Annular protofibrils are a structurally and functionally distinct type of amyloid oligomer. J Biol Chem 2009; 284: 4230-7.
[198] Noguchi A, Matsumura S, Dezawa M, *et al.* Isolation and characterization of patient-derived, toxic, high mass amyloid β-protein (Aβ) assembly from Alzheimer disease brains. J Biol Chem 2009; 284: 32895-905.

[199] Matsumura S, Shinoda K, Yamada M, *et al.* Two distinct amyloid β-protein (Aβ) assembly pathways leading to oligomers and fibrils identified by combined fluorescence correlation spectroscopy, morphology, and toxicity analyses. J Biol Chem 2011; 286: 11555-62.

[200] Cooper JA, Buhle EL, Jr., Walker SB, Tsong TY, Pollard TD. Kinetic evidence for a monomer activation step in actin polymerization. Biochemistry 1983; 22: 2193-202.

[201] Shen CL, Murphy RM. Solvent effects on self-assembly of β-amyloid peptide. Biophys J 1995; 69: 640-51.

[202] Lee S, Fernandez EJ, Good TA. Role of aggregation conditions in structure, stability, and toxicity of intermediates in the Aβ fibril formation pathway. Protein Sci 2007; 16: 723-32.

[203] Chimon S, Ishii Y. Capturing intermediate structures of Alzheimer's β-amyloid, Aβ(1–40), by solid-state NMR spectroscopy. J Am Chem Soc 2005; 127: 13472-3.

[204] Koudinov AR, Berezov TT, Koudinova NV. The levels of soluble amyloid β in different high density lipoprotein subfractions distinguish Alzheimer's and normal aging cerebrospinal fluid: implication for brain cholesterol pathology? Neurosci Lett 2001; 314: 115-8.

[205] Koudinov AR, Koudinova NV, Kumar A, Beavis RC, Ghiso J. Biochemical characterization of Alzheimer's soluble amyloid Beta protein in human cerebrospinal fluid: association with high density lipoproteins. Biochem Biophys Res Commun 1996; 223: 592-7.

[206] Kawarabayashi T, Shoji M, Younkin LH, *et al.* Dimeric amyloid β protein rapidly accumulates in lipid rafts followed by apolipoprotein E and phosphorylated tau accumulation in the Tg2576 mouse model of Alzheimer's disease. J Neurosci 2004; 24: 3801-9.

[207] Morishima-Kawashima M, Ihara Y. The presence of amyloid β-protein in the detergent-insoluble membrane compartment of human neuroblastoma cells. Biochemistry 1998; 37: 15247-53.

[208] Townsend M, Shankar GM, Mehta T, Walsh DM, Selkoe DJ. Effects of secreted oligomers of amyloid β-protein on hippocampal synaptic plasticity: a potent role for trimers. J Physiol 2006; 572: 477-92.

[209] Walsh DM, Klyubin I, Fadeeva JV, Rowan MJ, Selkoe DJ. Amyloid-β oligomers: their production, toxicity and therapeutic inhibition. Biochem Soc Trans 2002; 30: 552-7.

[210] Walsh DM, Townsend M, Podlisny MB, *et al.* Certain inhibitors of synthetic amyloid β-peptide (Aβ) fibrillogenesis block oligomerization of natural Aβ and thereby rescue long-term potentiation. J Neurosci 2005; 25: 2455-62.

[211] Walsh DM, Selkoe DJ. Aβ Oligomers – a decade of discovery. J Neurochem 2007.

[212] Dudai Y. Molecular bases of long-term memories: a question of persistence. Curr Opin Neurobiol 2002; 12: 211-6.

[213] Kojima N, Shirao T. Synaptic dysfunction and disruption of postsynaptic drebrin–actin complex: a study of neurological disorders accompanied by cognitive deficits. Neurosci Res 2007; 58: 1-5.

[214] Calabrese B, Shaked GM, Tabarean IV, *et al.* Rapid, concurrent alterations in pre- and postsynaptic structure induced by naturally-secreted amyloid-β protein. Mol Cell Neurosci 2007; 35: 183-93.

[215] Shrestha BR, Vitolo OV, Joshi P, *et al.* Amyloid β peptide adversely affects spine number and motility in hippocampal neurons. Mol Cell Neurosci 2006; 33: 274-82.

[216] McLaurin J, Golomb R, Jurewicz A, Antel JP, Fraser PE. Inositol stereoisomers stabilize an oligomeric aggregate of Alzheimer amyloid β peptide and inhibit Aβ-induced toxicity. J Biol Chem 2000; 275: 18495-502.
[217] Townsend M, Cleary JP, Mehta T, *et al.* Orally available compound prevents deficits in memory caused by the Alzheimer amyloid-β oligomers. Ann Neurol 2006; 60: 668-76.
[218] Snyder EM, Nong Y, Almeida CG, *et al.* Regulation of NMDA receptor trafficking by amyloid-β. Nat Neurosci 2005; 8: 1051-8.
[219] Calero M, Rostagno A, Matsubara E, *et al.* Apolipoprotein J (clusterin) and Alzheimer's disease. Microsc Res Tech 2000; 50: 305-15.
[220] Stine WB, Jr., Dahlgren KN, Krafft GA, LaDu MJ. *In vitro* characterization of conditions for amyloid-β peptide oligomerization and fibrillogenesis. J Biol Chem 2003; 278: 11612-22.
[221] Whitlock JR, Heynen AJ, Shuler MG, Bear MF. Learning induces long-term potentiation in the hippocampus. Science 2006; 313: 1093-7.
[222] Martin SJ, Grimwood PD, Morris RG. Synaptic plasticity and memory: an evaluation of the hypothesis. Annu Rev Neurosci 2000; 23: 649-711.
[223] Wang HW, Pasternak JF, Kuo H, *et al.* Soluble oligomers of β amyloid (1–42) inhibit long-term potentiation but not long-term depression in rat dentate gyrus. Brain Res 2002; 924: 133-40.
[224] Fong DK, Rao A, Crump FT, Craig AM. Rapid synaptic remodeling by protein kinase C: reciprocal translocation of NMDA receptors and calcium/calmodulin-dependent kinase II. J Neurosci 2002; 22: 2153-64.
[225] Chang L, Bakhos L, Wang Z, Venton DL, Klein WL. Femtomole immunodetection of synthetic and endogenous amyloid-β oligomers and its application to Alzheimer's disease drug candidate screening. J Mol Neurosci 2003; 20: 305-13.
[226] Tong L, Balazs R, Thornton PL, Cotman CW. β-Amyloid peptide at sublethal concentrations downregulates brain-derived neurotrophic factor functions in cultured cortical neurons. J Neurosci 2004; 24: 6799-809.
[227] Harris KM, Kater SB. Dendritic spines: cellular specializations imparting both stability and flexibility to synaptic function. Annu Rev Neurosci 1994; 17: 341-71.
[228] Carlisle HJ, Kennedy MB. Spine architecture and synaptic plasticity. Trends Neurosci 2005; 28: 182-7.
[229] Fiala JC, Spacek J, Harris KM. Dendritic spine pathology: cause or consequence of neurological disorders? Brain Res Brain Res Rev 2002; 39: 29-54.
[230] Tzingounis AV, Nicoll RA. Arc/Arg3.1: linking gene expression to synaptic plasticity and memory. Neuron 2006; 52: 403-7.
[231] Guzowski JF, Lyford GL, Stevenson GD, *et al.* Inhibition of activity-dependent arc protein expression in the rat hippocampus impairs the maintenance of long-term potentiation and the consolidation of long-term memory. J Neurosci 2000; 20: 3993-4001.
[232] Oddo S, Caccamo A, Tran L, *et al.* Temporal profile of amyloid-β (Aβ) oligomerization in an *in vivo* model of Alzheimer disease. A link between Aβ and tau pathology. J Biol Chem 2006; 281: 1599-604.
[233] Lambert MP, Viola KL, Chromy BA, *et al.* Vaccination with soluble Aβ oligomers generates toxicity-neutralizing antibodies. J Neurochem 2001; 79: 595-605.
[234] Seilheimer B, Bohrmann B, Bondolfi L, *et al.* The toxicity of the Alzheimer's β-amyloid peptide correlates with a distinct fiber morphology. J Struct Biol 1997; 119: 59-71.
[235] Williams AD, Sega M, Chen M, *et al.* Structural properties of Aβ protofibrils stabilized by a small molecule. Proc Natl Acad Sci USA 2005; 102: 7115-20.
[236] Mosmann T. Rapid colorimetric assay for cellular growth and survival: application to proliferation and cytotoxicity assays. J Immunol Methods 1983; 65: 55-63.

[237] Korzeniewski C, Callewaert DM. An enzyme-release assay for natural cytotoxicity. J Immunol Methods 1983; 64: 313-20.

[238] Haass C, Steiner H. Protofibrils, the unifying toxic molecule of neurodegenerative disorders? Nat Neurosci 2001; 4: 859-60.

[239] Sayre LM, Zelasko DA, Harris PL, *et al.* 4-Hydroxynonenal-derived advanced lipid peroxidation end products are increased in Alzheimer's disease. J Neurochem 1997; 68: 2092-7.

[240] Siegel SJ, Bieschke J, Powers ET, Kelly JW. The oxidative stress metabolite 4-hydroxynonenal promotes Alzheimer protofibril formation. Biochemistry 2007; 46: 1503-10.

[241] Johansson AS, Garlind A, Berglind-Dehlin F, *et al.* Docosahexaenoic acid stabilizes soluble amyloid-β protofibrils and sustains amyloid-β-induced neurotoxicity *in vitro*. FEBS J 2007; 274: 990-1000.

[242] Eriksen JL, Janus CG. Plaques, tangles, and memory loss in mouse models of neurodegeneration. Behav Genet 2007; 37: 79-100.

[243] Codita A, Winblad B, Mohammed AH. Of mice and men: more neurobiology in dementia. Curr Opin Psychiatry 2006; 19: 555-63.

[244] Cole GM, Frautschy SA. Alzheimer's amyloid story finds its star. Trends Mol Med 2006; 12: 395-6.

[245] Jacobsen JS, Wu CC, Redwine JM, *et al.* Early-onset behavioral and synaptic deficits in a mouse model of Alzheimer's disease. Proc Natl Acad Sci USA 2006; 103: 5161-6.

[246] Billings LM, Green KN, McGaugh JL, LaFerla FM. Learning decreases Aβ*56 and tau pathology and ameliorates behavioral decline in 3×Tg-AD mice. J Neurosci 2007; 27: 751-61.

[247] Lin H, Bhatia R, Lal R. Amyloid β protein forms ion channels: implications for Alzheimer's disease pathophysiology. FASEB J 2001; 15: 2433-44.

[248] Quist A, Doudevski I, Lin H, *et al.* Amyloid ion channels: a common structural link for protein-misfolding disease. Proc Natl Acad Sci USA 2005; 102: 10427-32.

[249] Arispe N, Pollard HB, Rojas E. Giant multilevel cation channels formed by Alzheimer disease amyloid β-protein [AβP-(1–40)] in bilayer membranes. Proc Natl Acad Sci USA 1993; 90: 10573-7.

[250] Arispe N, Rojas E, Pollard HB. Alzheimer disease amyloid β protein forms calcium channels in bilayer membranes: blockade by tromethamine and aluminum. Proc Natl Acad Sci USA 1993; 90: 567-71.

[251] Kawahara M, Arispe N, Kuroda Y, Rojas E. Alzheimer's disease amyloid β-protein forms Zn^{2+}-sensitive, cation-selective channels across excised membrane patches from hypothalamic neurons. Biophys J 1997; 73: 67-75.

[252] Kawahara M, Kuroda Y. Molecular mechanism of neurodegeneration induced by Alzheimer's β-amyloid protein: channel formation and disruption of calcium homeostasis. Brain Res Bull 2000; 53: 389-97.

[253] Sanderson KL, Butler L, Ingram VM. Aggregates of a β-amyloid peptide are required to induce calcium currents in neuron-like human teratocarcinoma cells: relation to Alzheimer's disease. Brain Res 1997; 744: 7-14.

[254] Rhee SK, Quist AP, Lal R. Amyloid β protein-(1–42) forms calcium-permeable, Zn^{2+}-sensitive channel. J Biol Chem 1998; 273: 13379-82.

[255] Hirakura Y, Lin MC, Kagan BL. Alzheimer amyloid Aβ1–42 channels: effects of solvent, pH, and Congo Red. J Neurosci Res 1999; 57: 458-66.

[256] Lin H, Zhu YJ, Lal R. Amyloid β protein (1–40) forms calcium-permeable, Zn^{2+}-sensitive channel in reconstituted lipid vesicles. Biochemistry 1999; 38: 11189-96.

[257] Bhatia R, Lin H, Lal R. Fresh and globular amyloid β protein (1–42) induces rapid cellular degeneration: evidence for AβP channel-mediated cellular toxicity. FASEB J 2000; 14: 1233-43.

[258] Kourie JI, Henry CL, Farrelly P. Diversity of amyloid β protein fragment [1–40]-formed channels. Cell Mol Neurobiol 2001; 21: 255-84.

[259] Kagan BL, Hirakura Y, Azimov R, Azimova R, Lin MC. The channel hypothesis of Alzheimer's disease: current status. Peptides 2002; 23: 1311-5.

[260] Lin MC, Kagan BL. Electrophysiologic properties of channels induced by Aβ25–35 in planar lipid bilayers. Peptides 2002; 23: 1215-28.

[261] Bahadi R, Farrelly PV, Kenna BL, *et al.* Cu^{2+}-induced modification of the kinetics of Aβ(1–42) channels. Am J Physiol Cell Physiol 2003; 285: C873-80.

[262] Alarcón JM, Brito JA, Hermosilla T, *et al.* Ion channel formation by Alzheimer's disease amyloid β-peptide (Aβ40) in unilamellar liposomes is determined by anionic phospholipids. Peptides 2006; 27: 95-104.

[263] Sokolov Y, Kozak JA, Kayed R, *et al.* Soluble amyloid oligomers increase bilayer conductance by altering dielectric structure. J Gen Physiol 2006; 128: 637-47.

[264] Demuro A, Mina E, Kayed R, *et al.* Calcium dysregulation and membrane disruption as a ubiquitous neurotoxic mechanism of soluble amyloid oligomers. J Biol Chem 2005; 280: 17294-300.

[265] Kayed R, Sokolov Y, Edmonds B, *et al.* Permeabilization of lipid bilayers is a common conformation-dependent activity of soluble amyloid oligomers in protein misfolding diseases. J Biol Chem 2004; 279: 46363-6.

[266] Lashuel HA, Petre BM, Wall J, *et al.* α-Synuclein, especially the Parkinson's disease-associated mutants, forms pore-like annular and tubular protofibrils. J Mol Biol 2002; 322: 1089-102.

[267] Kawahara M, Kuroda Y. Intracellular calcium changes in neuronal cells induced by Alzheimer's β-amyloid protein are blocked by estradiol and cholesterol. Cell Mol Neurobiol 2001; 21: 1-13.

[268] Dahlgren KN, Manelli AM, Stine WB, Jr., *et al.* Oligomeric and fibrillar species of amyloid-β peptides differentially affect neuronal viability. J Biol Chem 2002; 277: 32046-53.

[269] Scheuner D, Eckman C, Jensen M, *et al.* Secreted amyloid β-protein similar to that in the senile plaques of Alzheimer's disease is increased *in vivo* by the presenilin 1 and 2 and APP mutations linked to familial Alzheimer's disease. Nat Med 1996; 2: 864-70.

[270] Anderson DH, Talaga KC, Rivest AJ, *et al.* Characterization of β amyloid assemblies in drusen: the deposits associated with aging and age-related macular degeneration. Exp Eye Res 2004; 78: 243-56.

[271] Moore RA, Hayes SF, Fischer ER, Priola SA. Amyloid formation *via* supramolecular peptide assemblies. Biochemistry 2007; 46: 7079-87.

[272] Zhu YJ, Lin H, Lal R. Fresh and nonfibrillar amyloid β protein(1–40) induces rapid cellular degeneration in aged human fibroblasts: evidence for AβP-channel-mediated cellular toxicity. FASEB J 2000; 14: 1244-54.

[273] Buxbaum J. The amyloidoses. Mt Sinai J Med 1996; 63: 16-23.
[274] Buxbaum JN. The systemic amyloidoses. Curr Opin Rheumatol 2004; 16: 67-75.
[275] Gambetti P, Russo C. Human brain amyloidoses. Nephrol Dial Transplant 1998; 13 Suppl 7: 33-40.
[276] Bellotti V, Nuvolone M, Giorgetti S, *et al.* The workings of the amyloid diseases. Ann Med 2007; 39: 200-7.
[277] Glabe CG. Common mechanisms of amyloid oligomer pathogenesis in degenerative disease. Neurobiol Aging 2006; 27: 570-5.
[278] Layfield R, Cavey JR, Lowe J. Role of ubiquitin-mediated proteolysis in the pathogenesis of neurodegenerative disorders. Ageing Res Rev 2003; 2: 343-56.
[279] Betarbet R, Sherer TB, Greenamyre JT. Ubiquitin–proteasome system and Parkinson's diseases. Exp Neurol 2005; 191 Suppl 1: S17-27.
[280] Murray IVJ, Lee VMY, Trojanowski JQ. Synucleinopathies: A pathological and molecular review. Clin Neurosci Res 2001; 1: 445-55.
[281] Tompa P. Intrinsically unstructured proteins. Trends Biochem Sci 2002; 27: 527-33.
[282] Dyson HJ, Wright PE. Intrinsically unstructured proteins and their functions. Nat Rev Mol Cell Biol 2005; 6: 197-208.
[283] Conway KA, Lee SJ, Rochet JC, *et al.* Acceleration of oligomerization, not fibrillization, is a shared property of both α-synuclein mutations linked to early-onset Parkinson's disease: implications for pathogenesis and therapy. Proc Natl Acad Sci USA 2000; 97: 571-6.
[284] Ding TT, Lee SJ, Rochet JC, Lansbury PT, Jr. Annular α-synuclein protofibrils are produced when spherical protofibrils are incubated in solution or bound to brain-derived membranes. Biochemistry 2002; 41: 10209-17.
[285] Volles MJ, Lee SJ, Rochet JC, *et al.* Vesicle permeabilization by protofibrillar α-synuclein: implications for the pathogenesis and treatment of Parkinson's disease. Biochemistry 2001; 40: 7812-9.
[286] Volles MJ, Lansbury PT, Jr. Vesicle permeabilization by protofibrillar α-synuclein is sensitive to Parkinson's disease-linked mutations and occurs by a pore-like mechanism. Biochemistry 2002; 41: 4595-602.
[287] Fredenburg RA, Rospigliosi C, Meray RK, *et al.* The impact of the E46K mutation on the properties of α-synuclein in its monomeric and oligomeric states. Biochemistry 2007; 46: 7107-18.
[288] Takeda A, Hasegawa T, Matsuzaki-Kobayashi M, *et al.* Mechanisms of neuronal death in synucleinopathy. J Biomed Biotechnol 2006; 2006: 19365.
[289] Murali J, Jayakumar R. Spectroscopic studies on native and protofibrillar insulin. J Struct Biol 2005; 150: 180-9.
[290] Dzwolak W, Loksztejn A, Galinska-Rakoczy A, *et al.* Conformational indeterminism in protein misfolding: chiral amplification on amyloidogenic pathway of insulin. J Am Chem Soc 2007; 129: 7517-22.
[291] Dzwolak W, Loksztejn A, Smirnovas V. New insights into the self-assembly of insulin amyloid fibrils: an H–D exchange FT-IR study. Biochemistry 2006; 45: 8143-51.
[292] Grudzielanek S, Smirnovas V, Winter R. The effects of various membrane physical–chemical properties on the aggregation kinetics of insulin. Chem Phys Lipids 2007; 149: 28-39.
[293] Ahmad A, Uversky VN, Hong D, Fink AL. Early events in the fibrillation of monomeric insulin. J Biol Chem 2005; 280: 42669-75.

[294] Nettleton EJ, Tito P, Sunde M, *et al.* Characterization of the oligomeric states of insulin in self-assembly and amyloid fibril formation by mass spectrometry. Biophys J 2000; 79: 1053-65.
[295] Grudzielanek S, Velkova A, Shukla A, *et al.* Cytotoxicity of insulin within its self-assembly and amyloidogenic pathways. J Mol Biol 2007; 370: 372-84.
[296] Anguiano M, Nowak RJ, Lansbury PT, Jr. Protofibrillar islet amyloid polypeptide permeabilizes synthetic vesicles by a pore-like mechanism that may be relevant to type II diabetes. Biochemistry 2002; 41: 11338-43.
[297] Porat Y, Kolusheva S, Jelinek R, Gazit E. The human islet amyloid polypeptide forms transient membrane-active prefibrillar assemblies. Biochemistry 2003; 42: 10971-7.
[298] Jayasinghe SA, Langen R. Lipid membranes modulate the structure of islet amyloid polypeptide. Biochemistry 2005; 44: 12113-9.
[299] Knight JD, Hebda JA, Miranker AD. Conserved and cooperative assembly of membrane-bound α-helical states of islet amyloid polypeptide. Biochemistry 2006; 45: 9496-508.
[300] Meier JJ, Kayed R, Lin CY, *et al.* Inhibition of human IAPP fibril formation does not prevent β-cell death: evidence for distinct actions of oligomers and fibrils of human IAPP. Am J Physiol Endocrinol Metab 2006; 291: E1317-24.
[301] Lin CY, Gurlo T, Kayed R, *et al.* Toxic human islet amyloid polypeptide (h-IAPP) oligomers are intracellular, and vaccination to induce anti-toxic oligomer antibodies does not prevent h-IAPP-induced β-cell apoptosis in h-IAPP transgenic mice. Diabetes 2007; 56: 1324-32.
[302] Serpell LC. Alzheimer's amyloid fibrils: structure and assembly. Biochim Biophys Acta 2000; 1502: 16-30.
[303] Eisenberg D, Nelson R, Sawaya MR, *et al.* The structural biology of protein aggregation diseases: Fundamental questions and some answers. Acc Chem Res 2006; 39: 568-75.
[304] Kayed R, Head E, Thompson JL, *et al.* Common structure of soluble amyloid oligomers implies common mechanism of pathogenesis. Science 2003; 300: 486-9.
[305] Kelly JW. The alternative conformations of amyloidogenic proteins and their multi-step assembly pathways. Curr Opin Struct Biol 1998; 8: 101-6.
[306] Chiti F, Dobson CM. Protein misfolding, functional amyloid, and human disease. Annu Rev Biochem 2006; 75: 333-66.
[307] Stefani M, Dobson CM. Protein aggregation and aggregate toxicity: new insights into protein folding, misfolding diseases and biological evolution. J Mol Med 2003; 81: 678-99.
[308] Fezoui Y, Hartley DM, Walsh DM, *et al.* A *de novo* designed helix-turn-helix peptide forms nontoxic amyloid fibrils. Nat Struct Biol 2000; 7: 1095-9.
[309] Wang C, Huang L, Wang L, Hong Y, Sha Y. One-dimensional self-assembly of a rational designed β-structure peptide. Biopolymers 2007; 86: 23-31.
[310] Kammerer RA, Steinmetz MO. *De novo* design of a two-stranded coiled-coil switch peptide. J Struct Biol 2006; 155: 146-53.
[311] Guijarro JI, Sunde M, Jones JA, Campbell ID, Dobson CM. Amyloid fibril formation by an SH3 domain. Proc Natl Acad Sci USA 1998; 95: 4224-8.
[312] Litvinovich SV, Brew SA, Aota S, *et al.* Formation of amyloid-like fibrils by self-association of a partially unfolded fibronectin type III module. J Mol Biol 1998; 280: 245-58.
[313] Jiménez JL, Guijarro JI, Orlova E, *et al.* Cryo-electron microscopy structure of an SH3 amyloid fibril and model of the molecular packing. EMBO J 1999; 18: 815-21.

[314] Zurdo J, Guijarro JI, Dobson CM. Preparation and characterization of purified amyloid fibrils. J Am Chem Soc 2001; 123: 8141-2.

[315] Zurdo J, Guijarro JI, Jiménez JL, Saibil HR, Dobson CM. Dependence on solution conditions of aggregation and amyloid formation by an SH3 domain. J Mol Biol 2001; 311: 325-40.

[316] Carulla N, Caddy GL, Hall DR, *et al.* Molecular recycling within amyloid fibrils. Nature 2005; 436: 554-8.

[317] Chiti F, Bucciantini M, Capanni C, *et al.* Solution conditions can promote formation of either amyloid protofilaments or mature fibrils from the HypF N-terminal domain. Protein Sci 2001; 10: 2541-7.

[318] Polverino de Laureto P, Taddei N, Frare E, *et al.* Protein aggregation and amyloid fibril formation by an SH3 domain probed by limited proteolysis. J Mol Biol 2003; 334: 129-41.

[319] Chiti F, Webster P, Taddei N, *et al.* Designing conditions for *in vitro* formation of amyloid protofilaments and fibrils. Proc Natl Acad Sci USA 1999; 96: 3590-4.

[320] Tjernberg L, Hosia W, Bark N, Thyberg J, Johansson J. Charge attraction and β propensity are necessary for amyloid fibril formation from tetrapeptides. J Biol Chem 2002; 277: 43243-6.

[321] López De La Paz M, Goldie K, Zurdo J, *et al. De novo* designed peptide-based amyloid fibrils. Proc Natl Acad Sci USA 2002; 99: 16052-7.

[322] Relini A, Torrassa S, Rolandi R, *et al.* Monitoring the process of HypF fibrillization and liposome permeabilization by protofibrils. J Mol Biol 2004; 338: 943-57.

[323] Parbhu A, Lin H, Thimm J, Lal R. Imaging real-time aggregation of amyloid beta protein (1–42) by atomic force microscopy. Peptides 2002; 23: 1265-70.

[324] Poirier MA, Li H, Macosko J, *et al.* Huntingtin spheroids and protofibrils as precursors in polyglutamine fibrilization. J Biol Chem 2002; 277: 41032-7.

[325] Conway KA, Harper JD, Lansbury PT, Jr. Fibrils formed *in vitro* from α-synuclein and two mutant forms linked to Parkinson's disease are typical amyloid. Biochemistry 2000; 39: 2552-63.

[326] Calamai M, Taddei N, Stefani M, Ramponi G, Chiti F. Relative influence of hydrophobicity and net charge in the aggregation of two homologous proteins. Biochemistry 2003; 42: 15078-83.

[327] Bucciantini M, Giannoni E, Chiti F, *et al.* Inherent toxicity of aggregates implies a common mechanism for protein misfolding diseases. Nature 2002; 416: 507-11.

[328] Bucciantini M, Calloni G, Chiti F, *et al.* Prefibrillar amyloid protein aggregates share common features of cytotoxicity. J Biol Chem 2004; 279: 31374-82.

[329] Bucciantini M, Rigacci S, Berti A, *et al.* Patterns of cell death triggered in two different cell lines by HypF-N prefibrillar aggregates. FASEB J 2005; 19: 437-9.

[330] Cecchi C, Pensalfini A, Baglioni S, *et al.* Differing molecular mechanisms appear to underlie early toxicity of prefibrillar HypF-N aggregates to different cell types. FEBS J 2006; 273: 2206-22.

[331] Tartaglia GG, Pechmann S, Dobson CM, Vendruscolo M. Life on the edge: a link between gene expression levels and aggregation rates of human proteins. Trends Biochem Sci 2007; 32: 204-6.

[332] Calabrese MF, Eakin CM, Wang JM, Miranker AD. A regulatable switch mediates self-association in an immunoglobulin fold. Nat Struct Mol Biol 2008; 15: 965-71.

[333] Liu C, Sawaya MR, Cheng PN, *et al.* Characteristics of amyloid-related oligomers revealed by crystal structures of macrocyclic β-sheet mimics. J Am Chem Soc 2011; 133: 6736-44.

[334] Streltsov VA, Varghese JN, Masters CL, Nuttall SD. Crystal structure of the amyloid-β p3 fragment provides a model for oligomer formation in Alzheimer's disease. J Neurosci 2011; 31: 1419-26.

[335] Domanska K, Vanderhaegen S, Srinivasan V, *et al.* Atomic structure of a nanobody-trapped domain-swapped dimer of an amyloidogenic β2-microglobulin variant. Proc Natl Acad Sci USA 2011; 108: 1314-9.

[336] Laganowsky A, Liu C, Sawaya MR, *et al.* Atomic view of a toxic amyloid small oligomer. Science 2012; 335: 1228-31.

[337] Ecroyd H, Carver JA. Crystallin proteins and amyloid fibrils. Cell Mol Life Sci 2009; 66: 62-81.

[338] Thompson MJ, Sievers SA, Karanicolas J, *et al.* The 3D profile method for identifying fibril-forming segments of proteins. Proc Natl Acad Sci USA 2006; 103: 4074-8.

[339] Goldschmidt L, Teng PK, Riek R, Eisenberg D. Identifying the amylome, proteins capable of forming amyloid-like fibrils. Proc Natl Acad Sci USA 2010; 107: 3487-92.

[340] Greenwald J, Riek R. Biology of amyloid: structure, function, and regulation. Structure 2010; 18: 1244-60.

[341] Benzinger TL, Gregory DM, Burkoth TS, *et al.* Propagating structure of Alzheimer's β-amyloid$_{(10-35)}$ is parallel β-sheet with residues in exact register. Proc Natl Acad Sci USA 1998; 95: 13407-12.

[342] Tycko R. Solid-state NMR studies of amyloid fibril structure. Annu Rev Phys Chem 2011; 62: 279-99.

[343] Cheng PN, Liu C, Zhao M, Eisenberg D, Nowick JS. Amyloid β-sheet mimics that antagonize protein aggregation and reduce amyloid toxicity. Nat Chem 2012; 4: 927-33.

[344] Liu C, Zhao M, Jiang L, *et al.* Out-of-register β-sheets suggest a pathway to toxic amyloid aggregates. Proc Natl Acad Sci USA 2012.

[345] Griffith JS. Self-replication and scrapie. Nature 1967; 215: 1043-4.

[346] Prusiner SB. Novel proteinaceous infectious particles cause scrapie. Science 1982; 216: 136-44.

[347] Prusiner SB, Bolton DC, Groth DF, *et al.* Further purification and characterization of scrapie prions. Biochemistry 1982; 21: 6942-50.

[348] Prusiner SB. Prions. Proc Natl Acad Sci USA 1998; 95: 13363-83.

[349] Legname G, Baskakov IV, Nguyen HO, *et al.* Synthetic mammalian prions. Science 2004; 305: 673-6.

[350] Castilla J, Saá P, Hetz C, Soto C. *In vitro* generation of infectious scrapie prions. Cell 2005; 121: 195-206.

[351] Deleault NR, Harris BT, Rees JR, Supattapone S. Formation of native prions from minimal components *in vitro*. Proc Natl Acad Sci USA 2007; 104: 9741-6.

[352] Wang F, Wang X, Yuan CG, Ma J. Generating a prion with bacterially expressed recombinant prion protein. Science 2010; 327: 1132-5.

[353] Lansbury PT, Jr., Caughey B. The chemistry of scrapie infection: implications of the 'ice 9' metaphor. Chem Biol 1995; 2: 1-5.

[354] Saborio GP, Permanne B, Soto C. Sensitive detection of pathological prion protein by cyclic amplification of protein misfolding. Nature 2001; 411: 810-3.

[355] Soto C. Transmissible proteins: expanding the prion heresy. Cell 2012; 149: 968-77.

[356] Goedert M, Clavaguera F, Tolnay M. The propagation of prion-like protein inclusions in neurodegenerative diseases. Trends Neurosci 2010; 33: 317-25.

[357] Westermark GT, Westermark P. Prion-like aggregates: infectious agents in human disease. Trends Mol Med 2010; 16: 501-7.

[358] Angot E, Steiner JA, Hansen C, Li JY, Brundin P. Are synucleinopathies prion-like disorders? Lancet Neurol 2010; 9: 1128-38.

[359] Prusiner SB. Cell biology. A unifying role for prions in neurodegenerative diseases. Science 2012; 336: 1511-3.

[360] Kanouchi T, Ohkubo T, Yokota T. Can regional spreading of amyotrophic lateral sclerosis motor symptoms be explained by prion-like propagation? J Neurol Neurosurg Psychiatry 2012; 83: 739-45.

[361] Münch C, Bertolotti A. Self-propagation and transmission of misfolded mutant SOD1: prion or prion-like phenomenon? Cell Cycle 2011; 10: 1711.

[362] Münch C, O'Brien J, Bertolotti A. Prion-like propagation of mutant superoxide dismutase-1 misfolding in neuronal cells. Proc Natl Acad Sci USA 2011; 108: 3548-53.

[363] Lee SJ, Desplats P, Sigurdson C, Tsigelny I, Masliah E. Cell-to-cell transmission of non-prion protein aggregates. Nat Rev Neurol 2010; 6: 702-6.

[364] Lee SJ, Lim HS, Masliah E, Lee HJ. Protein aggregate spreading in neurodegenerative diseases: problems and perspectives. Neurosci Res 2011; 70: 339-48.

[365] Guest WC, Silverman JM, Pokrishevsky E, *et al.* Generalization of the prion hypothesis to other neurodegenerative diseases: an imperfect fit. J Toxicol Environ Health Part A 2011; 74: 1433-59.

[366] Luk KC, Kehm VM, Zhang B, *et al.* Intracerebral inoculation of pathological α-synuclein initiates a rapidly progressive neurodegenerative α-synucleinopathy in mice. J Exp Med 2012; 209: 975-86.

[367] Luk KC, Kehm V, Carroll J, *et al.* Pathological α-synuclein transmission initiates parkinson-like neurodegeneration in nontransgenic mice. Science 2012; 338: 949-53.

[368] Kane MD, Lipinski WJ, Callahan MJ, *et al.* Evidence for seeding of β-amyloid by intracerebral infusion of Alzheimer brain extracts in β-amyloid precursor protein-transgenic mice. J Neurosci 2000; 20: 3606-11.

[369] Meyer-Luehmann M, Coomaraswamy J, Bolmont T, *et al.* Exogenous induction of cerebral β-amyloidogenesis is governed by agent and host. Science 2006; 313: 1781-4.

[370] Watts JC, Giles K, Grillo SK, *et al.* Bioluminescence imaging of Aβ deposition in bigenic mouse models of Alzheimer's disease. Proc Natl Acad Sci USA 2011; 108: 2528-33.

[371] Eisele YS, Obermüller U, Heilbronner G, *et al.* Peripherally applied Aβ-containing inoculates induce cerebral β-amyloidosis. Science 2010; 330: 980-2.

[372] Eisele YS, Bolmont T, Heikenwalder M, *et al.* Induction of cerebral β-amyloidosis: intracerebral *versus* systemic Aβ inoculation. Proc Natl Acad Sci USA 2009; 106: 12926-31.

[373] Langer F, Eisele YS, Fritschi SK, *et al.* Soluble Aβ seeds are potent inducers of cerebral β-amyloid deposition. J Neurosci 2011; 31: 14488-95.

[374] Rosen RF, Fritz JJ, Dooyema J, *et al.* Exogenous seeding of cerebral β-amyloid deposition in βAPP-transgenic rats. J Neurochem 2012; 120: 660-6.

[375] Morales R, Duran-Aniotz C, Castilla J, Estrada LD, Soto C. *De novo* induction of amyloid-β deposition *in vivo*. Mol Psychiatry 2012; 17: 1347-53.

[376] Aguzzi A, Calella AM. Prions: protein aggregation and infectious diseases. Physiol Rev 2009; 89: 1105-52.

[377] Makarava N, Lee CI, Ostapchenko VG, Baskakov IV. Highly promiscuous nature of prion polymerization. J Biol Chem 2007; 282: 36704-13.

[378] Zhang B, Une Y, Fu X, *et al.* Fecal transmission of AA amyloidosis in the cheetah contributes to high incidence of disease. Proc Natl Acad Sci USA 2008; 105: 7263-8.

[379] Caughey B, Baron GS. Are cheetahs on the run from prion-like amyloidosis? Proc Natl Acad Sci USA 2008; 105: 7113-4.

[380] Lundmark K, Westermark GT, Nyström S, *et al.* Transmissibility of systemic amyloidosis by a prion-like mechanism. Proc Natl Acad Sci USA 2002; 99: 6979-84.

[381] Solomon A, Richey T, Murphy CL, *et al.* Amyloidogenic potential of foie gras. Proc Natl Acad Sci USA 2007; 104: 10998-1001.

[382] Larsson A, Malmström S, Westermark P. Signs of cross-seeding: aortic medin amyloid as a trigger for protein AA deposition. Amyloid 2011; 18: 229-34.

[383] Yan J, Fu X, Ge F, *et al.* Cross-seeding and cross-competition in mouse apolipoprotein A-II amyloid fibrils and protein A amyloid fibrils. Am J Pathol 2007; 171: 172-80.

[384] Paravastu AK, Qahwash I, Leapman RD, Meredith SC, Tycko R. Seeded growth of β-amyloid fibrils from Alzheimer's brain-derived fibrils produces a distinct fibril structure. Proc Natl Acad Sci USA 2009; 106: 7443-8.

[385] Qiang W, Yau WM, Tycko R. Structural evolution of Iowa mutant β-amyloid fibrils from polymorphic to homogeneous states under repeated seeded growth. J Am Chem Soc 2011; 133: 4018-29.

[386] Nath S, Agholme L, Kurudenkandy FR, *et al.* Spreading of neurodegenerative pathology *via* neuron-to-neuron transmission of β-amyloid. J Neurosci 2012; 32: 8767-77.

[387] Braak H, Braak E. Neuropathological stageing of Alzheimer-related changes. Acta Neuropathol 1991; 82: 239-59.

[388] Harris JA, Devidze N, Verret L, *et al.* Transsynaptic progression of amyloid-β-induced neuronal dysfunction within the entorhinal–hippocampal network. Neuron 2010; 68: 428-41.

[389] Braak H, Braak E, Yilmazer D, *et al.* Pattern of brain destruction in Parkinson's and Alzheimer's diseases. J Neural Transm 1996; 103: 455-90.

[390] Kai H, Shin RW, Ogino K, *et al.* Enhanced antigen retrieval of amyloid β immunohistochemistry: re-evaluation of amyloid β pathology in Alzheimer disease and its mouse model. J Histochem Cytochem 2012; 60: 761-9.

[391] Ono K, Takahashi R, Ikeda T, Yamada M. Cross-seeding effects of amyloid β-protein and α-synuclein. J Neurochem 2012; 122: 883-90.

[392] Lasagna-Reeves CA, Castillo-Carranza DL, Guerrero-Muoz MJ, Jackson GR, Kayed R. Preparation and characterization of neurotoxic tau oligomers. Biochemistry 2010; 49: 10039-41.

[393] Frost B, Jacks RL, Diamond MI. Propagation of tau misfolding from the outside to the inside of a cell. J Biol Chem 2009; 284: 12845-52.

[394] Clavaguera F, Bolmont T, Crowther RA, *et al.* Transmission and spreading of tauopathy in transgenic mouse brain. Nat Cell Biol 2009; 11: 909-13.

[395] Nonaka T, Watanabe ST, Iwatsubo T, Hasegawa M. Seeded aggregation and toxicity of α-synuclein and tau: cellular models of neurodegenerative diseases. J Biol Chem 2010; 285: 34885-98.

[396] Guo JL, Lee VM. Seeding of normal Tau by pathological Tau conformers drives pathogenesis of Alzheimer-like tangles. J Biol Chem 2011; 286: 15317-31.

[397] de Calignon A, Polydoro M, Suárez-Calvet M, *et al.* Propagation of tau pathology in a model of early Alzheimer's disease. Neuron 2012; 73: 685-97.
[398] Liu L, Drouet V, Wu JW, *et al.* Trans-synaptic spread of tau pathology *in vivo*. PLoS One 2012; 7: e31302.
[399] Braak H, Braak E. Staging of Alzheimer's disease-related neurofibrillary changes. Neurobiol Aging 1995; 16: 271-8; discussion 78-84.
[400] Guo JP, Arai T, Miklossy J, McGeer PL. Aβ and tau form soluble complexes that may promote self aggregation of both into the insoluble forms observed in Alzheimer's disease. Proc Natl Acad Sci USA 2006; 103: 1953-8.
[401] Hart PJ. Pathogenic superoxide dismutase structure, folding, aggregation and turnover. Curr Opin Chem Biol 2006; 10: 131-8.
[402] Lang L, Kurnik M, Danielsson J, Oliveberg M. Fibrillation precursor of superoxide dismutase 1 revealed by gradual tuning of the protein-folding equilibrium. Proc Natl Acad Sci USA 2012; 109: 17868-73.
[403] Kato S, Takikawa M, Nakashima K, *et al.* New consensus research on neuropathological aspects of familial amyotrophic lateral sclerosis with superoxide dismutase 1 (SOD1) gene mutations: inclusions containing SOD1 in neurons and astrocytes. Amyotroph Lateral Scler Other Motor Neuron Disord 2000; 1: 163-84.
[404] Bruijn LI, Becher MW, Lee MK, *et al.* ALS-linked SOD1 mutant G85R mediates damage to astrocytes and promotes rapidly progressive disease with SOD1-containing inclusions. Neuron 1997; 18: 327-38.
[405] Durham HD, Roy J, Dong L, Figlewicz DA. Aggregation of mutant Cu/Zn superoxide dismutase proteins in a culture model of ALS. J Neuropathol Exp Neurol 1997; 56: 523-30.
[406] Grad LI, Guest WC, Yanai A, *et al.* Intermolecular transmission of superoxide dismutase 1 misfolding in living cells. Proc Natl Acad Sci USA 2011; 108: 16398-403.
[407] Chia R, Tattum MH, Jones S, *et al.* Superoxide dismutase 1 and tgSOD1 mouse spinal cord seed fibrils, suggesting a propagative cell death mechanism in amyotrophic lateral sclerosis. PLoS One 2010; 5: e10627.
[408] Ravits J, Paul P, Jorg C. Focality of upper and lower motor neuron degeneration at the clinical onset of ALS. Neurology 2007; 68: 1571-5.
[409] Ravits JM, La Spada AR. ALS motor phenotype heterogeneity, focality, and spread: deconstructing motor neuron degeneration. Neurology 2009; 73: 805-11.
[410] Botelho HM, Leal SS, Cardoso I, *et al.* S100A6 amyloid fibril formation is calcium-modulated and enhances superoxide dismutase-1 (SOD1) aggregation. J Biol Chem 2012.
[411] Kim HJ, Chatani E, Goto Y, Paik SR. Seed-dependent accelerated fibrillation of α-synuclein induced by periodic ultrasonication treatment. J Microbiol Biotechnol 2007; 17: 2027-32.
[412] Danzer KM, Krebs SK, Wolff M, Birk G, Hengerer B. Seeding induced by α-synuclein oligomers provides evidence for spreading of α-synuclein pathology. J Neurochem 2009; 111: 192-203.
[413] Hansen C, Angot E, Bergström AL, *et al.* α-Synuclein propagates from mouse brain to grafted dopaminergic neurons and seeds aggregation in cultured human cells. J Clin Invest 2011; 121: 715-25.
[414] Allan LE, Petit GH, Brundin P. Cell transplantation in Parkinson's disease: problems and perspectives. Curr Opin Neurol 2010; 23: 426-32.
[415] Li JY, Englund E, Holton JL, *et al.* Lewy bodies in grafted neurons in subjects with Parkinson's disease suggest host-to-graft disease propagation. Nat Med 2008; 14: 501-3.

[416] Desplats P, Lee HJ, Bae EJ, *et al.* Inclusion formation and neuronal cell death through neuron-to-neuron transmission of α-synuclein. Proc Natl Acad Sci USA 2009; 106: 13010-5.
[417] Angot E, Steiner JA, Lema Tomé CM, *et al.* Alpha-synuclein cell-to-cell transfer and seeding in grafted dopaminergic neurons *in vivo*. PLoS One 2012; 7: e39465.
[418] Bae EJ, Ho DH, Park E, *et al.* Lipid peroxidation product 4-hydroxy-2-nonenal promotes seeding-capable oligomer formation and cell-to-cell transfer of α-synuclein Antioxid Redox Signal 2012: [Epub ahead of print].
[419] Braak H, Del Tredici K, Bratzke H, *et al.* Staging of the intracerebral inclusion body pathology associated with idiopathic Parkinson's disease (preclinical and clinical stages). J Neurol 2002; 249 Suppl 3: III/1-5.
[420] Braak H, Del Tredici K, Rüb U, *et al.* Staging of brain pathology related to sporadic Parkinson's disease. Neurobiol Aging 2003; 24: 197-211.
[421] Braak H, Ghebremedhin E, Rüb U, Bratzke H, Del Tredici K. Stages in the development of Parkinson's disease-related pathology. Cell Tissue Res 2004; 318: 121-34.
[422] Brundin P, Li JY, Holton JL, Lindvall O, Revesz T. Research in motion: the enigma of Parkinson's disease pathology spread. Nat Rev Neurosci 2008; 9: 741-5.
[423] Riess O, Krüger R, Schulz JB. Spectrum of phenotypes and genotypes in Parkinson's disease. J Neurol 2002; 249 Suppl 3: III/15-20.
[424] Surgucheva I, Sharov VS, Surguchov A. γ-Synuclein: seeding of α-synuclein aggregation and transmission between cells. Biochemistry 2012; 51: 4743-54.
[425] Bhattacharyya AM, Thakur AK, Wetzel R. Polyglutamine aggregation nucleation: thermodynamics of a highly unfavorable protein folding reaction. Proc Natl Acad Sci USA 2005; 102: 15400-5.
[426] Scherzinger E, Lurz R, Turmaine M, *et al.* Huntingtin-encoded polyglutamine expansions form amyloid-like protein aggregates *in vitro* and *in vivo*. Cell 1997; 90: 549-58.
[427] Gupta S, Jie S, Colby DW. Protein misfolding detected early in pathogenesis of transgenic mouse model of Huntington disease using amyloid seeding assay. J Biol Chem 2012; 287: 9982-9.
[428] Ren PH, Lauckner JE, Kachirskaia I, *et al.* Cytoplasmic penetration and persistent infection of mammalian cells by polyglutamine aggregates. Nat Cell Biol 2009; 11: 219-25.
[429] Rosas HD, Salat DH, Lee SY, *et al.* Cerebral cortex and the clinical expression of Huntington's disease: complexity and heterogeneity. Brain 2008; 131: 1057-68.
[430] Furukawa Y, Kaneko K, Matsumoto G, Kurosawa M, Nukina N. Cross-seeding fibrillation of Q/N-rich proteins offers new pathomechanism of polyglutamine diseases. J Neurosci 2009; 29: 5153-62.
[431] Vonsattel JP, DiFiglia M. Huntington disease. J Neuropathol Exp Neurol 1998; 57: 369-84.
[432] Deng YP, Albin RL, Penney JB, *et al.* Differential loss of striatal projection systems in Huntington's disease: a quantitative immunohistochemical study. J Chem Neuroanat 2004; 27: 143-64.
[433] Bellingham SA, Guo BB, Coleman BM, Hill AF. Exosomes: vehicles for the transfer of toxic proteins associated with neurodegenerative diseases? Front Physiol 2012; 3: 124.
[434] Marzo L, Gousset K, Zurzolo C. Multifaceted roles of tunneling nanotubes in intercellular communication. Front Physiol 2012; 3: 72.
[435] Morales R, Green KM, Soto C. Cross currents in protein misfolding disorders: interactions and therapy. CNS Neurol Disord Drug Targets 2009; 8: 363-71.

CHAPTER 13

Thin, Stubby or Mushroom: Spine Pathology in Alzheimer's Disease

Christian Tackenberg[1,2], Adnan Ghori[1] and Roland Brandt[1,*]

[1]Department of Neurobiology, University of Osnabrück, Barbarastrasse 11, 49076 Osnabrück, Germany and [2]Division of Psychiatry Research, University of Zurich, Wagistrasse 12, 8952 Schlieren, Switzerland

Abstract: Since their first description by Ramon y Cajal at the end of the 19th century, dendritic spines have been proposed as important sites of neuronal contacts and it has been suggested that changes in the activity of neurons directly affect spine morphology. In fact, since then it has been shown that about 90% of excitatory synapses end on spines. Data indicate that spines are highly dynamic structures and that spine shape correlates with the strength of synaptic transmission. Several mental disorders including Alzheimer's disease (AD) are associated with spine pathology suggesting that spine alterations play a central role in mental deficits. The aim of this review is to provide an overview about the current knowledge on spine morphology and function as well as about different experimental models to analyze spine changes and dynamics. The second part concentrates on disease-relevant factors that are associated with AD and which lead to spine alterations. In particular, data that provide evidence that Aβ oligomers influence spine morphology and function will be presented and the contribution of tau pathology will be discussed. The review ends with the discussion of potential mechanisms how disease-relevant factors influence dendritic spines and whether and how spine changes could be therapeutically suppressed or reversed.

Keywords: Alzheimer's disease, amyloid-beta, dendritic spines, NMDA receptor.

INTRODUCTION

A characteristic feature of neurons is their functional and structural differentiation into a signal-receiving (somatodendritic) and a signal-transducing (axonal) compartment. Dendrites can receive thousands of synaptic inputs from other

***Corresponding author Roland Brandt:** Department of Neurobiology, University of Osnabrück; Barbarastraße 11, D-49076 Osnabrück, Germany; Tel: (+49) (541) 969-2338; Fax: (+49) (541) 969-2354; E-mail: brandt@biologie.uni-osnabrueck.de

D.K. Lahiri (Ed)

neurons, which are then integrated and processed in a complex manner. Dendrites emenate from the cell body and develop a dendritic arbor specific for the respective neuron type.

Dendritic spines are postsynaptic morphological specializations at dendrites. They are formed by small protruding pieces of the dendritic membrane with the total volume ranging from less than 0.01 to 0.8 μm^3 [1]. Spines are the primary site of excitatory input and about 90% of the excitatory synapses in the mature brain end on spines. Mature dendrites have up to 10 spines/µm of dendrites. In total, a typical CA1 pyramidal cell of the hippocampus has approximately 30,000 spines with 50% of them located in stratum radiatum and 40% in stratum oriens [2]. Spines may function as a microcompartment for segregating postsynaptic responses [3]. Thus, changes in spines may not only be important for learning and memory but also for neurodegenerative processes involving changes in signal transduction such as those occurring in Alzheimer's disease.

Spine Shape and Function

Spines have various shapes but they all are essentially formed by a neck and head attached to a dendritic membrane. Three major classes based on the relative size of the spine head and neck can be distinguished [4] (Fig. **1**). *Thin spines* have a small head and a narrow neck (<0.6 µm in diameter). Their total length is greater than the neck diameter and the head is not bulbous. *Stubby spines* have no obvious constriction between the head and attachment to the shaft. *Mushroom spines* have a constricted narrow neck and a large irregular head (>0.6 µm in largest diameter).

Each functional spine consists of postsynaptic density (PSD) usually at the head where the synaptic junction is located. PSD is an electron-dense thickening of the membrane in which hundreds of components including receptors, cytoskeletal proteins and associated signalling molecules are involved in a number of signalling pathways controlling synaptic plasticity. PSD ranges in shape from a disc (macular PSD) or a perforated annulus (perforated PSD), to a highly irregular or segmented structure. Perforated PSDs are consistently associated with more α-amino-3-hydroxy-5-methyl-4-isoxazole receptors (AMPARs) than the non-perforated PSDs. Mushroom shaped spines are more likely to have perforated shaped PSD whereas thin spines contain macular PSD [5].

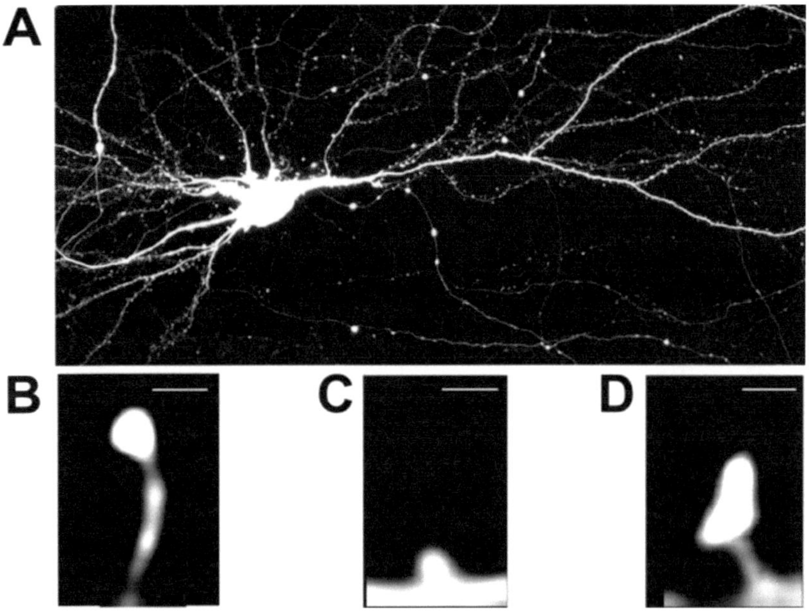

Figure 1: Visualization of dendritic spine morphology in organotypic slice preparations that have been infected with a eGFP coding viral vector. A. Overview of an infected CA3 pyramidal neuron, B. thin spine, C. stubby spine, D. mushroom spine. Scale bar, 25 µm (A), 0.5 µm (B-D).

Spines have an actin-based cytoskeleton. Occasionally, the larger CA3 dendritic spines have one or more microtubules within them [6]. Some pyramidal cell spines contain a structure called spine apparatus, an organelle formed by two or more disks of smooth endoplasmic reticulum (SER) separated by electron-dense material [7]. Large spines are associated with spine apparatus, whereas small spines are less likely to contain this structure. SER likely regulates the concentration of calcium in the spines. Therefore differently sized spines may have different ways of controlling calcium homeostasis [5].

There are several views how mature spines are formed. According to one hypothesis spines can form *de novo*. A filipodium shoots out of the dendrite, forms a contact with the presynapse and then collapses to become a short 1-2 µm mature spine [1]. In another hypothesis, spines are constantly formed and stabilized by the presynaptic partner into a functional spine of any morphology

[7]. However, data from many experiments suggest that no general path of spine formation may exist but that spines may form by different mechanisms.

The currently accepted opinion is that the spine functions as a microcompartment for segregating postsynaptic response [3]. In many studies, a correlation between the spine neck and the postsynaptic calcium response has been shown, proposing a spine as an unique calcium compartment [8], which could be important for the regulation of the phosphorylation of synaptic proteins that is necessary for synaptic plasticity [9]. Since large spines are more likely than smaller spines to contain SER, the calcium concentration may be regulated more tightly. In addition, large spines have larger PSDs, which anchor more AMPARs making the synapses functionally stronger than thin spines that contain predominantly N-methyl-D-aspartate glutamate receptors (NMDARs). From these features it has been suggested that mushroom spines represent more stable "memory" spines whereas thin spines could be "learning" spines.

The mechanism and relationship between spine alteration and learning and memory is still unclear. Experimental models to analyze spine dynamics and changes could contribute information, which would also be important for a better understanding of disease related impairment in spine function.

Experimental Approaches to Analyze spine Dynamics and Changes

In neurobiological investigations, several approaches have been used to analyze spine density, morphology, dynamics or function. Fixed cell cultures or tissues are appropriate to explore changes in density or morphology of populations of spines after exposure to putative spine effectors. In contrast, spine dynamics, *i.e.* change in spine shape, spine motility and the appearance or loss of spines over time can only be analyzed in living cell or tissue cultures or *in vivo*.

Classically, spines can be analyzed after Golgi-staining of brains and sectioning followed by light microscopy. While this method allows determining densities and morphological features of spine populations in brain regions of humans and animals, experimental manipulations are limited. The most simple culture model for spine analysis are differentiated, dissociated cortical or hippocampal primary neurons, which permit visualization of spines by standard microscopic techniques.

However, during culture preparation synaptic contacts are disrupted and have to be reformed *in vitro*. This re-establishment of synaptic contacts can be avoided by using organotypic hippocampal slice cultures, where neuronal connections remain largely intact and closely reflect *in vivo* conditions with respect to spine density and proportions of different spine types [10]. An additional advantage is the possibility to analyze distinct subregions which may differ in their connectivity. Spine density and morphology may be analyzed manually or automated with the latter having the advantage of avoiding a potential bias posed by the researcher. This approach is exemplified by the study of Shahani *et al.* [11], where spines in CA1 and CA3 neurons of fixed hippocampal slices were analyzed using the algorithm-based software 3DMA-Neuron [12, 13]. This software allows a semi-automated analysis of spine density, length, volume and shape as it divides spines into the three classes "mushroom", "stubby" or "thin"

One of the first live imaging studies used hippocampal primary neurons expressing GFP-actin [14]. With this approach, rapid actin-based changes in spine shape within seconds were shown. Such high spine dynamics were confirmed in a later study that reported morphological changes in less than a minute in hippocampal slice cultures [15]. Both experiments identified actin as a key player in spine dynamics since blocking of actin polymerization by cytochalasin D arrested spine motility. Interestingly, blocking of the actin-based motor myosin had no effect. Remarkably, highest spine dynamics were seen at the spine tip where the spine is in contact with the presynaptic bouton [16] suggesting a relation between synaptic transmission and spine motility. Interestingly, activation of AMPARs blocked motility rapidly but reversibly whereas NMDAR stimulation led to long-lasting effects which required 30 min to evolve [17, 18]. Thus, these results link actin-based spine dynamics to effects of glutamate receptor dependent activation such as long-term potentiation (LTP). NMDARs are also involved in the induction of long-term depression (LTD), the weakening of a synapse, by activating the actin depolymerizing factor cofilin through calcineurin [19-21].

Several research groups have analyzed changes in spine morphology that may be associated with LTP. Yang *et al.* [22] used acute hippocampal slice cultures and combined patch-clamp technique to induce LTP with two photon time-lapse imaging to analyze spine growth. They reported a rapid and persistent NMDAR dependent spine expansion after LTP induction. To study vesicle trafficking in pre- and postsynapses and the role of glutamate receptor exocytosis during LTP, dual channel time-lapse two-photon microscopy was used to simultaneously monitor receptor trafficking and spine morphology [23]. Chemical induction of LTP increased spine volume and enhanced AMPAR exocytosis whereas the density of NMDARs at the spine surface decreased. Interestingly, spine volume increased before accumulation of AMPARs on spine surface occurs, suggesting that spine expansion and glutamate receptor exocytosis follow distinct mechanisms. Contrary, in primary neurons, LTP triggered spine growth *via* relocalization and enhanced exocytotic travelling of endosomal vesicles. Blocking endosomal transport prevented LTP-induced increase in spine volume [24].

Two photon laser scan microscopy (2PLSM) offers also the possibility of investigating spine dynamics *in vivo.* Since biological tissue strongly scatters light, standard confocal imaging is inappropriate for deep imaging. Application of 2PLSM is a break through in deep tissue imaging and allows imaging several hundred micrometer deep in different tissues [25-27]. By creating a cranial window in the head of mice or rats, dendrites and spines in the cortex can be analyzed by 2PLSM up to several months [28]. However, analysis in the intact brain is restricted to the cortex but *via* special surgical preparations, cortical tissue above the hippocampus of anesthetized mice can be removed to permit two photon imaging of fluorescence labeled hippocampal CA1 pyramidal neurons *in vivo* [29].

Spine stability is developmentally regulated and increases during aging as determined from the fraction of persistent spines (lifetime longer than 8 days) in mice from different ages as determined by 2PLSM [30]. Interestingly, spine stability varied between different brain regions, which is probably due to the different capacity for experience-dependent plasticity. During a 1-month observation period of spine turnover in the visual cortex of mice, it was found that 73% of spines were stable in young mice whereas 96% were stable in old animals [31]. In the somatosensory cortex, spine stability increased from 35% to 73% during aging [30]. The results show that spines become remarkably stable during aging which may indicate a maturation of neuronal circuits and which may provide the structural basis for long-term memory. Thus, analyzing mechanisms of spine loss in aged animals could provide important information for the pathogenesis of neurodegenerative diseases.

Unlike confocal or two-photon microscopy, stimulated emission depletion (STED) microscopy is not fundamentally limited by diffraction and reaches resolutions of 60-80 nm [32], which is in the same range as the dendritic spine necks. STED imaging of dendritic spines of YFP-positive hippocampal neurons in organotypic slices revealed important structural parameters, such as the neck width and the curvature of the heads of spines, which are important for synaptic plasticity [33]. The 4-6 fold increase in resolution by STED offers new possibilities to analyze the dynamics of single spines in living tissue *e.g.* in respond to synaptic signals using voltage-sensitive dyes [34], as well as the detrimental effects of disease-relevant factors at nanoscale resolution.

Spine Pathology in AD

AD patients show changes in many brain regions with respect to axonal and dendritic morphology and neuron loss [35]. In addition, loss of synapses and dendritic spines is one of the common abnormalities found in human AD brains. In the acoustic cortex of patients with AD many distorted, dystrophic and degenerated dendritic spines were observed, which were intermixed with some giant spines [36]. The acoustic cortex was analyzed in order to determine a potential neuropathological correlate of the communication impairment in AD patients. These results suggest that spines become deformed during AD compared to normal aged brains. Synapse loss and spine alterations in selected brain regions appear to be an early event during the development of AD since already individuals with mild AD have much fewer synapses (55%) in the stratum radiatum of the CA1 subfield [37]. The reduction in synapses correlates well with tests for cognitive impairment indicating that spine and synapse alterations are structural correlates of cognitive decline in AD. Interestingly, a significant reduction in the number of dendritic spines was also observed in CA1-3 pyramidal neurons in patients with Down's syndrome before onset of AD [38]. Spine density was then further reduced in Down's patients with associated AD. However, it should be taken into account that neurons undergo morphological changes also during "normal" aging. The changes include a reduction in dendritic arborisation, dendritic lengths and a decrease in spine number, most likely representing a change in synaptic density [39]. Thus, it appears that spine alterations and loss of synapses are a common feature during normal aging and are pathologically enhanced during the course of AD. It will be interesting to know which molecular factors cause spine impairment in the disease and how these factors interact in order to develop therapeutic approaches to prevent spine pathology and age-related neuronal dysfunction.

Factors Involved in Spine Pathology

An important role of Aβ as a main factor in the pathogenesis of Alzheimer's disease is widely accepted and is also supported by familial mutations that affect Aβ production [40]. Aβ is produced by proteolytic cleavage from the amyloid precursor protein (APP) and aggregates to amyloid plaques, which constitute histopathological hallmarks of AD although the amount of plaques doesn't directly correlate with the degree of cognitive dysfunction in patients. Instead, elevated levels of soluble Aβ peptides [41, 42] and the number of neurofibrillary tangles (NFTs) [43] correlate with cognitive decline.

In several APP transgenic mouse lines cognitive deficits and amyloid plaques are found in the absence of substantial neurodegeneration [44, 45]. This observation led to the hypothesis that alteration of neuronal connectivity by Aβ may precede neurodegeneration for which other factors beside Aβ, *e.g.* tau protein, are required. Whether amyloid plaques or lower molecular weight Aβ oligomers are responsible for spine and synapse alterations is still a matter of debate. Evidence for plaque related spine alterations is given by the finding that within a radius of 40 μm around plaques in a plaque-forming mouse model (PS1/APP mouse line) dendrites show varicosity formation, sprouting and spine loss. Similar changes were seen in human post-mortem AD brain [46]. In another plaque-forming mouse line, Knafo *et al.* [47] found differential effects in plaque-near and plaque-free regions. Whereas dendrites crossing plaques showed a strong reduction in spine density and an increase in spine length, the volume of spine heads was only decreased in plaque-free regions. This suggests that both, amyloid plaques and Aβ oligomers, affect spines. Oligomeric Aβ may also weaken synapses without causing a complete loss of synaptic contacts. *In vivo* multiphoton imaging revealed no obvious pathology at ages before plaques appear but increased spine elimination combined with stable spine formation after onset of plaque formation. This resulted in spine loss in plaque-bearing mice [48]. Interestingly, a study by Jacobsen *et al.* [49] in the same mouse line reported decreased spine density and impaired LTP long before plaques appeared. While it may not be excluded that both plaques and Aβ oligomers contribute to synaptic alterations in AD, more studies focus now on oligomer-induced pathology. For example, several *in vitro* studies showed that Aβ oligomers caused a decrease in spine density [50, 51], impaired LTP [52, 53] and were responsible for alterations in spine morphology like an elongation of spines [54]. Support for Aβ oligomer-mediated spine pathology comes also from a study in which plaque-bearing APP transgenic mice having memory deficits were treated with an antibody against Aβ [55]. In these mice, memory improved although plaque levels remained unchanged. Another study using a different antibody and another mouse line came to similar results [56]. The data suggest that memory impairment is not only caused by plaques but also by more soluble Aβ species. Besides its effect on spine density and morphology, Aβ appears also to affect the motility of spines. Using two photon time lapse imaging of hippocampal neurons, Shrestha *et al.* [51] observed a strong decrease in spine motility in Aβ oligomer-treated cultures.

The number of different natural or synthetic Aβ oligomers species described in the literature is still increasing with several of the identified species having overlapping properties. Naturally secreted dimers and trimers but not monomers caused loss of dendritic spines [50] and impairment in LTP [52]. Amyloid beta-derived diffusible ligands (ADDLs) are natural or synthetic small soluble globular Aβ oligomers ranging from dimers to 24mers [57]. Treatment of cultures with ADDLs caused reductions in dendritic spine numbers [58] and inhibited LTP [59]. Aβ42 and mixture of 3:7 Aβ42:40 synthetic oligomers caused loss of synaptic proteins in primary neurons [60]. Other species of Aβ oligomers, *e.g.* Aβ*56 [61], have been described to cause memory impairment *in vivo*, however the direct effect on dendritic spines or synaptic transmission still has to be determined.

Besides amyloid plaques, AD is also characterized by the formation of neurofibrillary tangles composed of hyperphosphorylated and aggregated tau protein. The influence of tau modification on neuronal connectivity is still a matter of debate. Tau has been found in dendritic spines targeting Fyn kinase to NMDA receptors thereby affecting downstream signaling [62]. In hippocampal primary neurons overexpressed human tau induced a loss of spines [63]. In transgenic mice expressing tau mutants that differ in their aggregation propensity, tau also appeared to contributed to spine loss [64]. This is in contrast to other studies where a hyperphosphorylation-mimicking tau mutant (PHP tau) did not effect hippocampal spine density or morphology *ex vivo* or *in vivo* [11, 65]. In organotypic slice cultures the expression of human wt tau did not further increase Aβ-induced spine loss although tau was required for neuronal degeneration [66] indicating that spine alteration and neurodegeneration are affected differentially. In summary, contribution of tau to dendritic spine changes in AD models is controversial.

Currently, most data suggest that increased levels of Aβ - either in an oligomeric or plaque-like form - is the major factor that is responsible for disrupting synaptic connections in AD. This is also supported by the finding that familial AD mutations of the presenilins or APP shift the processing of APP to the amyloidogenic form of Aβ ($A\beta_{42}$) [67] whereas no tau mutations have been identified in AD. However, it cannot be excluded that other disease-related factors may affect dendritic spines.

Potential Mechanisms of AD-Related Spine Pathology

The mechanism of LTP and how Aβ may induce spine pathology is schematically depicted in Fig. **2**. Aβ-induced changes in density and morphology of spines may occur *via* direct binding of Aβ to excitatory synapses. In support of this hypothesis, ADDLs colocalized with PSD-95, a marker protein for excitatory synapses, in hippocampal primary neurons [68] and bound to or near NMDARs [54]. Preventing the synaptic targeting of ADDLs could abolish dendritic spine loss [58, 69]. Since NMDARs are essential for synapse function and LTP, Aβ-induced alterations such as a decrease in NMDAR density *via* increased endocytosis [70] could explain memory failure in AD. This is consistent with studies where NMDAR antibodies were reported to block ADDL binding [71] and NMDAR antagonists protected synapses and spines from ADDL induced toxicity [72]. The NMDA receptor forms a heterotetramer of two NR1 and two NR2 subunits, with NR2A and N2B being the main NR2 subunits in the hippocampus [73]. NR2A-containing NMDAR inhibition as well as NR2A-subunit knockout abolished Aβ-induced dendritic spine loss in organotypic slice cultures [74]. However, Aβ oligomers have also been shown to excessively activate extrasynaptically located NR2B-containing NMDARs in acute slices resulting in LTP inhibition [75]. Further, activation of NR2B-containing NMDARs by Aβ in primary neurons caused a loss of synaptophysin- and PSD-95 signals [76]. Recently, Kessels *et al.* [77] showed that Aβ-induced synaptic depression required the metabotropic NMDAR function on GluN2B-containing NMDARs. Besides NMDARs also AMPARs may be targets of Aβ. Hsieh *et al.* [78] showed that Aβ reduced AMPAR currents in hippocampal slice cultures. The surface density of AMPAR was decreased by increased endocytosis, along with a general decrease in spine density.

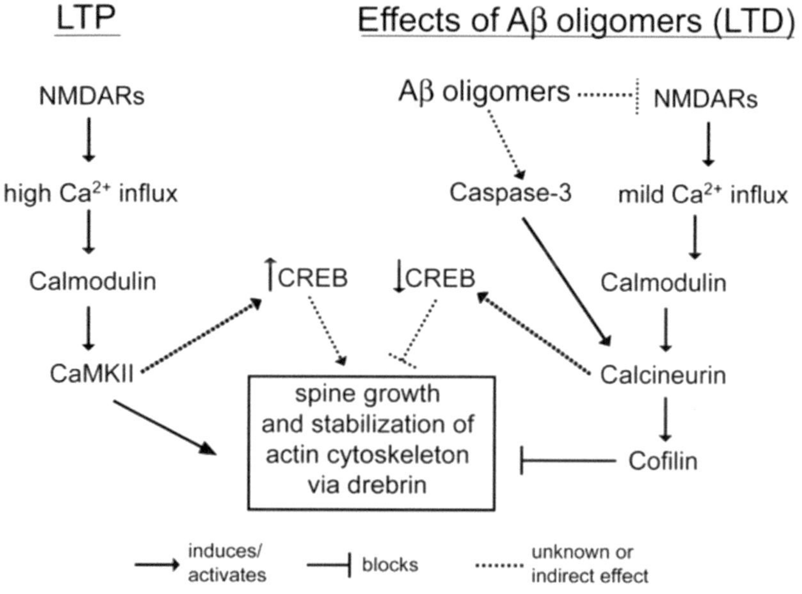

Figure 2: Schematic representation showing the mechanisms of LTP (left) and the pathways affected by Aβ oligomers (right). See text for details.

Caspase-3 is an important mediator of LTD [79]. Caspase-3 was found to be locally activated in dendritic spines from APP transgenic mice where it activated calcium-dependent phosphatase calcineurin [80], another key enzyme in LTD. Blocking either Caspase-3 or Calcineurin could abolish Aβ-induced LTP deficits

[81], reduce memory deficits in APP transgenic mice [80] or prevent dendritic spine loss in culture [66, 74].

As discussed previously, high spine motility appears to be coupled to the dynamic state of the actin cytoskeleton. Therefore, alterations of spine morphology and motility found after Aβ oligomer exposure may be caused by an effect on actin binding proteins. In fact, Aβ has been shown to downregulate the levels of the actin stabilizing protein drebrin A [82]. Similar results were obtained in mature hippocampal primary cultures [54]. This fits to data where it has been shown that drebrin A is decreased in brains of AD patients [83-85]. In other studies it has been shown that the actin depolymerizing factor cofilin becomes activated by Aβ [86]. Blocking cofilin and calcineurin both prevented Aβ-induced spine loss in hippocampal slices [50]. The effect of Aβ on dendritic spines could also be blocked by Rolipram in hippocampal slice cultures [51]. Rolipram, a phosphodiesterase inhibitor, stimulates the cAMP/PKA/CREB pathway that is involved in LTP and prevented Aβ-induced inhibition of CREB. Indeed, active CREB levels are decreased in AD patients [87, 88]. Interestingly, CREB is also essential for the formation of spines in culture [88] and becomes inactivated during LTD. These results are in agreement with a recent study from Shankar *et al.* [52], in which A[beta] oligomers induced LTD after 300 pulses at 1 Hz, whereas no LTD was observed as a result of this stimulus in the absence of Aβ. Similarly, in acute slice preparations from APP transgenic mice (arcAβ mice) a severe impairment of LTP was observed [53]. Taken together, the data suggest that Aβ may harm excitatory synapses by inducing a LTD-like signalling pathway accompanied by LTD-mediated spine retraction [89, 90].

It remains to be shown what downstream events finally regulate spine dynamics and shape, *e.g.* a potential involvement and interactions of different cytoskeletal elements. This information might be very helpful to develop effective therapeutic strategies.

Therapeutic Approaches

Current data suggest that spine pathology in Alzheimer's disease is mainly caused by Aβ. Thus, treatment strategies based on a reduction of Aβ, an increase of Aβ clearance or an inhibition of oligomerization appear to be most promising and have been covered in other review articles [91].

Besides addressing Aβ, factors that positively influence spine dynamics could also have therapeutic potential. A candidate could be the brain derived neurotrophic factor (BDNF). BDNF, which signals through its receptor TrkB, has been shown to modulate structural plasticity and spine development in different types of nerve cells including mature hippocampal neurons [92, 93]. BDNF and its receptor are expressed in brain regions exhibiting a high degree of plasticity, such as the hippocampus [94]. During cortical development levels of BDNF rise, which may be important for spine maintenance in adult brains [95]. Spine development was strongly dependent on protein synthesis linking it to LTP [96]. Application of small molecules that function as ligands for neurotrophin receptors (for review see [97]) may provide a new therapeutic strategy to positively influence spine dynamics and stabilize spines against disease-related loss.

Levels of sex hormones, such as testosterone and estradiol decrease with aging, which has been suggested to constitute a risk for cognitive decline and dementia [98, 99]. It has been shown that testosterone is required to maintain spine density in the CA1 region of the hippocampus in gonadectomized male rats [100] suggesting that it stabilizes spines. Also the steroid estradiol and neurosteroids such as pregnenolone sulfate increase spine strength in hippocampal neurons [101, 102]. At least in the case of estradiol, also increased spine density and involvement of NMDARs were observed [101, 103]. Thus, administration of sex hormones or affecting steroid signalling may constitute a neuroprotective strategy by stabilizing spines during neurodegeneration.

Recent data indicates that also microtubules may play an important role in regulating dendritic spine plasticity, especially in mushroom spines. This is suggested by the finding that knock-down of a microtubule plus-end binding protein in hippocampal primary neurons reduced spine number and microtubule-altering drugs affected BDNF-induced increase of spine density [104]. It is possible that microtubule-stabilizing agents such as taxol may prevent Aβ-induced spine loss during AD.

CONCLUSIONS

Many data show that spine morphology and dynamics are closely linked to learning and memory performance and that the spine loss observed in neurodegenerative diseases is causally linked to the devastating cognitive decline. Spines are regulated by multiple processes including NMDAR-dependent processes and actin dynamics. During AD, Aβ appears to have a key role in causing spine loss *via* multiple mechanisms. Attacking Aβ in its effects on spines or supporting spine dynamics may be effective in preventing AD-related spine loss, thus slowing down or even preventing disease progression.

ACKNOWLEDGEMENTS

We thank Lidia Bakota for helpful suggestions on the manuscript. This work was supported by grant BR 1192/11-1 of the Deutsche Forschungsgemeinschaft (DFG).

CONFLICT OF INTEREST

The authors confirm that this chapter content has no conflict of interest.

DISCLOSURE

This chapter is an update of our previous publication in CAR "Thin, Stubby or Mushroom: Spine Pathology in Alzheimer's Disease" published in 'CAR', Volume 6, Number 3, June, pp. 261 to 268.

REFERENCES

[1] Harris KM and Kater SB. Dendritic spines: cellular specializations imparting both stability and flexibility to synaptic function. Annu Rev Neurosci 17: 341-71 (1994)

[2] Fiala JC and Harris KM. Dendrite Structure. Oxford University Press: Oxford UK (1999)

[3] Sabatini BL, Maravall M and Svoboda K. Ca(2+) signaling in dendritic spines. Curr Opin Neurobiol 11: 349-56 (2001)

[4] Peters A and Kaiserman-Abramof IR. The small pyramidal neuron of the rat cerebral cortex. The perikaryon, dendrites and spines. Am J Anat 127: 321-55 (1970)

[5] Sala C. Molecular regulation of dendritic spine shape and function. Neurosignals. 11: 213-23 (2002)

[6] Sorra KE and Harris KM. Overview on the structure, composition, function, development, and plasticity of hippocampal dendritic spines. Hippocampus 10: 501-11 (2000)

[7] Nimchinsky EA, Sabatini BL and and Svoboda K. Structure and function of dendritic spines. Annu Rev Physiol. 64: 313-53 (2002)

[8] Korkotian E and Segal M. Structure-function relations in dendritic spines: is size important? Hippocampus 10: 587-95 (2000)

[9] Segal M. Dendritic spines and long-term plasticity. Nat Rev Neurosci. 6: 277-84 (2005)

[10] De Simoni A, Griesinger CB and Edwards FA. Development of rat CA1 neurones in acute *vs.* organotypic slices: role of experience in synaptic morphology and activity J Physiol 550: 135-47 (2003)

[11] Shahani N, Subramaniam S, Wolf T, Tackenberg C and Brandt R. Tau aggregation and progressive neuronal degeneration in the absence of changes in spine density and morphology after targeted expression of Alzheimer's disease-relevant tau constructs in organotypic hippocampal slices. J Neurosci 26: 6103-14 (2006)

[12] Koh IY, Lindquist WB, Zito K, Nimchinsky EA and Svoboda K. An image analysis algorithm for dendritic spines. Neural Comput 14: 1283-310 (2002)

[13] Sündermann F, Golovyashkina N, Tackenberg C, Brandt R and Bakota L. High-resolution imaging and evaluation of spines in organotypic hippocampal slice cultures. Methods Mol Biol 846: 277-93 (2012)

[14] Fischer M, Kaech S, Knutti D and Matus A. Rapid actin-based plasticity in dendritic spines. Neuron 20: 847-54 (1998)

[15] Dunaevsky A, Tashiro A, Majewska A, Mason C and Yuste R. Developmental regulation of spine motility in the mammalian central nervous system. Proc Natl Acad Sci U S A 96: 13438-43 (1999)

[16] Roelandse M, Welman A, Wagner U, Hagmann J and Matus A. Focal motility determines the geometry of dendritic spines. Neuroscience 121: 39-49 (2003)

[17] Ackermann M and Matus A. Activity-induced targeting of profilin and stabilization of dendritic spine morphology. Nat Neurosci 6: 1194-200 (2003)

[18] Brünig I, Kaech S, Brinkhaus H, Oertner TG and Matus A. Influx of extracellular calcium regulates actin-dependent morphological plasticity in dendritic spines. Neuropharmacology 47: 669-76 (2004)

[19] Mulkey RM, Endo S, Shenolikar S and Malenka RC. Involvement of a calcineurin/inhibitor-1 phosphatase cascade in hippocampal long-term depression. Nature 369: 486-488 (1994)

[20] Cummings JA, Mulkey RM, Nicoll RA and Malenka RC. Ca2 signaling requirements for long-term depression in the hippocampus. Neuron 16: 825- 833 (1996)

[21] Nagerl UV, Eberhorn N, Cambridge SB and Bonhoeffer T. Bidirectional activity-dependent morphological plasticity in hippocampal neurons. Neuron 44: 759 -767 (2004)

[22] Yang Y, Wang XB, Frerking M and Zhou Q. Spine expansion and stabilization associated with long-term potentiation J Neurosci 28: 5740-51 (2008)

[23] Kopec CD, Li B, Wei W, Boehm J and Malinow R. Glutamate receptor exocytosis and spine enlargement during chemically induced long-term potentiation. J Neurosci 26: 2000-9 (2006)

[24] Park M, Penick EC, Edwards JG, Kauer JA and Ehlers MD. Recycling endosomes supply AMPA receptors for LTP. Science 305: 1972-5 (2004)

[25] Denk W, Delaney KR, Gelperin A, Kleinfeld D, Strowbridge BW, Tank DW, *et al.* Anatomical and functional imaging of neurons using 2-photon laser scanning microscopy. J Neurosci Methods 54: 151-62 (1994)

[26] Denk W. Two-photon excitation in functional biological imaging. J Biomed Opt 1: 296-304 (1996)

[27] Denk W and Svoboda K. Photon upmanship: why multiphoton imaging is more than a gimmick. Neuron 18: 351-7 (1997)

[28] Alvarez VA and Sabatini BL. Anatomical and physiological plasticity of dendritic spines. Annu Rev Neurosci 30: 79-97 (2007)

[29] Mizrahi A, Crowley JC, Shtoyerman E and Katz LC. High-resolution *in vivo* imaging of hippocampal dendrites and spines. J Neurosci 24: 3147-51 (2004)

[30] Holtmaat AJ, Trachtenberg JT, Wilbrecht L, Shepherd GM, Zhang X, Knott GW, *et al.* Transient and persistent dendritic spines in the neocortex *in vivo*. Neuron 45: 279-91 (2005)

[31] Grutzendler J, Kasthuri N and Gan WB. Long-term dendritic spine stability in the adult cortex. Nature 420: 812-6 (2002)

[32] Loew LM and Hell SW. Superresolving dendritic spines. Biophys J 104: 741-3 (2013)

[33] Nägerl UV, Willig KI, Hein B, Hell SW and Bonhoeffer T. Live-cell imaging of dendritic spines by STED microscopy. Proc Natl Acad Sci 105: 18982-7 (2008)

[34] Yan P, Acker CD, Zhou WL, Lee P, Bollensdorff C, Negrean A, *et al.* Palette of fluorinated voltage-sensitive hemicyanine dyes. Proc Natl Acad Sci 109: 20443-8 (2012)

[35] Spires TL and Hyman BT. Neuronal structure is altered by amyloid plaques. Rev Neurosci. 15: 267-78 (2004)

[36] Baloyannis SJ, Costa V, Mauroudis I, Psaroulis D, Manolides SL and Manolides LS. Dendritic and spinal pathology in the acoustic cortex in Alzheimer's disease: morphological and morphometric estimation by Golgi technique and electron microscopy. Acta Otolaryngol 127: 351-4 (2007)

[37] Scheff SW, Price DA, Schmitt FA, DeKosky ST and Mufson EJ. Synaptic alterations in CA1 in mild Alzheimer disease and mild cognitive impairment. Neurology. 68: 1501-8 (2007)

[38] Ferrer I and Gullotta F. Down's syndrome and Alzheimer's disease: dendritic spine counts in the hippocampus. Acta Neuropathol. 79: 680-5 (1990)

[39] Dickstein DL, Kabaso D, Rocher AB, Luebke JI, Wearne SL and Hof PR. Changes in the structural complexity of the aged brain. Aging Cell 6: 275-84 (2007)

[40] Hardy J and Selkoe DJ. The amyloid hypothesis of Alzheimer's disease: progress and problems on the road to therapeutics Science 297: 353-6 (2002)

[41] McLean CA, Cherny RA, Fraser FW, Fuller SJ, Smith MJ, Beyreuther K, *et al.* Soluble pool of Abeta amyloid as a determinant of severity of neurodegeneration in Alzheimer's disease. Ann Neurol 46: 860-6 (1999)

[42] Lue LF, Kuo YM, Roher AE, Brachova L, Shen Y, Sue L, *et al.* Soluble amyloid beta peptide concentration as a predictor of synaptic change in Alzheimer's disease. Am J Pathol 155: 853-62 (1999)

[43] Braak H and Braak E. Neuropathological stageing of Alzheimer-related changes. Acta Neuropathol 82: 239-59 (1991)

[44] Irizarry MC, McNamara M, Fedorchak K, Hsiao K and Hyman BT. APPSw transgenic mice develop age-related A beta deposits and neuropil abnormalities, but no neuronal loss in CA1. J Neuropathol Exp Neurol 56: 965-73 (1997)

[45] Irizarry MC, Soriano F, McNamara M, Page KJ, Schenk D, Games D, *et al.* Abeta deposition is associated with neuropil changes, but not with overt neuronal loss in the human amyloid precursor protein V717F (PDAPP) transgenic mouse. J Neurosci 17: 7053-9 (1997)

[46] Grutzendler J, Helmin K, Tsai J and Gan WB. Various dendritic abnormalities are associated with fibrillar amyloid deposits in Alzheimer's disease. Ann N Y Acad Sci 1097: 30-9 (2007)

[47] Knafo S, Alonso-Nanclares L, Gonzalez-Soriano J, Merino-Serrais P, Fernaud-Espinosa I, Ferrer I, *et al.* Widespread Changes in Dendritic Spines in a Model of Alzheimer's Disease. Cereb Cortex ([Epub ahead of print] (2008))

[48] Spires-Jones TL, Meyer-Luehmann M, Osetek JD, Jones PB, Stern EA, Bacskai BJ, *et al.* Impaired spine stability underlies plaque-related spine loss in an Alzheimer's disease mouse model. Am J Pathol 171: 1304-11 (2007)

[49] Jacobsen JS, Wu CC, Redwine JM, Comery TA, Arias R, Bowlby M, *et al.* Early-onset behavioral and synaptic deficits in a mouse model of Alzheimer's disease. Proc Natl Acad Sci U S A 103: 5161-6 (2006)

[50] Shankar GM, Bloodgood BL, Townsend M, Walsh DM, Selkoe DJ and Sabatini BL. Natural oligomers of the Alzheimer amyloid-beta protein induce reversible synapse loss by modulating an NMDA-type glutamate receptor-dependent signaling pathway. J Neurosci 27: 2866-75 (2007)

[51] Shrestha BR, Vitolo OV, Joshi P, Lordkipanidze T, Shelanski M and Dunaevsky A. Amyloid beta peptide adversely affects spine number and motility in hippocampal neurons. Mol Cell Neurosci 33: 274-82 (2006)

[52] Shankar GM, Li S, Mehta TH, Garcia-Munoz A, Shepardson NE, Smith I, *et al.* Amyloid-beta protein dimers isolated directly from Alzheimer's brains impair synaptic plasticity and memory. Nat Med 14: 837-42 (2008)

[53] Knobloch M, Farinelli M, Konietzko U, Nitsch RM and Mansuy IM. Abeta oligomer-mediated long-term potentiation impairment involves protein phosphatase 1-dependent mechanisms. J Neurosci 27: 7648-53 (2007)

[54] Lacor PN, Buniel MC, Furlow PW, Clemente AS, Velasco PT, Wood M, *et al.* Abeta oligomer-induced aberrations in synapse composition, shape, and density provide a molecular basis for loss of connectivity in Alzheimer's disease. J Neurosci 27: 796-807 (2007)

[55] Dodart JC, Bales KR, Gannon KS, Greene SJ, DeMattos RB, Mathis C, *et al.* Immunization reverses memory deficits without reducing brain Abeta burden in Alzheimer's disease model. Nat Neurosci 5: 452-7 (2002)

[56] Kotilinek LA, Bacskai B, Westerman M, Kawarabayashi T, Younkin L, Hyman BT, *et al.* Reversible memory loss in a mouse transgenic model of Alzheimer's disease. J Neurosci 22: 6331-5 (2002)

[57] Klein WL. Synaptic targeting by A beta oligomers (ADDLS) as a basis for memory loss in early Alzheimer's disease. Alzheimers Dement 2: 43-55 (2006)

[58] De Felice FG, Vieira MN, Bomfim TR, Decker H, Velasco PT, Lambert MP, *et al.* Protection of synapses against Alzheimer's-linked toxins: insulin signaling prevents the pathogenic binding of Abeta oligomers. Proc Natl Acad Sci 106: 1971-6 (2009)

[59] Lambert MP, Barlow AK, Chromy BA, Edwards C, Freed R, Liosatos M, *et al.* Diffusible, nonfibrillar ligands derived from Abeta1-42 are potent central nervous system neurotoxins. Proc Natl Acad Sci 95: 6448-53 (1998)

[60] Kuperstein I, Broersen K, Benilova I, Rozenski J, Jonckheere W, Debulpaep M, *et al.* Neurotoxicity of Alzheimer's disease Aß peptides is induced by small changes in the Aß42 to Aß40 ratio. EMBO J 29: 3408-20 (2010)

[61] Lesné S, Koh MT, Kotilinek L, Kayed R, Glabe CG, Yang A, *et al.* A specific amyloid-beta protein assembly in the brain impairs memory. Nature 440: 352-7 (2006)

[62] Ittner LM, Ke YD, Delerue F, Bi M, Gladbach A, van Eersel J, *et al.* Dendritic function of tau mediates amyloid-beta toxicity in Alzheimer's disease mouse models. Cell 142: 387-97 (2011)

[63] Thies E and Mandelkow EM. Missorting of tau in neurons causes degeneration of synapses that can be rescued by the kinase MARK2/Par-1. J Neurosci 27: 2896-907 (2007)

[64] Eckermann K, Mocanu MM, Khlistunova I, Biernat J, Nissen A, Hofmann A, *et al.* The beta-propensity of Tau determines aggregation and synaptic loss in inducible mouse models of tauopathy. J Biol Chem 282: 31755-65 (2007)

[65] Hundelt M, Fath T, Selle K, Oesterwind K, Jordan J, Schultz C, *et al.* Altered phosphorylation but no neurodegeneration in a mouse model of tau hyperphosphorylation. Neurobiol Aging 32: 991-1006 (2011)

[66] Tackenberg C and Brandt R. Divergent pathways mediate spine alterations and cell death induced by amyloid-beta, wild-type tau, and R406W tau. J Neurosci 29: 14439-50 (2009)

[67] Scheuner D, Eckman C, Jensen M, Song X, Citron M, Suzuki N, *et al.* Secreted amyloid beta-protein similar to that in the senile plaques of Alzheimer's disease is increased *in vivo* by the presenilin 1 and 2 and APP mutations linked to familial Alzheimer's disease. Nat Med 2: 864-70 (1996)

[68] Lacor PN, Buniel MC, Chang L, Fernandez SJ, Gong Y, Viola KL, *et al.* Synaptic targeting by Alzheimer's-related amyloid beta oligomers. J Neurosci 24: 10191-200 (2004)

[69] Pitt J, Thorner M, Brautigan D, Larner J and Klein WL. Protection against the synaptic targeting and toxicity of Alzheimer's-associated Aß oligomers by insulin mimetic chiro-inositols. FASEB J 27: 199-207 (2013)

[70] Snyder EM, Nong Y, Almeida CG, Paul S, Moran T, Choi EY, *et al.* Regulation of NMDA receptor trafficking by amyloid-beta. Nat Neurosci 8: 1051-8 (2005)

[71] De Felice FG, Velasco PT, Lambert MP, Viola K, Fernandez SJ, Ferreira ST, *et al.* Abeta oligomers induce neuronal oxidative stress through an N-methyl-D-aspartate receptor-dependent mechanism that is blocked by the Alzheimer drug memantine. J Biol Chem 282: 11590-601 (2007)

[72] Calabrese B, Shaked GM, Tabarean IV, Braga J, Koo EH and Halpain S. Rapid, concurrent alterations in pre- and postsynaptic structure induced by naturally-secreted amyloid-beta protein. Mol Cell Neurosci 35: 183-93 (2007)

[73] Gambrill AC and Barria A. NMDA receptor subunit composition controls synaptogenesis and synapse stabilization. Proc Natl Acad Sci 108: 5855-60 (2011)

[74] Tackenberg C, Grinschgl S, Trutzel A, Santuccione AC, Frey MC, Konietzko U, *et al.* NMDA receptor subunit composition determines beta-amyloid-induced neurodegeneration and synaptic loss. Cell Death Dis 4:e608 (2013).

[75] Li S, Jin M, Koeglsperger T, Shepardson NE, Shankar GM and Selkoe DJ. Soluble Aß oligomers inhibit long-term potentiation through a mechanism involving excessive activation of extrasynaptic NR2B-containing NMDA receptors. J Neurosci 31: 6627-38 (2011)

[76] Liu J, Chang L, Roselli F, Almeida OF, Gao X, Wang X, *et al.* Amyloid-ß induces caspase-dependent loss of PSD-95 and synaptophysin through NMDA receptors. J Alzheimers Dis 22: 541-56 (2010)

[77] Kessels H W, Nabavi S and Malinow R. Metabotropic NMDA receptor function is required for ß-amyloid-induced synaptic depression. Proc Natl Acad Sci 110: 4033-8 (2013)

[78] Hsieh H, Boehm J, Sato C, Iwatsubo T, Tomita T, Sisodia S, *et al.* AMPAR removal underlies Abeta-induced synaptic depression and dendritic spine loss. Neuron 52: 831-43 (2006)

[79] Li Z, Jo J, Jia JM, Lo SC, Whitcomb DJ, Jiao S, *et al.* Caspase-3 activation *via* mitochondria is required for long-term depression and AMPA receptor internalization. Cell 141: 859-71 (2010)

[80] D'Amelio M, Cavallucci V, Middei S, Marchetti C, Pacioni S, Ferri A, *et al.* Caspase-3 triggers early synaptic dysfunction in a mouse model of Alzheimer's disease. Nat Neurosci 14: 69-76 (2011)

[81] Jo J, Whitcomb DJ, Olsen KM, Kerrigan TL, Lo SC, Bru-Mercier G, *et al.* Aß(1-42) inhibition of LTP is mediated by a signaling pathway involving caspase-3, Akt1 and GSK-3ß. Nat Neurosci 14: 545-7 (2011)

[82] Aoki C, Mahadomrongkul V, Fujisawa S, Habersat R and Shirao T. Chemical and morphological alterations of spines within the hippocampus and entorhinal cortex precede the onset of Alzheimer's disease pathology in double knock-in mice. J Comp Neurol 505: 352-62 (2007)

[83] Hatanpää K, Isaacs KR, Shirao T, Brady DR and Rapoport SI. Loss of proteins regulating synaptic plasticity in normal aging of the human brain and in Alzheimer disease. J Neuropathol Exp Neurol 58: 637-43 (1999)

[84] Shim KS and Lubec G. Drebrin, a dendritic spine protein, is manifold decreased in brains of patients with Alzheimer's disease and Down syndrome. Neurosci Lett 324: 209-12 (2002)

[85] Harigaya Y, Shoji M, Shirao T and Hirai S. Disappearance of actin-binding protein, drebrin, from hippocampal synapses in Alzheimer's disease. J Neurosci Res 43: 87-92 (1996)

[86] Maloney MT and Bamburg JR. Cofilin-mediated neurodegeneration in Alzheimer's disease and other amyloidopathies. Mol Neurobiol 35: 21-44 (2007)

[87] Yamamoto-Sasaki M, Ozawa H, Saito T, Rösler M and Riederer P. Impaired phosphorylation of cyclic AMP response element binding protein in the hippocampus of dementia of the Alzheimer type. Brain Res 824: 300-3 (1999)

[88] Murphy DD and Segal M. Morphological plasticity of dendritic spines in central neurons is mediated by activation of cAMP response element binding protein. Proc Natl Acad Sci U S A 94: 1482-7 (1997)

[89] Engert F and Bonhoeffer T. Dendritic spine changes associated with hippocampal long-term synaptic plasticity. Nature 399: 66-70 (1999)

[90] Maletic-Savatic M, Malinow R and Svoboda K. Rapid dendritic morphogenesis in CA1 hippocampal dendrites induced by synaptic activity. Science 283: 1923-7 (1999)

[91] Citron M. Alzheimer's disease: strategies for disease modification. Nat Rev Drug Discov 9: 387-98 (2010)

[92] Shimada A, Mason CA and Morrison ME. TrkB signaling modulates spine density and morphology independent of dendrite structure in cultured neonatal Purkinje cells. J Neurosci 18: 8559-70 (1998)

[93] Ji Y, Pang PT, Feng L and Lu B. Cyclic AMP controls BDNF-induced TrkB phosphorylation and dendritic spine formation in mature hippocampal neurons. Nat Neurosci 8: 164-72 (2005)

[94] Tapia-Arancibia L, Aliaga E, Silhol M and Arancibia S. New insights into brain BDNF function in normal aging and Alzheimer disease. Brain Res Rev 59: 201-20 (2008)

[95] Chakravarthy S, Saiepour MH, Bence M, Perry S, Hartman R, Couey JJ, *et al.* Postsynaptic TrkB signaling has distinct roles in spine maintenance in adult visual cortex and hippocampus. Proc Natl Acad Sci U S A. 103: 1071-6 (2006)

[96] Tanaka J, Horiike Y, Matsuzaki M, Miyazaki T, Ellis-Davies GC and Kasai H. Protein synthesis and neurotrophin-dependent structural plasticity of single dendritic spines. Science 1683-7 (2008)

[97] Longo FM, Yang T, Knowles JK, Xie Y, Moore LA and Massa SM. Small molecule neurotrophin receptor ligands: novel strategies for targeting Alzheimer's disease mechanisms. Curr Alzheimer Res 4: 503-6 (2007)

[98] Driscoll I and Resnick SM. Testosterone and cognition in normal aging and Alzheimer's disease: an update. Curr Alzheimer Res 4: 33-45 (2007)

[99] Xu H, Wang R, Zhang YW and Zhang X. Estrogen, beta-amyloid metabolism/trafficking, and Alzheimer's disease. Ann N Y Acad Sci 1089: 324-42 (2006)

[100] Leranth C, Petnehazy O and MacLusky NJ. Gonadal hormones affect spine synaptic density in the CA1 hippocampal subfield of male rats. J Neurosci 23: 1588-92 (2003)

[101] Pozzo-Miller LD, Inoue T and Murphy DD. Estradiol increases spine density and NMDA-dependent Ca2+ transients in spines of CA1 pyramidal neurons from hippocampal slices. J Neurophysiol. 81: 1404-11 (1999)

[102] Mameli M, Carta M, Partridge LD and and Valenzuela CF. Neurosteroid-induced plasticity of immature synapses *via* retrograde modulation of presynaptic NMDA receptors. J Neurosci 25: 2285-94 (2005)

[103] Woolley CS and McEwen BS. Estradiol regulates hippocampal dendritic spine density *via* an N-methyl-D-aspartate receptor-dependent mechanism. J Neurosci 14: 7680-7 (1994)

[104] Gu J, Firestein BL and Zheng JQ. Microtubules in dendritic spine development. J Neurosci 28: 12120-4 (2008)

CHAPTER 14

Planum Temporale Analysis *Via* a New Volumetric Method in Autoptic Brains of Demented and Psychotic Patients

Petr Zach[1,2,*], Zdena Krištofiková[1], Jana Mrzílková[2], Emerich Majer[3], Pavel Selinger[4], Filip Španiel[1], Daniela Řípová[1], Martina Kutová[2] and Jana Kenney[5]

[1]Prague Psychiatric Center, Czech Republic, [2]Institute of Anatomy, Third Faculty of Medicine, Charles University, Czech Republic, [3]Psychiatric Hospital Bohnice, Czech Republic, [4]Faculty Hospital Bulovka, Czech Republic, [5]Czech Academy of Science, Czech Republic

Abstract: Investigations of alterations in brain asymmetry often focus on the planum temporale of patients with schizophrenia. Data also suggest changes in laterality of demented patients associated with a more marked impairment of the left hemisphere. Our study was performed on autoptic brain tissue of 84 patients, out of which there were 25 nondemented nonpsychotic controls, 50 demented patients (34 Alzheimer disease, 9 multi - infarct dementia and 7 mixed-type dementia patients) and 9 people with schizophrenia. The plana temporalia were evaluated *via* a new volumetric method using dental resin matter. Areas, cortical thickness and volumes of the right and left planum temporale were evaluated without normalization to brain weight in 60 patients and with normalization in 24 people. In controls, a mild right/left laterality of areas, cortical thickness and volumes was found. Moreover, in control women the areas of the left planum temporale were smaller than those observed in control men. The shifts to left/right laterality of areas and volumes were found in all demented groups. In the more numerous Alzheimer group, the change in laterality of an area was associated with a mild decrease on the right and a mild increase on the left side. In contrast, marked but only bilateral area shrinkage as well as reduced cortical thickness and brain volumes were observed in schizophrenic patients.

Keywords: Brain laterality, dementia, planum temporale, schizophrenia, volumetry.

INTRODUCTION

The planum temporale (PT) is an area of the temporal lobe located on the superior

***Corresponding author Petr Zach:** Institute of Anatomy, Third Faculty of Medicine, Charles University at Prague, Ruská 87, Prague 10, 100 00, Czech Republic; Tel/Fax: +420267102508;
E-mail: zach.petr@post.cz

D.K. Lahiri (Ed)

surface of the superior temporal gyrus. The anterior portion of the PT is a part of the unimodal auditory association cortex (part of BA22) that surrounds the Heschl´s gyrus, whereas the posterior portion adjacent to the temporoparietal junction (other portions of BA22 and a part of BA39-40) is partially coextensive with the Wernicke's area, consisting of heteromodal association cortex [1, 2]. Cytoarchitecture has been studied to help describe the borders of the PT, but distribution of auditory association cortex is not altogether confluent with it. Although there is still a debate concerning the exact delineation of the PT, Pfeifer´s definition [3, 4] adapted by von Economo and Horn [5] is preferred at the present time.

Firstly, assessments of the PT area were carried out from photographs of post-mortem brains and studies using magnetic resonance and computer tomography followed. In the past, post-mortem studies concentrated only on measurement of the length of the PT and this tendency was also seen in magnetic resonance studies. Later studies have measured the PT volume taking into account cortical depth.

The PT area in the healthy human brain appears to be predominantly left/right (L/R) lateralized [6, 7]. Same asymmetry was also shown in Situs inversus totalis, a rare condition in which all visceral organs are arranged as mirror images [8]. The lateralization in a normal population lies along a continuum. This continuum (normal distribution) is skewed to the L in the normal population, with a few brains strongly asymmetrical towards the R [9]. Despite difficulties with an exact relationship between handedness on the PT size, there is a general agreement that R-handers demonstrate a significant leftward asymmetry of the PT in comparison to L-handed subjects, whose plana temporalia are usually either symmetrical or tend towards rightward asymmetry [10-12]. Similar results in recent studies with apes suggest that leftward asymmetries in the PT were present in the common ancestor of chimpanzees and humans [13-15].

Little systematic anatomical research has been done into the effect of sex on structural differences in the PT. One such study reported that females show more frequent reversals of PT asymmetry (*i.e.*, R>L) [16]. Another study supported this finding [17]. One study shows R/L asymmetry of the temporal region also in healthy males [18]. The mechanism of hand and language lateralization inheritance appears to be multiple and independent [19].

Functional neuroimaging studies indicate that the PT has a predominantly language related function. One study demonstrated that the L PT becomes activated equally to tones and words during passive listening and even greater activation was observed during active listening [20]. A further study reports that the PT shows greater activation bilaterally during a tone task compared with a semantic decision task [21], although another study has shown significant activation in the PT, particularly in the R hemisphere, when listening to a variety of acoustic stimuli [22]. New findings support a heterogeneous model of the PT, with functionally distinct regions for auditory spatial perception and sensory-motor response [23]. Patients with a variety of lesions near or including the PT have been shown to exhibit a number of associated auditory discrimination and speech comprehension deficits [24-26].

Data suggest atrophy of the medial and lateral parts of the temporal lobe in patients with Alzheimer disease (AD) when compared to the age-matched controls [27]. Moreover, the changes in temporal-parietal cortices appear to be lateralized. Namely, a spreading wave of grey matter loss occurs in both hemispheres, however, L-hemisphere regions are affected earlier and more severely [28, 29]. Nevertheless, another study performed on the post-mortem brain tissue reported either bilateral reduction of the PT volume in AD patients when compared to the controls or no gender-dependent differences in both groups [30]. In contrast to AD, laterality of the PT has not been evaluated yet in patients with multi-infarct dementia (MID). Microanatomical measures shows correlation between cortical minicolumn thinning and loss of cognitive ability in MCI and AD [31].

Investigation of PT size or asymmetry differences in schizophrenic (SCHIZ) patients when compared with controls has yielded contradictory results. In the first-episode of disease, bilateral volumetric deficits but no differences in PT asymmetry were observed in patients when compared to the controls [32] but another study reported the marked reduction only in the L PT volume [33]. In chronic SCHIZ patients, reversed asymmetry (R/L) of the PT [*e.g.*, 34-37], bilateral reduction [38] or no changes when compared to the controls [for review, see 9, 29] were observed. Recent study comparing neuronal density and size of PT did not show significant effect of schizophrenia [39], but more sensitive laminar measurements proved the thinner upper layers of the caudal PT [40]. Research with antipsychotic naive people found a significant relationship between grey matter reductions of the superior temporal gyrus and first-episode psychosis [41]. Another study observes increased severity of positive symptoms including auditory hallucinations [42].

As mentioned above, the PT structure has a curved rather than planar surface. Besides, its anatomical borders have not been unequivocally determined. A vast majority of recent studies dealing with the PT were done only by magnetic resonance or computer tomography and there does not seem to be any recent purely anatomical study that would focus on measuring the area and volume of the PT in autoptic human brains. Thus the aims of the present study are as follows: 1) to create reliable anatomical methodology for measurement of the PT area and volume in autoptic human brains, and 2) to evaluate alterations in laterality of demented or psychotic patients compared to nondemented nonpsychotic controls.

MATERIALS AND METHODS

Histological Analysis of the Brains and Diagnosis

In total, 84 human brains with *post-mortem* delays shorter than 24 hours were analyzed. Beside the PT, five other brain areas from both hemispheres were dissected and used for histological analysis. These include three neocortex areas (*gyrus frontalis medius, gyrus temporalis superior et medius* and *lobulus parietalis inferior*), one area of hippocampus (*cornu Ammoni et gyrus parahippocampalis*) and one of cerebellum (*lobulus semilunaris inferior*). We used the same histological examination methods and diagnostic criteria as in our previous study [43]. Briefly, the clinical diagnosis of AD was confirmed *via* a silver stain technique based upon the distribution of numerous senile plaques and neurofibrillary tangles. The criteria were consistent with those used in the classification of Mirra [44]. Subsequently, the samples were divided into five groups: nondemented nonpsychotic controls (patients without marked signs of dementia or psychosis, number of senile plaques and tangles corresponding to normal aging), AD (clinically diagnosed dementia, number of senile plaques and tangles in given areas of the cortex and hippocampus higher than would be expected for age), MID (clinically diagnosed dementia, vascular changes, neuropathologic lesions and gliosis, number of senile plaques and tangles corresponding to normal aging), MIX (clinically diagnosed dementia, changes due to the AD and MID simultaneously) and SCHIZ (clinically diagnosed schizophrenia, number of senile plaques and tangles corresponding to normal aging). Information concerning handedness of our patients was not available to us.

PT Delineation and Dissection

Literature offers more than one working definition of the PT area anatomical delineation. We have selected the most widely accepted anatomical definition according to two studies of Pfeifer [3, 4] and von Economo and Horn [5]. Briefly, anterior border of the PT is defined as the transverse sulcus located dorsally to the transverse Heschl´s gyrus, where the transverse sulcus originates from the retroinsular region. The situation, where two Heschl´s gyri are on the R side and one Heschl´s gyrus is on the L side, is considered normal anatomy. Sometimes the Heschl´s gyrus is divided into anterior and posterior sections by an additional ´transverse sulcus´, called the sulcus intermedius of Beck arising from the lateral border. If, however, there is a second or a third transverse sulcus arising separately from the retroinsular region, then there should be by definition two or more Heschl´s gyri. The posterior boundary of the PT is complicated by asymmetries in the temporal lobe and the Sylvian fissure. As most others investigators we have used an arbitrary cut-off point, where the horizontal Sylvian fissure either terminates or bifurcates into the posterior descending ramus and/or posterior ascending ramus. The lateral border has been uniformly defined as coincident with the superolateral margin of the *superior temporal gyrus*. Since the PT resembles an isosceles triangle with its apex pointing medially, the medial border is theoretically located where the anterior border heading posteromedially meets the posterior border heading anteromedially behind the insula.

PT areas cuts from L and R hemisphere were carefully dissected with sharp knife and placed into 8% paraformaldehyde solution.

Volumetric Analysis of the PT

60 out of the 84 analysed human brains were used for determination of areas, cortical thickness and volumes of the PT and were not normalized to brain weight. The remaining 24 brains were used for determination of areas normalized to brain weights and of alterations in cytoarchitecture (data not shown, the experiments are still in progress). The group totally included 25 nondemented nonpsychotic controls, 50 demented patients (34 AD, 9 MID and 7 MIX) and 9 psychotic patients with different clinical subsets of SCHIZ.

Dental Resin Impression of the PT Area

We washed the PT samples in water and placed them on glass Petri dishes. We covered by means of a small brush the whole surface of the samples with a liquid phase of condensation curing polysiloxane impression material (STOMAFLEX CRÈME (SC)), a substance conventionally used in dental medicine. We made sure that liquid phase penetrated into all irregularities on the PT surfaces. The SC polymerized and formed a thin impression layer on the samples (mask), which we then carefully removed *via* forceps and put back on Petri dishes. This way created masks of the PT surfaces were noted for irregular 3D shape. Using scissors, we have cut masks in order to obtain several pieces with almost ideal 2D surface. All 2D pieces from one PT were placed between two glass slides normally used in microscopy. Images of these slides were acquired by means of digital camera Olympus 5050 attached to standard PC.

The PT Cortical Width Measurement

The PT brain samples were washed by distilled water and placed again on Petri dishes. Then five 4-5 mm thick slices were carefully obtained using a sharp knife from the following parts of every PT sample: transition to the Sylvian fissure, transition to *gyrus temporalis superior*, transition to the posterior part of the PT, where tissue continues to ascending or descending *rami*, the second Heschl´s gyrus, if present and the center of the area dorsal to the second Heschl´s gyrus. Knife cuts were done perpendicularly to the PT cortex in selected parts, so that slices on the cut sides would have reliably exposed cortical width and subcortical white matter for further examination. Slices were placed on anti reflexive white paper and photographed with digital camera (Olympus C-5050, light for photographing was obtained from Intralux 6000-1) into standard PC. The photographed pictures were analyzed using software Image J.31. Cortical thickness in the samples was measured manually with mouse pointer.

Computer Measurement of the PT Dental Resin Impressions

Slides with 2D SC masks together with a millimeter scale were photographed with a digital camera on tripod (Olympus C-5050). We exported the pictures from the digital camera to the software Image J.31 program in a TIFF format and set the measurement scale. Then we delineated the PT SC masks images with a mouse pointer and the software computed the PT area in mm^2. Cortical thickness and PT area data were applied to calculate the volume of the PT.

Statistical Analysis

Lateralization index of the PT was obtained as (L-R)/(L+R). To evaluate the experimental data, BMDP statistical software was used [45]. For global analysis, ANOVA with repeated measures (program 2V) and one-way ANOVA (program 7D) were applied. Student´s t-test (pooled variance) was calculated with respect to controls (* $p < 0.05$, ** $p < 0.01$, *** $p < 0.001$) or to AD (+ $p< 0.05$, ++ $p < 0.01$). Data in charts are presented as mean values ± S.D.

RESULTS

We obtained totally 25 brains of nondemented nonpsychotic control patients, 15 of whom were men (Tables **1** and **3**). Nonpsychiatric (n = 22, especially people with carcinoma) as well as neurological/psychiatric patients (Parkinsonism, n = 2 and oligophrenia, n = 1) were included in the study. We observed a mild R/L laterality of the areas (Tables **2**, **4**, **5** and **6**) and of cortical thickness or volumes (Table **2**). In control women, L sides of PT area were generally smaller when compared to control men, however, global tests did not indicate statistically significant differences (Table **5**).

There was totally 34 people in the AD group, who were further classified according to plaque density (sparse, n = 3, moderate, n = 9 and frequent, n = 22). 14 of the patients were men (Tables **1** and **3**). In most cases, the plaque density did not differ between hemispheres, although in a few patients it was higher in the L than R hemisphere. The group with pure MID consisted totally of 9 people (5 men and 4 women) and the MIX group only of 7 people (5 men and 2 women) with sparse or moderate plaque density (Table **1**). Mild shifts to L/R laterality of the PT areas (Tables **2**, **4** and **6**) and volumes (Table **2**) were observed in all demented groups but statistically significant changes supported by global tests were found especially in the more numerous AD group. The shifts were associated with a moderate shrinkage in the R and a mild increase in the L sides of PT area (Table **6**). In addition, a pronounced reduction of cortical thickness in the L side of the PT was found in the MIX group (Table **2**). Normalization of areas to brain weight did not significantly influence the differences between the AD and the control groups (see results of ANOVA with repeated measures, Table **4**).

Table 1: Characteristics of patiens, where brain tissue, the areas, cortical heights and volumes of the PT were determined without normalization

Groups	**n**	**Sex (M/F)**	**Age (years)**	**Cause of Death**
Controls	16	11/5	68.0 ± 13.3	6xM, 2xCI, BP, A, MI, TC, BI, HC, P, U
AD	19	10/9	79.9 ± 7.9***	13xCI, 2xBP, U, MI, ChP, EXS
MID	9	5/4	80.6 ± 3.6**	8xCI, BP
MIX	7	5/2	79.7 ± 6.6**	6xCI, BP
SCHIZ	9	5/4	68.7 ± 10.5	4xBP, 3xCI, 2xPE
	60		ANOVA: p = 0.0007	

Sex: M – men, F – women; Causes of death: M – malignancy, CI - cardiac insufficiency, BP - bronchopneumonia, A – alcoholism, MI - myocardial infarct, TC - tumorous cachexia, BI - brain infarct, HC - hepatocirrhosis, P - peritonitis, U - uremia, ChP - cholecyst perforation, EXS - exsanguination, PE – pulmonary embolism; Student´s t-test was calculated with respect to controls (**p < 0.01, *** p < 0.001).

SCHIZ group consisted of 9 patients, 5 of whom were men (Table **1**). Clinical diagnoses indicated residual (n = 4), chronic (n = 3) and paranoid (n = 2) phase of the disease. In patients with SCHIZ, marked but only bilateral alterations in areas, cortical thickness and volumes of the PT were found when compared to controls (Table **2**). Beside these, we observed shape abnormalities of the PT (Fig. **1**).

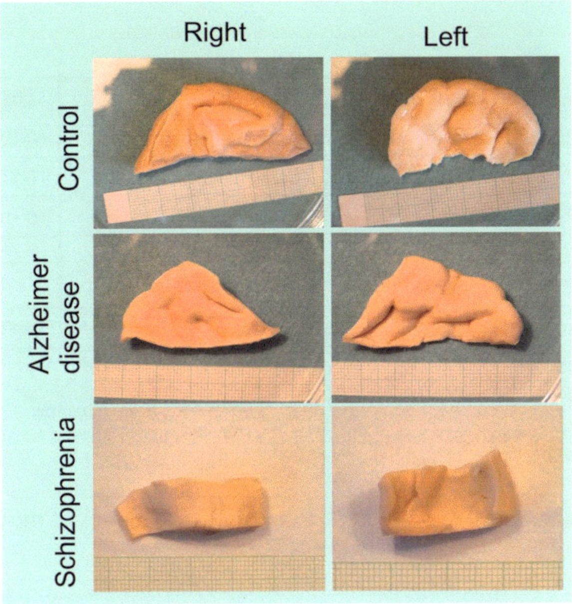

Figure 1: The right and left PT of controls or of Alzheimer disease and schizophrenic patients. Typical examples of shape of the right and left PT of controls, Alzheimer diesease and schizophrenic patients (from above down, attached is millimeter scale).

Table 2: Alterations in the areas, cortical heights and volumes of the PT without normalization (patients of Table **1**)

Groups	**R**	**L**	**L-R/L+R**
i) Area	**mm^2**	**mm^2**	
Controls	1216.9 ± 396.6	1182.6 ± 487.9	-0.034 ± 0.183
AD	1044.1 ± 240.5	1195.2 ± 274.8	+0.067 ± 0.117*
MID	962.0 ± 472.5	1084.4 ± 403.4	+0.082 ± 0.111*
MIX	1031.0 ± 333.6	1223.1 ± 430.1	+0.086 ± 0.102
SCHIZ	690.2 ± 335.1***+	719.1 ± 288.1**++	+0.034 ± 0.129
ANOVA:	p = 0.0161	p = 0.0297	p = 0.1523
ii) Cortical Height	**mm**	**mm**	
Controls	3.154 ± 0.372	3.030 ± 0.334	-0.019 ± 0.082
AD	2.875 ± 0.511	2.777 ± 0.364	-0.014 ± 0.077
MID	2.810 ± 0.533	2.943 ± 0.519	+0.024 ± 0.068
MIX	2.795 ± 0.364	2.404 ± 0.299***+	-0.075 ± 0.052
SCHIZ	2.622 ± 0.714*	2.545 ± 0.441**	-0.005 ± 0.107
ANOVA:	p = 0.1305	p = 0.0033	p = 0.1958

Table 1: contd….

iii) Volume	mm^3	mm^3	
Controls	3850.6 ± 1381.6	3591.8 ± 1530.7	-0.052 ± 0.209
AD	2979.9 ± 800.4*	3293.0 ± 763.2	+0.053 ± 0.130
MID	2854.4 ± 1884.7	3252.4 ± 1532.4	+0.105 ± 0.153*
MIX	2946.7 ± 1144.1	2993.7 ± 1195.6	+0.012 ± 0.085
SCHIZ	1676.0 ± 653.5 ***++	1801.8 ± 730.8 ***++	+0.029 ± 0.174
ANOVA:	p = 0.0023	p = 0.0118	p = 0.1792

ANOVA with repeated measures i) for area: groups - $F(4,55) = 3.44$, $p = 0.0141$, laterality – $F(1,55) = 5.31$, $p = 0.0250$, interaction – $F(4,55) = 1.30$, $p = 0.2820$, ii) for for cortical height: groups – $F(4,55) = 3.56$, $p = 0.0119$, laterality – $F(1,55) = 2.70$, $p = 0.1062$, interaction – $F(4,55) = 1.15$, $p = 0.3439$ and iii) for volume: groups – $F(4,55) = 4.92$, $p = 0.0018$, laterality – $F(1,55) = 0.76$, $p = 0.3871$, interaction – $F(4,55) = 0.87$, $p = 0.4865$; Student´s t-test was calculated with respect to controls (* $p< 0.05$, **$p < 0.01$, *** $p < 0.001$) or to patients with AD (+ $p< 0.05$, ++ $p < 0.01$).

Table 3: Characteristics of patients in which brain tissue of the areas of the PT were normalized to brain weight

Groups	n	Sex (M/F)	Age (years)	Brain Weight (g)	Cause of Death
Controls	9	4/5	76.1 ± 15.7	1103.3 ± 102.7	5xCI, 2xA, BP, H
AD	15	4/11	77.9 ± 7.9	1157.3 ± 178.7	12xCI, 3xBP
	24	8/16	ANOVA: p = 0.7178	ANOVA: p = 0.4189	

Sex: M – men, F – women; Causes of death: CI – cardiac insufficiencia, A – asphyxia, BP – bronchopneumonia, H – hepatocirrhosis.

DISCUSSION

New Volumetric Method

The SC substance, when in liquid phase, is capable of replicating the surface pattern of the PT, including fissures, twists and other irregularities, and after polymerization it creates an ideal rubber mask of the surface. Then, with a little skill, it is possible to flatten the whole imprint, or to separate the problematic parts that stick out with scissors. Then, the irregularities and nonlinear shape of the PT surface became easy to be evaluated, in contrast to more complicated methods of former *post-mortem* brain analyses [*e.g.*, 24]. We believe that SC could be potentially used for imprints of not only the PT area, but also of other cortical surface regions that are hard to measure. When histological analysis of the brain tissue is performed, both area and volumes can be evaluated.

When compared to highly expensive imaging techniques, further advantages of the method are as follows. In volumetry studies, delineation methodologies used in the imaging techniques (magnetic resonance, computer tomography) fit basically into the two categories. Firstly, there is manual delineation of structures of interest, based on direct recognition by investigator eye. The second approach is voxel-based volumetry. Delineation of structures of interest is done automatically by computer. Distinguishing mark is there grey scale of pixels (voxels) ranging from white to dark. There are many structures, where this grey scale gradient serves well, since these structures have more or less sharp anatomical boundaries with contrast white-dark pixel (voxel) transitions. Among these structures belongs *e.g.* the hippocampus. On the other hand, many cortical areas of the human brain are anatomically defined within context of neuronal cytoarchitecture (for example subdivisions of the medial frontal cortex or parietal cortex). When delineating these structures *via* imaging techniques, we have to approximate selected regions, often taking into the account well visible surrounding structures or areas. Our volumetric method can be a good substitute in the cases when imaging techniques have problems with exact delineation of rather cytoarchitectonically defined parts of brain cortex.

Although we did not observe marked alterations between our data without and with normalization to brain weight (Table **4**), we recommend using it to eliminate possible sex- or age-dependent differences. However, area or volume of the brain at the level of the *commissura anterius* could be used to normalization, too.

Table 4: The areas of the PT without normalization to brain weight when compared to the normalized (patients of Table **3**)

	i) Without Normalization			**ii) Normalized**	
Groups	**R** mm^2	**L** mm^2	**L-R/L+R**	**R** mm^2/g	**L** mm^2/g
Controls	936.9±106.5	873.4±226.0	-0.045±0.112	0.853±0.104	0.790±0.177
AD	952.6±225.8	1026.7±309.6	+0.030±0.157	0.827±0.170	0.901±0.296
ANOVA	p = 0.8473	p = 0.2108	p = 0.2284	p = 0.6778	p = 0.3232

ANOVA with repeated meaures: i) for areas without normalization: groups – $F(1,22) = 1.05$, $p = 0.3164$, laterality – $F(1,22) = 0.01$, $p = 0.9291$, interaction – $F(1,22) = 1.34$, $p = 0.2594$; ii) for normalized areas: groups – $F(1,22) = 0.34$, $p = 0.5665$, laterality – $F(1,22) = 0.01$, $p = 0.9186$, interaction – $F(1,22) = 1.70$, $p = 0.2062$.

CONTROLS

We have found the mild R/L asymmetries in area, cortical thickness and volume of the PT (*i.e.*, negative indexes of laterality on average, see Tables **2**, **4**, **5** and **6**) in the nondemented nonpsychotic controls. The results are not in a good accord with many data in literature reporting L/R asymmetry [*e.g.*, 6, 7], however, they can be supported by another studies [*e.g.*, 18]. Discrepancies can be associated *e.g.* with differences in PT delineation derived from various definitions of the PT borders. It results sometimes in incorporation of adjacent areas (*gyrus temporalis superior*, *posterior ascending ramus* and *posterior descending ramus*). Moreover, even if area delineation is comparable, there are still differences in morphological settings of the PT as obvious from naked eye observations of the PT and sometimes only approximation of PT borders is possible. And finally, we suppose that differences between R and L sides of the PT are too small on average to correctly evaluate laterality of healthy controls in relation to their low number in our study.

Although global statistical analysis did not support pronounced sex-dependent differences in the controls, borderline results of ANOVA with repeated measures and significant result of pair wise t-test did not exclude it (Table **5**). It seems that R area of the PT is bigger than L area in women which could be associated with enhanced reversal asymmetry in women when compared to men. The result is in a good accord in literature [16].

Table 5: The areas of the PT without normalization of all controls

Sex	n	R mm^2	L mm^2	L-R/L+R
M	15	1186.1 ± 391.4	1198.6 ± 483.2	-0.013 ± 0.177
F	10	1011.0 ± 252.3	880.4 ± 269.4*	-0.075 ± 0.126
	25	ANOVA: p = 0.2246	ANOVA: p = 0.0718	ANOVA: p = 0.3523

Sex: M – men, F – women; ANOVA with repeated measures: sex – $F(1,23) = 3.17$, $p = 0.0881$, laterality – $F(1,23) = 0.72$, $p = 0.4063$, interaction – $F(1,23) = 1.05$, $p = 0.3163$; Student´s t-test was calculated with respect to controls (*$p<0.05$).

DEMENTED GROUPS

We have observed generally shifts to L/R laterality in area, cortical height of volume of the PT in all demented groups, however, global statistical analysis supported it only in the case of AD (Tables **2** and **6**). A more detailed analysis of the PT area revealed the mild decrease in the R side but the mild increase in the L side in AD group when compared to the controls (Table **6**). As our experiments evaluating changes in PT cytoarchitecture are not yet terminated, we can only speculate about the reasons. Firstly, the R side of the PT could be more damaged by neurodegenerative processes in AD especially *via* atrophy. This finding is however in contradiction with works reporting a more pronounced damage of the dominant, *i.e.* L hemisphere, in the majority of cases [29]. Secondly, the L side of the PT could be more afflicted through processes of inflammation and gliosis leading among others to increased area and volume [46]. And finally, both sides of the PT could be impaired but antagonistic changes should occur in the R and L hemisphere. Histological analysis did not reveal marked laterality in the plaque densities in the hippocampal or cortical areas, nevertheless, the L hemisphere was impaired in a higher degree in same cases (data not shown).

Table 6: The areas of the PT without normalization of all controls and all patients with AD

Groups	**n Sex (M/F)**	**R mm^2**	**L mm^2**	**L-R/L+R**
Controls	25 15/10	1116.1 ± 347.7	1071.3 ± 434.4	-0.038 ± 0.158
AD	34 14/20	1003.7 ± 235.2	1120.9 ± 298.4	+0.051 ± 0.135*
	59 29/30	ANOVA: $p = 0.1440$	ANOVA: $p = 0.6055$	ANOVA: $p = 0.0246$

Sex: M – men, F – women; ANOVA with repeated measures: groups – $F(1,57) = 0.17$, $p = 0.6811$, laterality – $F(1,57) = 0.80$, $p = 0.3752$, interaction – $F(1,57) = 4.00$, $p = 0.0504$; Student´s t-test was calculated with respect to controls (*$p<0.05$).

SCHIZOPHRENIA

We have found the reduction in the PT area, cortical thickness and volume in patients with SCHIZ (Table **2**) in accordance with most previously published studies [9, 29, 49]. However, bilateral decreases were not followed by significant changes in laterality, in contrast to some studies [*e.g.*, 32-35]. Nevertheless, our results can be supported by the others [*e.g.*, 36].

Our most prominent findings in SCHIZ patients, *i.e.* the striking shape abnormalities of the PT on both sides were observed when compared to the controls or to patients with AD (the typical examples are shown in Fig. **1**). Sometimes the abnormalities were different in the L and R PT within one brain. Moreover, it was often extremely difficult to estimate borders of these PT areas by application of anatomical delineation mentioned above, since the superior part of the temporal lobe was of almost rectangular shape, often without Heschl´s gyri and/or visible transition to the Sylvian fissure. Therefore, a question arises whether estimation of the PT area in patients with SCHIZ can be reliable.

PT AS A MARKER OF HANDEDNESS

Although the left hemisphere is dominant for language in the majority of people (approximately 96% of R- and 73% of L-handers show L-hemisphere language localization), the dominant hemisphere or handedness should be determined to correctly evaluate brain laterality *e.g.* at biochemical level. In human *autoptic* tissue, the relevant information is often not accessible, data however suggest that volumetric asymmetry of the PT could be used as a possible marker since the degree of its laterality is higher in R- than in L-handers [for review, see 29].

We used our new method to evaluate laterality of mitochondrial enzyme 17β-hydroxysteroid dehydrogenase type 10 [47] or of nitric oxide mediator system [48] in the hippocampus of people with AD, MID and SCHIZ. However, no marked correlation was found on the controls. The negative result suggests that there is no simple relationship between *e.g.* asymmetry of endothelial nitric oxide synthase and handedness or more universally either between laterality at biochemical/volumetric level or between laterality of various brain regions. Nevertheless, it is important to point out that the number of our control samples was too small to reveal subtle links. On the other hand, the volumetric asymmetry of the PT sensitively reflected alterations due to pathological processes [47, 48].

CONCLUSIONS

Our new volumetric method using SC dental resin matter is relatively simple and cheap when compared to imaging techniques. It is also sufficiently precise but cannot be used in experiments *in vivo*. Besides confirming the alterations in the PT of SCHIZ patients previously described in the literature, our results demonstrate for the first time changes in laterality of the PT in demented patients, statistically significant especially in the AD group. Causes leading to these changes will be evaluated in our future research. Information about the degree of PT lateralization could be used as a supplementary source of data in situations where information concerning handedness is missing, such as in already dead subjects.

ACKNOWLEDGEMENTS

We would like to express gratitude for the excellent help of our laboratory technician Ludmila Horáková. The research was performed under the 260045/SVV/2014 grant of the Czech Republic, grant P 304/12/G069 from the Grant Agency of the Czech Republic and the Research Project Charles University in Prague, PRVOUK 34.

CONFLICT OF INTEREST

The authors confirm that this chapter content has no conflict of interest.

DISCLOSURE

This chapter is an update of our previous publication in CAR "Planum Temporale Analysis Via a New Volumetric Method in Autoptic Brains of Demented and Psychotic Patients" published in 'CAR', Volume 6, Number 1, February, pp. 69 to 76.

ABBREVIATIONS

AD = Clinically diagnosed dementia, number of senile plaques and tangles in given areas of the cortex and hippocampus higher than would be expected for age

L = Left

MID = Clinically diagnosed dementia, vascular changes, neuropathologic lesions and gliosis, number of senile plaques and tangles corresponding to normal aging

MIX = Clinically diagnosed dementia, changes due to the AD and MID simultaneously

PT = Planum temporale

R = Right

SC = Stomaflex creme (polysiloxane substance)

SCHIZ = Clinically diagnosed schizophrenia, number of senile plaques and tangles corresponding to normal aging

REFERENCES

[1] Pearlson GD. Superior temporal gyrus and planum temporale in schizophrenia: A selective review. Prog Neuro-Psychoph 21: 1203-1229 (1997).

[2] Mesulam MM. Behavioral neuroanatomy. Principles of Behavioral and Cognitive Neurology. Oxford University, New York, p. 1-120 (2000).

[3] Pfeifer RA. Mylogenetisch - anatomische untersuchungen uber das korticale ende untersuchungen end der heorleitung. Acad Wiss Berlin, p. 37 (1920).

[4] Pfeifer RA. In: 'Pathologie der Hoerstrahlung und der corticalen Hoesphare. Handbuch der Neurologie'. (Ed: Bumke O and Foerster O), Springer Verlag Berlin', p. 523-626 (1936).

[5] Von Economo C, Horn L. Uber windungsrelief mabe und Rindenarchitektonic der supratemporal flache, ihre individuellen und seitenunterschiede. Neuropsychiatrie 30: 678-757 (1930).

[6] Geschwind N, Lewitsky W. Human brain: left - right asymmetries in temporal speech regions. Science 161: 186-187 (1968).

[7] Galaburda AM, Corsiglia J, Rosen GD, Sherman GF. Planum temporale asymmetry, reappraisal since Geschwind and Levitsky. Neuropsychol 25: 853-868 (1987).

[8] Ihara A, Hirata M, Fujimaki N, Goto T, Umekawa Y, Fujita N, *et al.* Neuroimaging study on brain asymmetries in situs inversus totalis. J Neurol Sci 288: 72-78 (2010)

[9] Shapleske J, Rossell SL, Woodruff PWR, David AS. The planum temporale: a systematic, quantitative review of its structural, functional and clinical significance. Brain Res Rev 29: 26-49 (1999).

[10] Steinmetz H, Volkmann J, Jancke L, Freund HJ. Anatomical left-right asymmetry of language related temporal cortex is different in left handers and right handers. Ann Neurol 29: 315-319 (1991).

[11] Foundas AL, Leonard CM, Gilmore R, Fennell E, Heilman KM. Planum temporale asymmetry and language dominance. Neuropsychol 32: 1225-1231 (1994).

[12] Habib M, Robichon F. Neuroanatomical correlates of hemispheric specialization. Rev Neuropsychol 12: 87-127 (2002).

[13] Hopkins WD, Nira TM. Planum temporale surface area and grey matter asymmetries in chimpanzees (Pan troglodytes): The effect of handedness and comparison with findings in humans. Behav Brain Res 208: 436-443 (2010).

[14] Gilissen EP, Hopkins WD. Asymmetries of the parietal operculum in chimpanzees (Pan troglodytes) in relation to handedness for tool use. Cereb Cortex 23: 411-422 (2013).

[15] Hopkins WD, Pilger JF, Storzc R, Ambrosec A, Hofd PR, Sherwood CC. Planum temporale asymmetries correlate with corpus callosum axon fiber density in chimpanzees (Pan troglodytes) Behav Brain Res 234: 248-254 (2012).

[16] Wada J, Clarke R, Hamm A. Cerebral hemispheric asymmetry in humans. Cortical speech zones in 100 adult and 100 infant brains. Arch Neurol 32: 239-246 (1975).

[17] Witelson SF, Kigar DL. Sylvian fissure morphology and asymmetry in men and woman - bilateral differences in relation to handedness in men. J Comp Neurol 323: 326-340 (1992).

[18] Bilder RM, Wu H, Bogerts B, Degreef G, Ashtari M, Alvir JM, *et al.* Absence of regional hemispheric volume asymmetries in first - episode schizophrenia. Am J Psychiatry 151: 1437-1447 (1994).

[19] Tzourio-Mazoyer N, Simon G, Crivello F, Jobard G, Zago L, Perchey G, *et al.* Effect of familial sinistrality on planum temporale surface and brain tissue asymmetries. Cereb Cortex 20: 1476-1485 (2010).

[20] Binder JR, Frost JA, Hammeke TA, Rao SM, Cox RW. Function of the left planum temporale in auditory and linguistic processing. Brain 119: 1239-1247 (1996).

[21] Binder JR. Neuroanatomy of language processing studied with functional magnetic resonance. Clin Neurosci 4: 87-94 (1997).

[22] Johnsrude IS, Paus T, Zatorre RJ, Perry DW, Ward GP, Evans AC. The location of auditory activation foci relative to Heschl's gyri. Neuroimage 5: 177-201 (1997).

[23] Isenberg AL, Vaden KI Jr., Saberi K, Muftuler LT, Hickok G. Functionally distinct regions for spatial processing and sensory motor integration in the planum temporale. Hum Brain Mapp 33: 2453-2463 (2012).

[24] Praamstra P, Hagoort P, Maassen B, Crul T. Word deafness and auditory cortical function - A case history and hypothesis. Brain 114: 1197-1225 (1991).

[25] Caplan D, Gow D, Makris N. Analysis of lesions by MRI in stroke patients with acoustic - phonetic processing deficits. Neurology 45: 293-298 (1995).

[26] Alsop DC, Detre JA, D'Esposito M, Howard RS, Maldjian JA, Grossman M, *et al.* Functional activation during an auditory comprehension task in patients with temporal lobe lesions. Neuroimage 4: 55-59 (1996).

[27] Visser PJ, Verhey FRJ, Hofman PAM, Scheltens P, Jolles J. Medial temporal lobe atrophy predicts Alzheimer's disease in patients with minor cognitive impairment. J Neurol Neurosur Ps 72: 491-497 (2002).

[28] Thompson PM, Mega MS, Woods RP, Zoumalan CI, Lindshield CJ, Blanton RE, *et al.* Cortical change in Alzheimer's disease detected with a disease-specific population-based brain atlas. Cereb Cortex 11: 1-16 (2001).

[29] Toga AW, Thompson PM. Mapping Brain Asymmetry. Nat Rev Neurosci 4: 37-48 (2003).

[30] Harasty JA, Halliday GM, Kril JJ, Code C. Specific temporoparietal gyral atrophy reflects the pattern of language dissolution in Alzheimer's disease. Brain 122: 675-86 (1999).

[31] Chance SA, Clover L, Cousijn H, Currah L, Pettingill R, Esiri MM. Microanatomical correlates of cognitive ability and decline: normal ageing, MCI, and Alzheimer's disease. Cereb Cortex 21: 1870-1878 (2011).

[32] Steen RG, Mull C, McClure R, Lieberman JA. Brain volume in first-episode schizophrenia - systematic review and meta-analysis of magnetic resonance imaging studies. Brit J Psychiat 188: 510-518 (2006).

[33] Hirayasu Y, McCarley RW, Salisbury DF, Tanaka S, Kwon JS, Frumin M, *et al.* Planum temporale and Heschl gyrus volume reduction in schizophrenia - A magnetic resonance imaging study of first- episode patients. Arch Gen Psychiat 57: 692-699 (2000).

[34] Falkai P, Bogerts B, Schneider T, Greve B, Pfeiffer U, Pilz K, *et al.* Disturbed planum temporale asymmetry in schizophrenia. A quantitative post-mortem study. Schizophr Res 14: 161-176 (1995).

[35] Petty RG, Barta PE, Pearlson GD, McGilchrist IK, Lewis RW, Tien AY, *et al.* Reversal of asymmetry of the planum temporale in schizophrenia. Am J Psychiat 152: 715-721 (1995).

[36] Sommer I, Ramsey N, Kahn R, Aleman A, Bouma A. Handedness, language lateralization and anatomical asymmetry in schizophrenia: Meta-analysis. Brit J Psychiat 178: 344-351 (2001).

[37] Kawasaki Y, Suzuki M, Takahashi T, Nohara S, McGuire PK, Seto H, Kurachi M. Anomalous cerebral asymmetry in patients with schizophrenia demonstrated by voxel-based morphometry. Biol Psychiat 15: 793-800 (2008).

[38] Mosnik DM, Tranel AP, Oleary DS, Andreasen NC. Left-hemisphere language dominance in schizophrenic-patients and normal controls - a study of anatomical and functional asymmetries. Schizophr Res 15: 30-31 (1995).

[39] Smiley JF, Rosoklija G, Mancevski B, Pergolizzi D, Figarsky K, Bleiwas C, *et al.* Hemispheric comparisons of neuron density in the planum temporale of schizophrenia and nonpsychiatric brains. Psych Res 192: 1-11 (2011).

[40] Smiley JF, Rosoklija G, Mancevski B, Mann JJ, Dwork AJ, Javitt DC. Altered volume and hemispheric asymmetry of the superficial cortical layers in the schizophrenia planum temporale. Eur J Neurosci 30: 449-463 (2009).

[41] Takahashi T, Wood SJ, Yung AR, Walterfang M, Phillips LJ, Soulsby B, *et al.* Superior temporal gyrus volume in antipsychotic-naive people at risk of psychosis. Br J Psychiatry 196: 206-211 (2010).

[42] Oertel V, Knöchel C, Rotarska-Jagiela A, Schönmeyer R, Lindner M, van de Ven V, *et al.* Reduced laterality as a trait marker of schizophrenia—evidence from structural and functional neuroimaging. J Neurosci 30: 2289 -2299 (2010).

[43] Zach P, Kristofikova Z, Majer E, Selinger P. Alterations in the planum temporale in patients with Alzheimer disease estimated *via* a new volumetric method. In 'New Trends in Alzheimer and Parkinson Related Disorders' (Eds: Fisher A, Hanin I, Memo M, Stocchi F), Medimond, Bologna, p. 171-176 (2005).

[44] Mirra SS, Heyman A, McKeel D, Sumi SM, Crain BJ, Brownlee LM, *et al.* The consortium to establish a registry for Alzheimer´s disease (CERAD). 2. standardization of the neuropathologic assessment of Alzheimer´s disease. Neurology 4: 479-486 (1991).

[45] Dixon WJ. BMDP Statistical Software Manual. University of California Press, Berkeley, p. 1-220 (1990).

[46] Miller DH. Biomarkers and surrogate outcomes in neurodegenerative disease: Lessons from multiple sclerosis. NeuroRx 1: 284-294 (2004).
[47] Hovorkova P, Kristofikova Z, Horinek A, Ripova D, Majer E, Zach P, *et al*. Lateralization of 17beta-hydroxysteroid dehydrogenase type 10 in hippocampi of demented and psychotic patients. Dement Geriatr Cogn Disord 26: 193-198 (2008).
[48] Kristofikova Z, Kozmikova I, Hovorkova P, Ricny J, Zach P, Majer E, *et al*. Lateralization of hippocampal nitric oxide mediator system in people with Alzheimer disease, multi-infarct dementia and schizophrenia. Neurochem Int 53: 118-125 (2008).
[49] Vita A, de Peri L, Deste G, Sacchetti E. Progressive loss of cortical gray matter in chizophrenia: a meta-analysis and meta-regression of longitudinal MRI studies. Transl Psychiatry 2: e190 (2012).

CHAPTER 15

Experience and Perspectives of Caregivers of Spouses with Mild Cognitive Impairment

Yueh-Feng Y. Lu[1,*] and Joan E. Haase[2]

[1]Adult Health Nursing, Indiana University School of Nursing, 1111 Middle Drive, NUW407, Indiana University School of Nursing, Indianapolis, IN 46202, USA and [2]Emily Holmquist Professorship in Pediatric Oncology Nursing, Indiana University School of Nursing, Indianapolis, 1111 Middle Drive, NUE421, Indiana University School of Nursing, Indianapolis, IN 46202, USA

Abstract: Purpose: To describe commonalities of the lived experience of being a spouse caregiver of a person with mild cognitive impairment (MCI).

Design and Methods: The Colaizzi method of empirical phenomenology was used for interviewing and analyzing data obtained from 10 spouse caregivers of persons with MCI.

Results: Four major themes were found and labeled: (a) Putting the Puzzle Pieces Together-There Really is Something Wrong; (b) A Downward Spiral into a World of Silence; (c) Consequences to Caregivers of Living in a World of Silence; (d) Taking Charge of Care.

Implications: The findings of this study provided data rich in implications for interventions to help caregivers to gain awareness, information, and skills to more effectively deal with and adjust to the caregiving of their spouse with MCI over the long-term.

Keywords: Caregiver perspectives, caregiving issues, mild cognitive impairment, stress and coping.

INTRODUCTION

Most family caregiver studies have focused on family caregivers of persons with

***Corresponding author Yueh-Feng Y. Lu:** Indiana University School of Nursing, NU W407, 1111 Middle Drive, Indianapolis, IN 46202-5107, USA; Tel: 317-278-2042; E-mail: yuelu@iupui.edu

D.K. Lahiri (Ed)

Alzheimer Disease (AD), but few studies have discussed family caregivers' lived experience with their loved one with mild cognitive impairment (MCI). The transitional phase between healthy cognitive aging and dementia has been specified as MCI and has received much attention in recent years. MCI is a syndrome recognized as a cognitive decline greater than expected for an individual's age and educational level that interferes with functioning performance, but without other symptoms that would warrant a diagnosis of AD [1, 2].

Mild cognitive impairment now is considered to be the predementia stage of AD. Almost 20% of American older adults experience MCI and the conversion rate to AD for MCI patients is significantly higher than for healthy older adults (12% per year *vs.* 1-6%) [3-6]. MCI is associated with significant morbidity; potential economic loss to the individual, family, and society; and frustration and distress in caregivers [7-9]. Many studies have found that MCI adversely affects the patient's cognitive, emotional, and behavioral functioning [8, 10, 11]. When married individuals develop MCI, they and their spouse caregivers must cope with uncertainty in dealing with symptoms, diagnosis, prognosis, the relationship with each other and with others in family, and the necessity of making future plans [7, 9]. Depressive symptoms are common in elderly persons with MCI [12, 13] and although some persons with MCI may not progress to AD, MCI can still result in a heavy personal burden that may have an effect on family caregivers, particularly spouse caregivers [7-9, 11]. Spouse caregivers of persons with MCI are at the beginning stage of experiencing caregiver burden and lower quality in the marital relationship that could put them at risk of developing depression [8, 14]. Recent studies found that the prevalence of depressed mood among informal caregivers was 24.6% (95% confidence interval, 21.5-27.7) [15]. Understanding family caregivers' lived experience with those persons who are at an increased risk of developing dementia is an important area in order to develop early and effective interventions. With a rapidly aging population, an increasing number of persons suffering from AD, and a shrinking caregiving cohort, suggests a critical need for interventions targeted at the beginning stage of MCI and at caregivers. At this early stage of cognitive decline, patients and their caregivers may have a critical window to develop important self-management skills that may prevent premature disability and disengagement. Developing self-management skills may improve the quality of life for both MCI patients and their family caregivers, thereby saving billions of dollars for our society [16, 17].

Over several decades many studies have extensively examined AD family caregiver burden and caregivers' experience of living with a spouse with AD [18, 19], but few have described the experience of family caregivers of persons being diagnosed and living with MCI from the perspective of the spouse caregiver. Understanding the process of caregiving for spouse family caregivers will be an important guide for future intervention. This report was part of a larger study that focused on family caregivers of persons with MCI by describing and analyzing their needs, concerns, decision-making process, self-management skills, relationships, and other factors that might influence their quality of life. In this paper we focus on the caregivers' experience of living with a spouse with MCI and describe, from an empirical phenomenological perspective, the commonalities of the experience of living with a spouse diagnosed with MCI. The results of this study may be useful to guide health care providers in creating supportive care interventions for caregivers and their spouses with MCI.

DESIGN AND METHODS

The design of this portion of the larger study was based on empirical phenomenology conducted through interviews with 11 spouse caregivers of persons with MCI. Empirical phenomenology is useful to describe the commonality of a phenomenon across experiences, in this case caregivers' experiences. This commonality is referred to as the essential structure of the experience, whereby the key factors common across caregivers are elucidated [20].

Sampling Methods

The purposive sample of 11 spouse caregivers of persons with MCI was recruited through the Alzheimer Disease Center Clinic in Indiana. The in-depth nature of the phenomenological interview method lends itself well to small sample sizes [21]. To determine the sample size for this study, we used the criterion of redundancy, which is met when themes identified during the ongoing data analysis are repeated and no new themes emerge.

Caregivers were English-speaking adults, aged 20 or older, and who had identified themselves as the primary caregiver for their spouse who had a medical diagnosis of MCI for at least 12 months. The diagnosis of MCI was made on the basis of clinical examination by a geriatric neurologist and/or neuropsychologist, using criteria consistent with the guidelines established by Petersen and colleagues [22]. To be included in the study, each caregiver had to be willing and able to describe his or her experience of living with their spouse diagnosed with MCI.

Data Collection

Approval for this study was obtained from the Institutional Review Board at Indiana University and informed consent was obtained prior to each interview. Data were collected from caregivers of the spouse with MCI in private rooms at the caregiver's home or in the hospital clinic. The open-ended interviews lasted 45 - 90 minutes and were conducted by one of two doctoral researchers. Efforts were made to reduce distractions or interruptions during the interviews. Caregivers were clearly eager to tell their story and were interviewed until they felt they had provided a full description of their experience. Each interview started with a broad data-generating question provided to caregivers at least 7 days prior to the interview: "Please tell me about your experiences that led up to your spouse was diagnosed with mild cognitive impairment and your experiences since your spouse being diagnosed." After caregivers described their experiences, additional descriptive questions were asked to understand their concerns and needs related to living with their spouses with mild cognitive impairment. Examples of additional questions are: "What are the things that have helped you deal with your spouse's mild cognitive impairment?" and "Please tell me about your concerns of living with your spouse since the diagnosis of MCI."

Data Analysis and Interpretation

Each interview was audiotaped. After the audiotapes were professionally transcribed, the data were analyzed using a step-by-step procedure adapted from Colaizzi's phenomenological method [23]. First, familiarity with the experience as a whole was gained by listening to the taped interviews and reading transcriptions for accuracy. Second, significant statements were identified, restated, and formulated into meanings by the first author. Third, the formulated meanings were discussed in meetings with research team members until consensus was reached by the research team. Fourth, themes were extracted from the formulated meanings. Fifth, extracted themes were organized into a hierarchy of themes across all caregiver data. Sixth, theme clusters and categories were examined and adjusted until consensus was reached during meetings of the research team. Seventh, an exhaustive narrative description of the experience that incorporated all themes was developed. Finally, the essential structure of the experience was developed.

Several strategies were used to ensure the validity, value, and credibility of the results. Prior to data collection, the interviewers conducted practice interviews and received peer critique to ensure a consistent approach to the interview process. Data analysis and validation were done as a team. For example, theme categories were derived separately by members of the research team then compared. The few discrepancies were discussed until 100% agreement was achieved.

FINDINGS

Sample

Of the 11 spouse caregivers of persons with MCI, interview data from only 10 (5 male and 5 female) were included in the data analysis, because we found that one female family caregiver's responses to the interview questions were frequently unrelated to questions asked and we could not discern any context to meaningfully tie her comments to focus of our study. The age of the 10 participants ranged from 47 to 87 (mean 72, SD = 11.22) years and the time since spouse's diagnosis ranged from 1.5 to 4.5 years (mean = 2.5, SD = 0.8). All caregivers were Caucasian and married, with four in their second marriage. Seven had some college or higher education. All caregivers had a history of employment, with one still working in a full-time position, five working in part-time positions, and four retired. Most caregivers reported having some savings and having no financial burden. Two caregivers lived in retirement communities and 8 lived in their own house. Most of the caregivers (n = 8) reported that their household income was just enough to meet their monthly needs or having some money left over, but two reported that they were not making enough money to meet their monthly needs.

Results

A total of 1618 significant statements about the experience of living with a spouse diagnosed with MCI were extracted from the data and analyzed. Table **1** shows the resulting four major theme categories and corresponding theme clusters. Each caregiver described the spouse's memory loss as a gradual and slow process with the following themes: (a) Putting the Puzzle Pieces Together- There Really is Something Wrong; (b) A Downward Spiral into a World of Silence; (c) Consequences of living in a World of Silence and Loss; (d) Taking Charge of Care.

The following is a detailed description of the themes related to each category. Pseudonyms are used throughout the results section.

Table 1: The Lived Experience of having a Spouse with MCI

Major Theme	Cluster Cluster
Putting the puzzle pieces together: There really is something wrong	a. Short-term memory declining b. Difficulty in engaging in some familiar tasks c. Behavioral changes d. Emotional changes e. Changes in social activity engagement
A downward spiral into a world of silence	a. Best friend is gone b. My world is shrinking c. Rollercoaster distress
Consequences to caregivers of living in a world of silence	a. Taking on increasing obligation b. Decision-making challenge c. High cost to quality of life
Taking charge of care	a. Knowing major needs and concerns b. Finding care strategies

PUTTING THE PUZZLE PIECES TOGETHER: THERE REALLY IS SOMETHING WRONG

Through a process of "putting the puzzle pieces together", caregivers gradually became aware that their spouse's cognitive impairment was long lasting and progressive. Susan: "Well, it is not something that came on all of a sudden. I mean it's just kind of a slowly developing process." As caregivers puzzled over the reality of memory problems, they eventually sought outside confirmation by seeking medical assessment. Beth: "I knew he was having memory problems years ago… For a long time I thought it was work and stress… I could see something was not quite right and it got down to where I eventually said, "John, maybe you should get tested." Through this gradual awareness process they eventually came to the conclusion that there really was something wrong.

Categories associated with this process of "Putting the Puzzle Pieces Together'' included short-term memory decline, difficulty in engaging in familiar tasks, behavioral changes, emotional changes, and changes in social activity engagement. Short-term memory decline was one of the early signs of mild cognitive impairment. Beth: "He couldn't remember the things we just talked about 30 minutes ago." Patients' struggles to remember dates, individuals' name, or appointments were commonly reported by caregivers. Caregivers realized that their spouses were having difficulty in engaging in previously familiar tasks such as putting household items away, changing light bulbs, preparing dinner, or using "the to-do list" as usual. Joyce: "He realized that he couldn't do things that he easily had done before. Simple things like…[handyman activities] and then all at once he couldn't figure out how to do those anymore. It was very frustrating to him." As caregivers realized that their spouses were having difficulty in performing activities as usual, they gradually began to take over tasks and responsibilities. Beth: "He used to cook… I have him do the dishes. It's hard for him to figure out where they… I'll just have to tell him where they go. Just leave them out and I'll put them away." It often took caregivers awhile to realize their spouse's financial management capabilities had lessened. David: "She sent several checks to unknown companies… she was cheated by some bad persons several times."

Caregivers also described their spouses' changes in behavior, emotional responses, and social activity engagement. Repeatedly asking questions was a common behavioral change. Joyce: "… he was forgetting more than what I thought was normal… Repeating things a lot, telling you the same things several times a day and there was some depression over this."

Emotional changes commonly found by caregivers included their spouses getting easily upset or angry and feeling irritable, worried, or sad as a consequence of having difficulty in remembering or doing what used to be familiar tasks. Joyce: "He has become a bit more childish. Sometimes when he really can't do things that he used to do before, he gets angry. And the anger that comes out, now that is hard to deal with." Caregivers also realized that their spouse had difficulty in understanding the complex context or difficulty in following conversation while conversing with multiple parties and would then withdraw from social interaction. Joyce: "Sometimes it's embarrassing because when there are people around he recedes back to his office. He is not comfortable being around large groups … It is hard to carry on a conversation for him because people talk about politics, they talk about the war, they talk about everything and he doesn't retain what he has heard.''

A DOWNWARD SPIRAL INTO A WORLD OF SILENCE

Caregivers experienced their own downward spiral into a world of silence as they put the pieces of the puzzle together. They described that their world was lost without any obvious warning signs. The characteristics of their loss were like a spiral in that the patients' days of what seemed like normal aging increasingly became more markedly signs of MCI. Beth: "I didn't know it was going on either. I was thinking that maybe he just doesn't do that for me anymore or I don't know. It was hard for me to detect that at the beginning." Categories associated with this process of a downward spiral into a world of silence included (a) My Best Friend is Gone, (b) My World is Shrinking, and (c) Rollercoaster Distress.

<u>Best friend is gone</u>. As memory worsened, caregivers experienced unwanted and uncontrollable changes in both the intimate and functional aspects of their relationship with the patients. Beth: "My best friend [husband] has been gone. He is part of me, but he is no longer the same person… He knows me better than anybody. I just don't want to lose him … I really miss him."

The caregiver/patient dyads in the study had been married over 40 years and traditional roles were the norm. For wives, their husbands were most often the key decision maker. As the husbands' executive functions declined, spouse caregivers had to take on decision-making roles for a wide range of issues. Phyllis: "…taking over someone's life, making decisions for them, not telling them the whole truth every time, that was a terrible thing for me.''

Caregivers also experienced less effective communication and increasing misunderstanding and conflict with their spouse that was associated with the progression of memory problems and the spouse adjusting to the need for supervision. David: "She has that feeling that I'm against her and I'm not… The other day I said something to her about "Would you want me to help you with your meds?" "No! You've taken enough stuff away from me already."

My world is shrinking. Caregivers also experienced a shrinking world, including shrinking spaces, activities, finances, and social relationships. The aspects of the caregivers' world that were shrinking included moving to more manageable housing, shifting to communities that were unfamiliar, compacting life routine, dwindling financial resources, and devastating relationship changes. Caregivers' concerns for a manageable living space, and safe environment, as well as financial pressures, led them to reluctantly and often prematurely begin the process of selling their own home or business and moving into a smaller house, condo, or retirement community. Beth: "So we sold our business and in September we moved out of the house because it was too big. It was too much of a financial burden." Although most participants carefully selected and planned for relocation, the process of adjustment to a new environment/community was challenging and stressful.

Daily life routines were shrinking as the spouse's condition resulted in decreased engagement in volunteer activities, leisure activities, and/or personal hobbies. Finances also often were shrinking because of patients' MCI-related early retirement or the need to meet the demands of caregiving. Beth: "Since this came on his memory, we had to get rid of our business. My husband was the owner of a business."

Caregivers also experienced shrinking social relationships with extended family members and friends. Beth: "Most people when they find out about this, they don't know how to ask about it. They don't understand he has memory problem… they don't realize how difficult it is."

Rollercoaster distress. As caregivers became more aware of their spouse's condition, they intermittently experienced unpredictable periods of heightened emotional distress as they observed the consequences of their spouse's functional decline. The range of distressful emotions was linked to the situations and included shock, anger, guilt, anxiety, frustration, sadness, loneliness, helplessness, worry, and uncertainty. Beth: "I felt guilty and overwhelmed and I felt frustrated, people didn't understand". For example, caregivers described extreme frustration and anger when finding that someone was taking advantage of their spouse; they felt sad when seeing their loved one unable to do familiar tasks. Joyce: "It hurts (crying). I watch him try to do the simplest thing… And it is hard. It is hard to watch him, but there is nothing you can do, really."

Caregivers reached a tipping point in their ability to cope with the level of stress related to caregiving. Phyllis: "I've run out of the ability to cope and that's where I am right now." Caregivers also experienced emotional distress and frustration with family members and other significant friends who could not understand the situation. "Why can't you still do this? He looks fine!" In the midst of distress, caregivers looked for and held on to anything positive in the situation. David: "The diagnosis at that time was mild cognitive impairment, which it still is. A huge relief because still today there are many times that I ask myself (Am I just imagining this?)".

CONSEQUENCES TO CAREGIVERS OF LIVING IN A WORLD OF SILENCE

Caregivers experienced the consequences of living in a world of silence brought on by their spouse's memory loss. These included (a) Taking on Increased Obligations, (b) Decision-Making Challenge, and (c) High Cost to Quality of Life.

Taking on increasing obligations. As caregivers worked through the realization that the patient had gradually declined in cognitive and functional ability, they gradually took on more obligations to help the patients continue to be able to function for as long as possible. Joyce: "[providing care] is not something that I can't do for him. I want to take care of him as long as I can--and no matter what."

Caregivers increasingly provided more detailed help to enable the patient to remain engaged in daily activities. Beth: "If I tell him or give him directions, he's fine. But left alone it's like he's floundering. He doesn't know what to do next. It was that way in the beginning, [I'd say] 'call me with questions' and he'd call me back with another question and I knew that was another thing that I thought [he would need help with]."

Decision-making challenges. Stepping in to make multiple decisions for the patient was challenging for caregivers, especially financial and legal decisions, when these were usually previously done by the patient. Phyllis: "... I did all the legal work, all the financial work, everything. I did it all. And so when I get discouraged sometimes I think you know the answer to the question why am I the person who has to do this. The answer to that question is because I see what's happening and I'm capable of doing it. It's not easy. I don't want to do it but something has to be done."

High cost to quality of life. Even at the stage of mild impairment, caregivers experienced a high cost to the quality of their life, including the quality of both married and personal life. Phyllis: "So it was very costly. It was costly to my marriage; it was costly personally to me because it made me feel lonely."

TAKING CHARGE OF CARE

Caregivers gradually began to take charge as part of their long journey of caregiving. During this journey, they gradually identified their major needs and concerns and found the care strategies that worked best for them and their spouse.

Knowing major concerns and needs. Caregivers' major concerns and needs included (a) information related to MCI (b) establishing effective communication skills, (c) developing caregiving skills, and (d) managing emotional distress for their spouse and for themselves.

Most caregivers reported that one of their major needs and concerns was searching for current information regarding the meaning of neuropsychological tests results at the diagnosis of MCI, especially related to prognosis. They also needed current information on pharmacological and non-pharmacological treatments. They expected the information to be provided by their health care providers. They also stated that being understood by the health providers was very important for them. Chris: "…it is really important to me to be able to talk, to understand, and listen [to health care providers]." They also had financial concerns associated with their spouse's increasing inability to manage finances, the costly new medications prescribed for their spouse, and the need to adjust their work situation to assure their spouse's safety in all settings.

They also had concerns and needs regarding establishing effective communication skills. These concerns were centered on the need to minimize misunderstanding and to retain or regain a trusting relationship. Beth: "At first he thought I was treating him like a little kid and so we had our battles. I'm just trying to help you… He knows that helps him and he doesn't take offense with me anymore." Caregivers experienced concerns about communicating using "white lies" because of the conflict between inner values and reality. Phyllis: "I did the preparation for our income taxes and sent them to our accountant because I would rather have him be angry with me for an hour about doing that than have him anxious and agitated for a week while he is trying to put those figures together unsuccessfully. So I have changed my definition of what is ethical behavior and I trust God understands that, … I can't tell him everything I've done and everything I'm going to do every time, every day. I can't do it. I just don't have the energy to do it or to cope with the results of it."

Caregivers also had a litany of caregiving skills they need to develop. These skills included: 1) managing their spouse's emotional distress. Joyce: "I think the hardest part for me is… I don't want to ever make him feel like he is less of a person, or I don't want to degrade him or embarrass him"; 2) assessing performance capacity, dealing with driving safety issues; 3) strategies to assure that their spouse was not being cheated when handling money. Matthew: "I really dread the day when she won't be able to have her checkbook…when she won't be able to drive… because I know how she's going to react and she's going to be very bitter, very bitter"; 4) making long-term care plans, Phyllis: "I've had a lot of family experience with dementia…I made the decision about when they needed to be in in-care."; 5) keeping their spouse involved with usual life routine activities, Beth: "He doesn't know what to do for the whole day and needs someone to guide him. My concern is how I'm going to keep him busy…"; and, 6) dealing with their spouse's behavior (*e.g.*, repeating questions, sleeping problem, misplacing items).

Finding care strategies. All caregivers gradually found new strategies to cope with their spouse's functional deficits. These included: building a reminder system (*e.g.*, using to-do lists, calendars with large print, listing important contact phone numbers in visible places), engaging in some pleasurable activities together (*e.g.*, attending Sunday service, eating out with good old friends), giving adequate time for their spouse to communicate, having a pet (dog) as company, moving into a retirement condo to allow more time to focus on their spouse, minimizing financial cheating by controlling unwanted mail, and being mindful of ways to manage their own emotional distress and health needs.

Most caregivers also recognized their stress was associated with patients' emotional distress and behavior problems (*e.g.*, repeating questions, misplaced items, withdrawing from significant social events and others). Gradually, they developed new coping strategies in dealing with these stressors. Phyllis: "…I'm learning how on a daily basis to say I know what I need to do today. If I get to the end of the day and I need to, I go to a movie or just go to the grocery store and look at greeting cards…" Even when relocation was not a caregiver's preferred action, he or she began to realize and appreciate the good results from the relocation. Susan: "Since we moved here I don't have the responsibility of doing the outdoor work…I just feel sort of free…I feel very comfortable…"

ESSENTIAL STRUCTURE OF LIVING EXPERIENCE WITH SPOUSE WITH MILD COGNITIVE IMPAIRMENT

The essential structure of the experience of being a spouse caregiver of a person with mild cognitive impairment (MCI) began as a long process of trying to put the puzzle pieces together to get a picture of the spouse's progression of memory impairment. As part of the process, caregivers became aware of their spouse's memory decline through the declines in their spouse's abilities, behavioral and emotional changes, and social interactions. This awareness and the actual multiple changes in the patient and the responses of others led caregivers to a downward spiral into a world of silence. That world was characterized as shrinking and accompanied by great waves of distress, loneliness, lost relationships, and diminished interactions. As consequences of living in a world of silence, caregivers took on increasing obligations, were challenged to make many decisions alone, and paid for these choices in diminished quality of life for themselves. Gradually, they made their way through this world to begin to take charge of what they could, gaining knowledge about each concern and identifying specific strategies to address them.

DISCUSSION

An examination of each of the major theme categories and comparison of the findings with existing literature is presented in the discussion section. The limitations of this study and clinical implications for practice are also presented.

Putting the Puzzle Pieces Together

Becoming aware of the spouse's mild memory problem and putting the puzzle pieces together was a lengthy and confusing process. Even though caregivers had previous in-depth understanding of their spouse, they initially lacked awareness and knowledge of what was happening to their spouse. All caregivers experienced difficulty in sorting out the differences between the signs of memory decline, normal aging, and working stress. Findings from our study of caregivers of MCI patients are similar to the pattern of becoming aware of the memory problem that was in the literature for AD caregivers at the early stage [7, 19]. The literature indicates that caregivers try to define and sort out their spouse's unusual behaviors, research the conclusion that their spouse's behaviors are not normal and are problematic, and figure out what to do next. The specific troublesome behaviors in our study are similar to those found in a recent study that described caregivers' concerns that patients were "asking the same questions over and over again", "losing or misplacing things", and had "trouble remembering recent things" [8], as well as "getting angry easily" and "were less engaged in social activities than usual."

A Downward Spiral into a World of Silence

Even at this earliest stage of MCI, the caregivers experienced behavioral stressors similar to those in the literature. This indicates that there is a variety of behaviors exhibited as part of MCI impairment that are both frequently occurring and distressing to spousal caregivers [8, 14]. Still at this stage of cognitive impairment, caregivers gradually experienced loss of intimacy in their relationship, loss of communication with spouse, loss of the hoped-for future, and loss of social and recreational interactions. These losses are similar to those found in caregiving studies of those persons in the advanced stage of cognitive impairment [24-26]. Caregivers in this study experienced similar emotional responses to patients' behaviors as did caregivers of patients with dementia, and these responses were robust predictors of distress outcomes for family caregivers [7, 14, 27]. Our study found that caregivers experienced a wide range of distressful emotions such as shock, anger, guilt, anxiety, frustration, sadness, loneliness, helplessness, and uncertainty that were associated with spouses' symptoms of cognitive impairment, behavior changes, and functional deficits that were similar to those of caregivers of patients with AD [28, 29]. However, they also felt relieved that their spouse was not diagnosed with AD and that the deterioration in signs and symptoms of cognitive impairment would only gradually occur over several years [7, 14, 30].

Consequences to Caregivers of Living in a World of Silence

Similar to previous studies, our findings showed that caregivers first realized the changes in their spouse's behaviors and performance capability, then followed with a reflection on the changes that had occurred [7, 31]. The caregivers gradually recognized their quality of life was significantly affected by their spouse's cognitive impairment, but at the same time, they gradually began to take on roles and activities that were usually performed by their spouse as they experienced an increased sense of obligation to take care of their spouse. Most of the caregivers met the challenges in making decisions for the patients. Some decision-making required new knowledge and skills, or professional assistance, such as selling property (house or husband's company), relocating to retirement housing, filing taxes, and selecting treatment.

Taking Charge of Care

Previous studies also support our findings that caregivers need information regarding the diagnosis and treatment of MCI. These studies indicate that brief information and support-oriented therapies are associated with modest reductions in caregiver emotional distress [28, 32, 33]. Therefore, providing brief information and early support-oriented therapies for caregivers and patients at the early stages of MCI may minimize later emotional distress.

Some recent caregiving intervention studies found that caregiving skill-building treatment interventions were more effective than standard care in reducing caregiver distress in dealing with the care receiver's agitated symptoms over time, but were equally effective to standard care in improving caregiver management skills over time [34, 35]. Since MCI patients are more aware of their own deficits and experience fewer specific troublesome behaviors than AD patients, providing early intervention on caregiving knowledge and skill-building may help build caregiving confidence to prevent or minimize patients' problem behaviors and obtain better outcomes with less cost over time.

Compared to previous studies in caring for persons with dementia [36], the caregivers of this study reported fewer and less multifaceted safety concerns than AD caregivers. With the need to focus on fewer concerns, interventions to improve safety may be more easily implemented and learned by caregivers in the early stages of MCI, when the issues are less complex. In the literature, there are no reliable measures of driving capability and little is known about how to manage driving cessation for MCI patients. Previous studies reported that the driving issues most difficult to manage were AD patients who were not aware of the need to make changes [37]. Since MCI patients are more aware of their decision, it might be an optimum opportunity for caregivers and patients to make balanced and mutually agreed-upon decisions relative to driving that are based on patients' strengths and limitations at this stage of cognitive impairment. They might also discuss future scenarios when driving would not be safe and this could make it easier for the caregiver to have the resolve to tell the patient to stop driving when that time comes.

STRENGTHS, LIMITATIONS, AND IMPLICATIONS

The strengths of this study include a nearly equal gender representation of spouse caregivers and the fact that the participants were living independently in various settings such as their own home or a retirement community. Limitations in this study are a lack of diversity in socioeconomic status and ethnicity and a lack of a longitudinal perspective on patients' progress. Future studies should include more minority subjects from varied socioeconomic status and multiple interview time points along the various stages of caregiving memory loss progresses. Our study showed that there is a critical need to develop an early intervention that can help MCI patient-caregiver dyads modify behavior, compensate for deficits, and minimize negative outcomes from conflicts associated with those deficits. The perspectives provided by the caregivers in this study are rich in implications for finding interventions to help caregivers gain awareness, information, and learn skills to more effectively deal with and adjust to caring for their MCI spouse over time.

ACKNOWLEDGMENT

The authors thank all caregivers and their spouses with mild cognitive impairment who participated, as well as Dr. Martin R. Farlow and the research team of Indiana University Alzheimer Center Clinic Core that helped in recruitment process. Funding was provided by the National Institute of Aging, Indiana Alzheimer Disease Center, grant # P30AG10133, and the first author was supported through a National Research Service Award Institutional Research Training Grant, PHS T32 NR07066, National Institute of Nursing Research, and Indiana University School of Nursing.

CONFLICT OF INTEREST

The authors confirm that this chapter content has no conflict of interest.

DISCLOSURE

This chapter is an update of our previous publication in CAR "Experience and Perspectives of Caregivers of Spouse with Mild Cognitive Impairment" published in 'CAR', Volume 6, Number 4, August, pp. 384 to 391.

REFERENCES

[1] Alzheimer Association. Alzheimer's disease facts and figures. 2012 Alzheimer's Disease Facts and Figures [Internet]. 1-72 (2012).

[2] Ward A, Arrighi HM, Michels S, Cedarbaum JM. Mild cognitive impairment: Disparity of incidence and prevalence estimates. Alzheimer's & Dementia: J the Alzheimer's Association 8:14-21 (2012).

[3] Busse A, Bischkopf J, Riedel-Heller SG, Angermeyer MC. Subclassifications for mild cognitive impairment: prevalence and predictive validity. Psychol Med 33:1029-1038 (2013).

[4] Davatzikos C, Bhatt P, Shaw LM, Batmanghelich KN, Trojanowski JQ. Prediction of MCI to AD conversion, *via* MRI, CSF biomarkers, and pattern classification Neurobiol Aging 32:2322 e19-27 (2011).

[5] DeCarli C. Mild cognitive impairment: Prevalence, prognosis, etiology, and treatment. Lancet Neurol 2:15-21 (2003).

[6] Unverzagt FW, Gao S, Baiyewu O, Ogunniyi AO, Gureje O, Perkins A, *et al.* Prevalence of cognitive impairment: data from the Indianapolis Study of Health and Aging. Neurol 57:1655-1662 (2001).

[7] Blieszner R, Roberto KA. Care partner responses to the onset of mild cognitive impairment. Gerontolo 50:11-22 (2011).

[8] Garand L, Dew MA, Urda B, Lingler JH, DeKosky ST, Reynolds III CF. Marital quality in the context of mild cognitive impairment. Western J Nurs Res 29:976-992 (2007).

[9] Lu YYF, Haase JE, Farran CJ. Perspective of persons with mild cognitive impairment: Sense of being able. Alzheimer's Care Quarterly 8:45-86 (2007).

[10] Burton CL, Straussa E, Bunceb D, Huntera MA, Hultscha DF. Functional abilities in older adults with mild cognitive impairment. Gerontol 55:570-581 (2009).

[11] Frank L, Lloyd A, Flynn JA, Kleinman L, Matza LS, Margolis M, *et al.* Impact of cognitive impairment on mild dementia patients and mild cognitive impairment patients and their informants. Intern Psych 18:151-162 (2006).

[12] Apostolova LG, Cummings JL. Neuropsychiatric manifestations of mild cogntiive impairment: A systematic review of the literature. Dement Geriatr Cogn Disord. 25:115-116 (2008).

[13] Lopez OL, Jagust WJ, Dulberg C, Becker JT, DeKosky ST, Fitzpatrick A, *et al.* Risk factors for mild cognitive impairment in the cardiovascular health study. Arch Neurol 60:1394-1395 (2003).

[14] Garand L, Dew MA, Eazor LR, DeKosky ST, Reynolds CF, 3rd. Caregiving burden and psychiatric morbidity in spouses of persons with mild cognitive impairment. Intern J Geria Psych 20:512-22 (2005).

[15]. Lu Y-F, Austrom M, Perkins S, Bakas T, Farlow RM, He F, *et al.* Depressed mood in Informal Caregivers of Persons with Mild Cognitive Impairment. American J Alzheimer's Disease & Other Dement 22:273-285 (2007).

[16] Kinsella GJ, Mullaly E, Rand E, Ong B, Burton C, Price S, *et al.* Early intervention for mild cognitive impairment: A radomized clinical trial. J Neurolo Neurosurg & Psych 80:730-736 (2009).

[17] Ryan KA, Weldon A, Huby NM, Persad C, Bhaumik AK, Heidebrink JL, *et al.* Caregiver support service needs for patients with mild cognitive impairment and Alzheimer disease. Alzheimer Disease & Associated Disord 24:171-176 (2010).

[18] Chappell NL, Reid RC. Burden and well-being among caregivers: Examining the distinction. The Gerontol 42:772-780 (2002).

[19] Perry J. Wives giving care to husbands with Alzheimer's disease: A process of interpretive caring. Res in Nurs & Health 25: 307-316 (2002).

[20] Girogi A. The theory, practice and evaluation of the phenomenological methods as a qualitative research procedure. J Phenomenolo Psychol 28:235-260 (1997).

[21] Boss P, Dahl C, Kaplan L. The use of phenomenology for family therapy research. The search for meaning. Sprenkle DH, Moon SM, editors. New York: Guilford 83-105 (1996).

[22] Petersen RC, Parisi JE, Dickson DW, Johnson K, Knopman DS, Boeve BF, *et al.* Neuropathologic features of amnestic mild cognitive impairment. Arch Neurol 63:665-672 (2006).

[23] Colaizzi PF. Psychological research as the phenomenologist view it. (Eds) IRSVMK, editor. New York: Oxford University Press 48-71 (1978).

[24] Donaldson C, Tarrier N, Burns A. Determinants of caregivers stress in Alzheimer's disease. Intern J Geria Psychi 134:248-256 (1998).

[25]. Lawerence RH, Tennstedt SL, Assmann SF. Quality of caregiver. Care recipient relationship: Does it offset negative consequences of caregiving for family caregivers?. Psycholol Aging 13:150-158 (1998)

[26] Walker RJ, Pomeroy EC. Depression or gried? The experience of caregiver of people with dementia. Health Social Work 21:247-254 (1996).

[27] Beeson RA. Loneliness and depression in spousal caregivers of those with Alzheimer's disease *vs.* non-caregiving spouses. Arch Psychi Nurs 17:135-143 (2003).

[28] Schulz R, Beach SR, Cook TB, Martire LM, Tomlinson JM, Monin JK. Predictors and consequences of perceived lack of choice in becoming an informal caregiver. Aging Mental Health 16:712-721 (2012).

[29] Zarit SH, Femia EE. A future for family care and dementia intervention research? Aging and Mental Health 12:5-13 (2008).

[30] Clare L. Awareness in early-stage Alzheimer's disease: A review of methods and evidence. British J Clinil Psychol 43:177-196 (2004).

[31] Perry J, O'Connor D. Preserving personhood: (Re)membering the spouse with dementia. Family Relations 51:55-62 (2002).

[32] Mittelman MS, Roth DL, Haley WE, Zarit SH, Mittelman MS, Roth DL, *et al.* Effects of a caregiver intervention on negative caregiver appraisals of behavior problems in patients with Alzheimer's disease: results of a randomized trial. J Gerontolo Series B-Psycholo Sci & Social Sci 59: 27-34 (2004).

[33] Schulz R, Burgio L, Burns R, Eisdorfer C, Gallagher-Thompson D, Gitlin LN, *et al.* Resources for Enhancing Alzheimer's Caregiver Health (REACH): overview, site-specific outcomes, and future directions. Gerontolog 43:514-520 (2003).

[34] Farran CJ, Gilley DW, McCann JJ, Bienias JL, Lindeman DA, Evans DA. Efficacy of behavioral interventions for dementia caregivers. Western J Nurs Res 29:944-960 (2007).

[35] Farran CJ, Staffileno BA, Gilley DW, McCann JJ, Yan Li, Castro CM, *et al.* A lifestyle physical activity intervention for caregivers of persons with Alzheimer's disease. American J Alzheimer's Disease & Other Dement 23:132-142 (2008).

[36] Jean L, Bergeron M, Thivierge S, Simard M. Cognitive intervention program for individuals with mild cognitive impairment: Systematic review of the literature. American J Geria Psychi 18:281-296 (2010).

[37] Ott BR, Anthony D, Papandonatos GD, D'Abreu A, Burock J, Curtin A, *et al.* Clinician assessment of the driving competence of patients with dementia. J American Geria Soci 53:829-33 (2005).

Index

D.K. Lahiri (Ed)

E

F

G

L

M

O

P

Q

R

S

Made in the USA
Las Vegas, NV
03 November 2026

57424452R00276